$\mathcal{R}$ecognizing Health and Illness

Pathology for Massage Therapists and Bodyworkers

Health Positive! Publishing

Lawrence, Kansas 66046

PRINTED IN THE UNITED STATES OF AMERICA

ISBN 0-9658690-0-8

Printed on recycled paper.

Contents

Chapter 3, Part 2

CHAPTER 4

Chapter 5

Chapter 9

Chapter 10

Chapter 11, Part 1

Chapter 11, Part 2

Chapter 12, Part 1

Chapter 12, Part 2

Appendix

This book is dedicated with boundless love

to my daughter Adria

and to all the children.

May we grow in a world that's full of peace,

collaboration, and sufficiency for all.

Acknowledgments

A special thank you is extended to all the people who generously shared their time and attention with me during this project. This includes the illustrator Dian Hauser, the proofreader Diane Bourgeois, the layout designer Susan Wolfe, the graphic consultants Laurie Martin-Friedman and Mindy Wheeler, and the students in the pathology classes at Johnson County Community College and BMSI Institute in Overland Park, Kansas. A million thanks for your input, encouragement, and patience!

Also, I would not have been able to complete this book without the steadfast love, support and inspiration of my deep friends, Chris Fire Heart and Nadereh Nasseri. Chris kept me fed, clothed, and massaged through four intense months of writing, teaching and practice. Then she drew the sea turtle for the book's cover. Nadereh took me out for coffee, walks, and conversation. They cared for my soul and kept me laughing, and they are treasures in my life.

The following people read parts of the manuscript and gave me their professional input. Thanks go to each one.

Andy Bernay-Roman, RN, MS, LMT
President, Spectrum Healing Associates
North Palm Beach, Florida

Annette Chamness, NCTMB
Touched for Life by Chamness
Morton Grove, Illinois

Cheryl Chapman, RN, NCTMB
Instructor, Bodywork & Massage for Cancer & AIDS
Springfield, New Jersey

Ralph R. Stephens, LMT, NCTMB
Ralph R. Stephens Seminars
Cedar Rapids, Iowa

Preface

Pathology is the study of the nature of diseases and the structural and functional changes produced by them. Massage therapists/bodyworkers are ethically and legally responsible for recognizing clients' deviations from normal health, knowing if bodywork is indicated or contraindicated, and, if contraindicated, referring the client to the appropriate health practitioner.

The purpose of this book is to help the reader form a knowledge base upon which s/he can build a safe and ethical practice. It is not intended to account for the various advanced studies in massage/bodywork that may, in some cases, inform and empower therapists to work beyond the contraindications and limits described herein.

This book is written from the perspective of bridging current mainstream American medical language and theory with current bodywork language and theory. The glossary has been designed to define the words that may be unfamiliar to you, but some prior study of human anatomy, physiology, and kinesiology is assumed. References and resources for further study are given at the end of each chapter.

At present, there is little consensus as to what bodywork is appropriate in a given client situation, and there are few published research studies available for guidance. Massage therapists/bodyworkers are encouraged to read a variety of professional journals and text-books, attend conferences, and reference the Internet to continually develop their knowledge as the profession's knowledge evolves.

It is the author's intention to equally acknowledge and address bodyworkers and massage therapists in this text. However, she found it cumbersome to always include both terms, and she hopes that the reader will be able to mentally edit and insert whichever term s/he prefers. Moreover, the author has used the term "bodywork" to refer to work that physically touches, moves or directs the movement of the physical body. In this book the author has not specifi-cally addressed issues related to bodywork (or "energy work") that does not involve physical touch or movement.

Chapter 1

HUMAN HEALTH, DISABILITY AND DISEASE

How do you define *health? disability? disease?* Most people define these words in terms of how they feel inside and/or how they function. However, there are many, many theories of what causes health and disease. The distinctions between mental, emotional, spiritual and physical health and illness are not absolute. Most theories suggest that health and illness form a continuum, and most of us are somewhere in the middle of that continuum most of the time. *Pathology* is the study of the nature of diseases and the structural and functional changes produced by them. Massage therapists/bodyworkers have an ethical and legal responsibility not to do harm (for an example, see AMTA Code of Ethics, **Appendix A**).

If a client's condition becomes worse and he/she thinks your bodywork contributed to that deterioration, you can be sued, and the burden of your defense rests on you. If you have followed the client's physician's recommendation, you are generally less likely to lose the case. However, the courts hold each professional person liable for their acts, so, if the court finds evidence that your bodywork probably did contribute to the client's harm, you can be held liable for that contribution, even if there was a physician's OK. This is one reason why it is so important that you learn as much as you can about how the body/mind works and how your bodywork affects it.

Each bodyworker's decisions about which techniques s/he uses in any given situation will be based on his/her own education, experience, and style. This book will not try to point to any one set of techniques. Techniques will be mentioned only to illustrate ways you might apply the book's instructions in your everyday practice.

HEALTH

A well-known American medical dictionary provides this definition of health: "a condition in which all functions of the body and mind are normally active" (Taber's, 1989). The World Health Organization (WHO) defines health as "a state of complete physical, mental or social well-being and not merely the absence of disease or infirmity." These two definitions are widely used in today's American healthcare professions, supplemented by a theory called Maslow's Hierarchy of Needs.

Maslow's theory says that people are most healthy and whole when they have been able to meet their needs. Maslow proposed that there is an order, or hierarchy, of human needs, with some being more fundamental than others. A pyramid is used to represent this progression (see illustration on next page). According to Maslow's theory, if the needs at the bottom of the pyramid are not met, it is very hard to give attention to the needs higher up.

Another well-known theory is called Holistic (or Wholistic) Health. This theory is an amalgam of many theories, developed over millennia of time, by communities in many different cultures. This theory proposes that people are intricate beings who experience life through facets of *mind, body, spirit,* and *emotion*, and whatever affects the person affects all the facets. For example, touching the body influences the mind, emotion and spirit, and being emotionally "touched" affects the body, mind and spirit. According to this theory, all the parts of a human being function in concert, so the study and healing of any dysfunction must be viewed in relation to its meaning for the whole person. The Holistic Health theory does not mean simply giving herbs or other complementary treatments, such as massage, to a

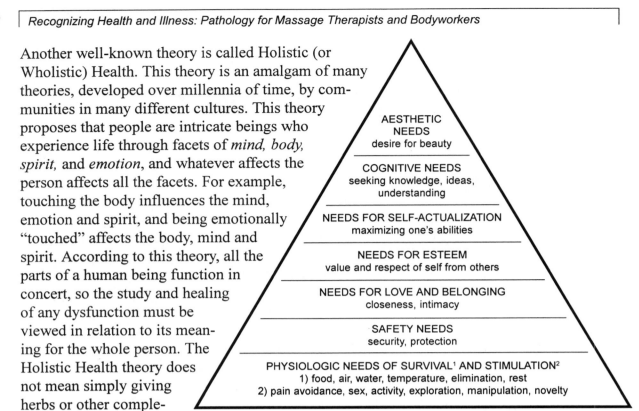

AESTHETIC
NEEDS
desire for beauty

COGNITIVE NEEDS
seeking knowledge, ideas,
understanding

NEEDS FOR SELF-ACTUALIZATION
maximizing one's abilities

NEEDS FOR ESTEEM
value and respect of self from others

NEEDS FOR LOVE AND BELONGING
closeness, intimacy

SAFETY NEEDS
security, protection

PHYSIOLOGIC NEEDS OF SURVIVAL[1] AND STIMULATION[2]
1) food, air, water, temperature, elimination, rest
2) pain avoidance, sex, activity, exploration, manipulation, novelty

Table 1.   Maslow's Hierarchy of Needs

person in place of pharmaceuticals or surgery. In order to be holistic, the practitioners and client work together (*collaborate*) to identify and give attention to what is occurring in all facets of the whole person. In this book, the terms *body/mind* or *whole person* are used as condensed terms for the whole mind/body/spirit/emotion human being.

DISABILITY

A *disability* can be defined as a limited function in any aspect of the body/mind. Some disabilities are visible and some are "invisible" or not obvious to observers. Common disabilities include: paralysis, retardation, phobia, chronic depression, epilepsy, bulimia, amputation, asthma, hearing loss, arthritis, diabetes, substance abuse, blindness, and brain and spinal cord injuries. Certain learning disabilities and extremes in physical size may also be disabling. The National Council of Disability estimates that there are 49 million Americans with disabilities. That is approximately one person in five.

The single most important difference between disabled and non-disabled people is that people with disabilities have to adapt to an environment designed for the non-disabled. In many cases, if the environment was designed to accommodate them, their disabilities would be much less important.

People sometimes feel uncomfortable around a person who has a disability. This discomfort usually comes from inexperience and ignorance, because we do not know what to do or say to this person who appears different from us. If you do not know what to say or do, it is your responsibility to find out. The best source of information is the client. Ask the client to explain his/her situation and what assistance, if any, might be needed. It is very important to focus on the person who has the disability rather than on the disability itself. Patronization, overcompensation, and insensitivity are common barriers to a therapeutic relationship. The bodyworker is responsible for his/her behavior and communication. **Appendix B** has some guidelines that may help you.

Most people with disabilities can benefit from bodywork. Before beginning, ask each client if s/he has any conditions which are currently affecting his/her health or functioning, and always get his/her *consent,* or permission, for your work. Think about the positioning requirements and style of your work. Your standard techniques may not be appropriate in all cases. If you are unsure if your approach will be appropriate for a client, describe your work and discuss it with the client before the massage. Let the client know you will modify your work or stop at any time if so requested by the client.

DISEASE

Disease literally means a lack of ease. It can include any group of symptoms distinct from normal health conditions or any impaired performance of a vital function. Common American medical theory is that disease occurs in the physical facet, at the cellular level, and develops along a physical course. Many other disease theories exist, including theories proposing that disease occurs first in the spiritual facet and develops into emotional, mental and/or physical manifestations; or that the mental facet is the starting place, or that the emotional facet is. What is your personal theory about how disease occurs? Do you believe the same theory accounts for mental and emotional illnesses? What about accidents? Birth defects?

Currently, there is no theory known to hold true in all cases. Until such a theory exists, each person deserves to have his/her beliefs valued and respected. Your beliefs about health, disability and disease will create the image and experience of your practice, and will attract clients with similar beliefs. When you consciously inspect, question, and deepen your personal values, knowledge and beliefs about health and illness, you can more consciously create the practice and personal health that you want.

If you remain unconscious or confused about your own theories, that will also be communicated to your clients and to the public. If you have not already done so, take the time to read, attend workshops, and talk with other bodyworkers about theories of health and illness in which you are interested. Keep a journal or file of ideas that interest you and resources you can explore for deeper learning.

According to the predominant American medical theories, the human body constantly strives to maintain a balanced internal environment or *homeostasis* in the midst of ever-changing conditions. For example, when excess acidity or alkalinity develops in the blood or body fluids, the body/mind tells the kidneys to correct the imbalance. Another example is the way an even internal temperature is maintained despite drastically changing environmental temperatures.

The naming of a disease or illness is its *diagnosis*. The cause of the disease is its *etiology*. Only physicians are licensed to diagnose illnesses and determine etiologies. Radiology (x-rays), ultrasound (high-frequency sound waves), nuclear medicine (CT scans, MRIs, etc.), and laboratory tests are some of the methods physicians use to diagnose illnesses. When a cause is not known for a disease, it is said to be *idiopathic*.

A *sign* is some evidence of illness that an observer can see, hear, touch, or smell. For instance a bruise can be seen, a hypertonic muscle can be touched, a cough can be seen and heard, and halitosis can be smelled. A *symptom* is some evidence of illness that an observer can not see. Symptoms are reported and described by the client, for instance pain and nausea are usually symptoms. However, in some cases you can see body posturing that is a sign of pain or nausea.

Many signs and symptoms of illness are the body/mind's responses to a challenge and can be important mechanisms for correcting an unhealthy situation. For example, coughing and sneezing are reflex actions of the respiratory system that aid in ridding the nose and throat of irritants. Vomiting is a reflex action of the digestive system to empty its contents. Inflammation helps prevent the spread of infection by barricading it and attempting to overcome the pathogenic or toxic substances present. This is why unhealthy situations can not be corrected merely by alleviating symptoms. In a bodywork practice, it is very important that clients are encouraged to acknowledge their symptoms and consult with a health or healing practitioner of their choice so that the underlying cause of the problem can be identified.

If a disease is expected to develop and run its course quickly, it is called *acute*. Once it lasts six months or more, it is generally called *chronic*. Chronic illnesses have periods of *remission* when the signs and symptoms temporarily leave, and *exacerbation* when the signs and symptoms increase again. An illness's predicted course and outcome is its *prognosis*. The prognosis can also be an estimate of chance for recovery. A group of symptoms and signs related to one another by a pattern of anatomic, physiologic, or biochemical events is called a *syndrome*. Syndromes usually do not have a known etiology (cause) but form a descriptive framework for investigation.

> **Do you know what the leading causes of death are in the U.S.?** Heart disease, cancer, and stroke are the top three accounting for almost two-thirds of U.S. deaths according to 1994 statistics. The other top ten causes of death, in order, are: chronic obstructive pulmonary diseases, accidents, pneumonia and influenza, diabetes, HIV, suicide, and chronic liver disease. (Monthly Vital Statistics Report, Vol. 43, No. 13, Annual Summary of Births, Marriages, Divorces and Deaths: United States, 1994.) *Editor's note: As of 8/16/97 these are the most current statistics available.*

The identification of the causes (etiologies) of disease is outside the scope of bodywork practice. However, it is important that bodyworkers recognize the common signs and symptoms and **risk factors** for disease. Risk factors are conditions that make a negative event more likely, but they are not necessarily the cause. The major categories of risk factors for disease include: genetics, age, diet, exercise, lifestyle, stress, environment, and preexisting illnesses. The effects of genetics on health will be reviewed in Chapter 11. The effects of diet will be reviewed in Chapter 10. The effects of exercise and lifestyle will be reviewed in Chapter 4. The effects of stress are reviewed in Chapter 2, and the effects of aging are presented next.

GENERAL EFFECTS OF AGING

Aging means becoming older or maturing. Aging is what we do every day we are alive. For our first four decades, aging brings us more coordination, agility, language, thinking, and problem-solving skills. After about forty, aging begins to bring some losses in function. As far as we know now, this is considered "normal" in most European/American populations. However, in some other cultures, peak health is reached much later, in the 50's and 60's. Just like health, no current theory of aging holds true for all people. To date we have very little research about aging, and most of the aging research we have comes from looking at aging people who are sick rather than looking at those who are healthy.

Most gerontologists define the category "elderly" as beginning at age 70, however, many people younger than 70 exhibit elderly attitudes, behaviors, and physiology, and many people over 70 display a much younger Self. Because of this, it is best to focus on the person more than the age. All people, regardless of age or physical condition, need safe caring touch, and people who live alone are often most in need.

However, there are some differences that you can expect to see when working with older adults. The most common changes in people over 65 years old include:

- decreased immune responses
- slower responses to stimuli
- decreased secretions of all types
- decreased reserve energy
- decreased abilities to adapt to stressors
- decreased vascular and connective tissue elasticity

The proportions of the major body components change as follows: At age 25, the average American body is 15% fat, 17% muscle, 6% bone, 42% intracellular water and 20% extracellular water. At age 75, the average American body is 30% fat, 12% muscle, 5% bone, 33% intracellular water and 20% extracellular water. More specific changes due to aging will be included in this book as each body system is reviewed, except for the sensory changes, which are reviewed here.

People over age 70 generally have an 80% reduction in taste buds, especially for sweet and sour tastes. They often have a decrease in saliva and a decreased sense of smell, making food less appealing. They require less food, but good nutrition is more important than ever because the smaller quantity requires the food to be of higher quality in order to get all the essential nutrients.

There is a general decrease in near vision at about age 40 and a decrease in peripheral vision at about age 60, along with a slowed ability in the pupil to adapt to changes in light. There is often a decreased ability to hear high-pitched sounds and consonants, making "red," "bed," and "dead" all sound similar, and an increase in the amount and thickness of ear wax, making hearing more difficult. A decreased sensation of touch is common, as well as a generally slowed reflex arc and decreased peripheral nerve conduction.

Other common changes are that people over the age of 70 require less sleep and sleep lighter with less REM sleep. They also often have a decreased sense of body position in space, making little shifts in balance difficult to correct, so falls occur more often.

It is important that you know the basic signs and symptoms of aging and are able to be sensitive and supportive to older clients (and to yourself, as you age). In 1900, people over age 65 made up only 4% of the American population. By 2000, they will make up about 13%, and by 2030 they will be about 22%. The most rapid increases will be among those people who are 85 years and older. (Healthy People 2000: 1992) Always *refer* clients to another health professional when you are unsure if a change is normal or not (see page 27).

ASSESSING HEALTH CONDITIONS

Assessment is the collection and interpretation of information provided by the client, any referring health professionals, and your own observation. Assessment is methodically paying attention to what a client presents at this moment in time, to gather the information you need, so that you can give appropriate and effective bodywork. Assessment begins when you first see the client and is continual and on-going throughout each session. The components of an assessment are: 1) a *health history*, 2) *observation*, and 3) *palpation*.

HEALTH HISTORY

Each assessment begins with a review of the client's health history. A *health history* is a record of past health events, including illnesses, accidents, and surgeries. In the medical and psychiatric professions, the health history also includes major illnesses within the client's family, but that information is not generally needed in bodywork.

Most health histories are written by the client on their first visit, using a form that you provide (see example next page). Many bodyworkers refer to this as an "intake form." It may also include a statement of consent for bodywork. A written health history on each client is very important for two reasons. First, writing about oneself helps the client be more consciously connected with the components of his/her health. An increased self-awareness can often facilitate an increase in self-responsibility. Second, if your practice is ever reviewed in a court of law, your liability is limited to the information you were given by the client. Having written records documents and limits your responsibility.

There are five important questions to ask on a health history form. These are:

1) what are the client's past surgeries, illnesses and accidents,
2) what is his/her current problem or concern,
3) is s/he under a health practitioner's care? (The term "health practitioner" can include: MD, DO, chiropractor, nurse practitioner, social worker, psychologist, psychiatrist, dentist, podiatrist, herbalist, nutritionist, naturopath, shaman, etc.),
4) what condition is being treated, and
5) what is the therapy, medication, or supplementation being used?

Once you have a client's health history, you will review it at each visit, before giving body-work, so that your memory about this person is refreshed. Ask the client if anything has changed since the last time you saw him/her and, if so, add notes to update your information.

OBSERVATION AND PALPATION

Observation is looking and listening carefully with attention to detail. *Palpation* is the process of examining the body by applying one's hands to the body surface. The observation and palpation components of assessment can be best described by this process: look, listen, feel; look, listen feel; look, listen, feel. Remember that assessment begins when you first see the client and is continual and on-going throughout each session.

<u>Looking</u> includes inspecting the client's posture, gait, behavior, breathing, skin, and range of motion. Pay particular attention to how the client talks, moves and breathes. Do these things suggest stress? Relaxation? Function? Dysfunction? Ease? Disease?

<u>Listening</u> includes hearing both what is said to you and how it is said. It includes asking respectful, attentive questions before, during and after the bodywork, and waiting for the answers. Open-ended questions encourage sharing of information. The question "Have you ever had professional bodywork?" only asks for a "yes" or "no" answer. The question "What is your experience with professional bodywork?" invites a much more informative answer.

There are four important questions to ask each client. First, before any work begins, ask:

1) What do you want from this massage?
   (The client's answer becomes the <u>goal</u> of the session.)
2) What increases or decreases your problem?
3) What have you been doing about the problem?

Then, during the session, it is important to ask:

4) How does this feel right now?

Health Positive! Bodywork
1510 E. 1584 Road, Lawrence, KS 66046
913-555-1761

Name_____ Phone (h) _____ (w) _____

Address_____ City _____ St _____ Zip _____

Age _____ Date of birth _____ M ❑ F ❑ Referred by _____

Health Insurance Co. _____ ID # _____

Insurance address _____

Ins. phone _____ Occupation _____

What is you main area of pain (or concern)? _____

When did you first notice this? _____ What brought it on? _____

What aggravates it?_____ What relieves it? _____

Has there been a medical diagnosis? Y❑ N❑ If so, what? _____

Are you currently consulting with any health care practitioners? Y❑ N❑ If so, who?_____

Please list previous surgeries, illnesses, accidents, or conditions that may be affecting your current health or functioning: _____

_____

Person to notify in case of an emergency: _____

IMPORTANT Please indicate if you have any of the following conditions because, if so, standard massage therapy techniques might not be appropriate:

❑High blood pressure ❑Osteoporosis ❑Diabetes ❑AIDS ❑Acute infection
❑Swelling/edema ❑Recent injury ❑Cancer ❑Fever ❑Pregnancy
❑Prescription medication(s) _____

I understand that I am responsible for payment which is due at the end of each appointment unless other arrangements have been made in advance.

Date _____ Signature _____

The answers to these questions will help you form the boundaries of your work.

Feeling includes physical palpation of the client's body, feeling for lumps, tightness, looseness, spring, etc. It also includes intuitive feeling, in whatever ways that happens for you.

Recording Observation and Palpation Information

One of the best ways to organize, record and communicate the information you get from observation and palpation is to divide it into two categories: *subjective* and *objective*. These categories are the same ones described earlier as symptoms (subjective) and signs (objective). *Subjective* information (symptoms) is information that is known directly only by the person who experiences it, for instance, fear, pain, anxiety, joy, etc. *Objective* information (signs) is information that can be sensed or measured by an observer, for instance, a wart, bruise, or range of motion.

Assessments are best when they include both subjective and objective information. Written assessment notes, even if they are only a few short phrases, are important to the bodyworker because:

- it is very hard to remember personal details about each client between visits, and a written record makes recall easier, and
- being able to look back over time helps you see the progress (or lack of) that the client has made.
- written records are required for insurance claims, law suits, etc.

In hospitals and other clinical settings, assessments done by bodyworkers are written and discussed as a part of the total treatment plan. Most clinical settings have some system of documentation that all the health professionals use. A common system is called SOAP charting in which "S" is the subjective information, "O" is the objective information, "A" is the application or treatment that you gave the client, and "P" is the plan for future treatments. Even if you work in your own, solo practice, making brief notes that follow this format will yield a wealth of information for your use.

> **TIP**: One way to significantly increase your learning and effectiveness as a bodyworker is to ask your clients to rate their subjective experiences on a scale. This helps you because:
>
> - it gives you a clearer idea of what the client is describing,
> - it communicates to the client that you are really interested in understanding their experience, which helps build trust, and
> - by asking for a rating before the bodywork session and again afterwards, both you and the client can easily evaluate whether or not the session was helpful (see sample scales below).

Scales can be used to rate pain, pressure, nausea, anxiety, or any other subjective experience (symptom).

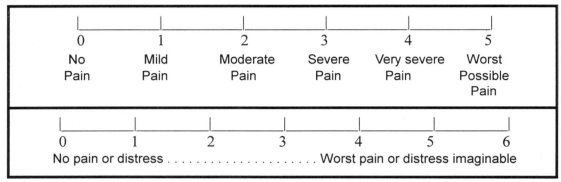

Table 2   Sample Pain Scales

Special Focus: Assessing Pain

One of the most common reasons people choose to receive bodywork is to reduce or eliminate pain. In order to effectively relieve pain, it helps to know how to assess it. One of the most effective ways to assess pain is to organize your questions around the following four areas: 1) *location*, 2) *duration*, 3) *intensity* and 4) *quality*.

- To assess the *location*, you can ask the client to show you where he/she hurts.
- To assess *duration*, you can ask when the client first noticed the pain and whether the pain is steady or comes and goes.
- To assess *intensity*, you can ask the client to rate the pain on a scale, e.g.. mild, moderate, severe, or 0 to 5, with 0 being no pain and 5 being the worst pain imaginable. For example: the client rates his/her neck pain as a 3 prior to the bodywork, and after the work rates the neck pain as a 0. This helps you both to realize the usefulness of the work.
- To assess *quality*, you can ask the client to describe how the pain feels, for instance, sharp, dull, aching, burning, stabbing, constant, intermittent, squeezing, cramping, pressing, etc.
- Another useful question is "What increases or decreases the pain?"

With experience and advanced instruction, you will learn how these descriptors can indicate different origins of pain.

THE CLIENT'S GOAL

As mentioned earlier, it is very important to ask the client "What do you want from this bodywork?" The client's answer is usually what you could call the goal for the session. If a client answered "I do not know," it would be appropriate to clarify what information you are seeking. For instance, you can say that some people get bodywork to help them relax, some to reduce pain and stiffness, some to receive safe, nurturing touch, etc. This gives the client a place to start, and makes it easier to add their own feelings.

Next, remember your scope of practice, the indications and contraindications for your work, and your education and experience. If a client wants something that you are not comfortable doing, it is important that you communicate this tactfully and directly. One example of this might be if a client asked you to "pop" her back, which is outside the scope of basic massage practice. If you and the client are unable to reach a mutually comfortable understanding of the session's goal, then it is better for both of you to know that and deal with it in the beginning.

INDICATIONS AND CONTRAINDICATIONS

An *indication* is any persuasive reason to do an action. For example, if you are considering doing effleurage to the client's erector spinae, you will mentally ask yourself if there is some indication, or persuasive reason, to do it. Perhaps you have learned that effleurage on the erector spinae is safe and relaxing to most clients.

From the knowledge base being developed in professional bodywork, we know that there are persuasive reasons to give bodywork for a variety of situations, some examples include muscle tense (hypertonic) muscles, weak (hypotonic) muscle tone, kinetic pain, chronic pain, muscle spasm, joint stiffness, sluggish circulation, constipation, headache, insomnia, low self-esteem, failure to thrive, depression, and chronic anxiety. When we talk about doing bodywork in these situations, we say the bodywork is indicated.

On the other hand, if there are any persuasive reasons to avoid the action under consideration, we say the bodywork is *contraindicated*. For example, a contraindication to doing effleurage to the erector spinae might be the existence of "shingles" on the client's back.

Lists or sets of contraindication guidelines are available from a variety of sources including the massage therapy regulations in some states, however, there is no clear agreement among them. Therefore, it is important that you make your own informed decisions in this area, based on your study, your practice, and all the additional resource information you can get. The continual and on-going study of indications and contraindications is a requirement for true professionalism. The goal of this book is to help you establish a knowledge base upon which you can build your understanding and eventual expertise about indications and contraindications in your practice.

There are two main types of contraindications discussed in this book: 1) *local contraindications* and *systemic contraindications*.

Local contraindications are those that relate to a specific area of the body so that bodywork can be given to the person except for the specific location of injury or problem. An example would be a case where the client had a large bruise. If there are no other problems, bodywork is indicated for this client, with a local contraindication in the area of the bruise.

Systemic contraindications are those that prevent all bodywork to the client. These situations require the attention of a health practitioner to assess the client's condition, diagnose the problem, and give an opinion about whether bodywork would be safe or not. An example would be a case where the client has cold, bluish hands and feet and difficulty breathing when lying flat. It is not within your scope of practice to determine the cause of the client's problems. However, there are persuasive reasons for not doing bodywork on this client until his/her condition has been assessed by a qualified health practitioner and you have received an opinion from that person that bodywork would not be harmful.

Another example is when a client is taking daily prescription medication. It is not your sole responsibility to decide whether your bodywork will effect this client positively or negatively. This responsibility is the client's, based on information gathered from his/her medical practitioner and other consultants, including you, the bodyworker.

In order to give the client accurate information, you are responsible for knowing some of the basics of how medication affects the body and how bodywork may interact with these effects. This book will give you information about general classes of medicines, including *anti-inflammatories*, *muscle relaxants*, *anti-coagulants*, and *analgesics* (see **Index**). The author recommends that you also consult a current prescription drug reference book when a client is taking a medication you are unfamiliar with.

MAKING REFERRALS TO OTHER HEALTH PROFESSIONALS

It is essential that you know what is within and outside your own scope of practice. Review your local, state, and professional association guidelines for this information. When your assessment uncovers conditions for which massage either is not indicated or is contraindicated, it is important that you refer the client. A *referral* is a recommendation that the client seek the advice of another health care practitioner. Clients generally appreciate being referred when you can not help them. Whenever possible, it is best to refer the client to his/her primary care physician or other health practitioner s/he is currently consulting. A *physician* (usually an MD or DO) is a person who has successfully completed a prescribed course of study in an officially recognized school and is licensed to practice medicine by the State. A *primary care physician* is the physician who provides periodic check-ups and makes the first assessment and diagnosis of illnesses. S/he may refer the person to a specialist or coordinate the person's care within a multi-disciplinary team (see table below for descriptions of different health care professionals).

If the client has no current relationship with a health care practitioner, give him/her a specific practitioner's name, or business card, if you know one. However, this approach depends on you or someone you trust having some personal experience or knowledge of the practitioner's skill and integrity because your client is trusting your guidance. If the client has a good experience with that person it will reflect on you, and if they have a negative experience it will also, to some extent, reflect on you. The best practice is to develop a network of health care practitioners whom you know and trust, and who trust you and will refer clients to you in return.

If you have no knowledge or experience with a specific practitioner, it is usually best not to name one, and to refer your client to a general category of practice instead. In either case, be sure to give the client one of your business cards or brochures to give to the professional they will be seeing so that the other practitioner can contact you easily, if desired.

The following is a partial list of typical health practitioners, their training and area of expertise. This list is only intended to be a general guide and may not reflect the unique preparation and skills of any individual.

LICENSED OR CERTIFIED PHYSICAL HEALTH PRACTITIONERS

TITLE	EDUCATION	COMMON TREATMENT
General MD	BS + MD (4 yrs) + R (2-3 yrs)	exam, diagnosis, medications
Specialist MD	BS + MD (4 yrs) + R (4-6 yrs)	exam, medication, and/or surgery
Dr. of Osteopathy	BS +DO (4 yrs) +R (3 yrs)	exam, diagnosis, medications
Chiropractor	BS + 1-2 yrs	spinal exam and adjustment
Nurse practitioner	BS + MS (2 yrs)	exam, diagnosis, medication
Dentist	BS + MD (4 yrs)	dental exam, medication, treatment
Podiatrist	BS + MD (4 yrs) + R (1-2 yrs)	foot exam, medication, treatment
Dietician	BS + MS (2 yrs)	teaching and individualized diets
Naturopath	BS + 4 yrs	exam, diagnosis, naturopathic treatment
Physicians' Asst.	BS + 1-2 yrs	exam, simple diagnosis, medications

Table 3

BS = Bachelor of Science degree   MD = Medical Doctor   DO = Dr. of Osteopathy
MS = Master of Science degree   PhD = Doctor of Philosophy   R = residency

LICENSED OR CERTIFIED MENTAL HEALTH PRACTITIONERS

TITLE	EDUCATION	COMMON TREATMENT
Psychiatrist	BS + MD + R (4 yrs)	psychiatric diagnosis & medications
Psychoanalyst	BS + MS + R (2 yrs)	explores & analyzes thought process
Psychologist	BS + PhD (4-5 yrs)	self-understanding & skill development
Social Worker	BS + MS (2 yrs)	strengthens interpersonal/social support
Marriage and Family Therapist	BS + MS or PhD (2-5 yrs)	interpersonal skills development
Nurse Practitioner	BS + MS (2 yrs)	diagnosis, medication, skill development

Table 4

BS = Bachelor of Science degree   MD = Medical Doctor   R = residency
MS = Master of Science degree   PhD = Doctor of Philosophy

Making a referral requires honesty, sensitivity and tact. For instance, if you noticed a mole on a client's back that had the signs of malignancy, the client might feel very frightened if you say "There's a big mole on your back, and it looks cancerous. You'd better see a doctor right away." A more helpful approach might be to say "Did you know you have a mole right here? (Touch the adjoining area.) Have you had it checked by a doctor? It is larger than a pencil eraser, has irregular borders, and it is two different colors. It would be a good idea to have it checked as soon as you can." Remember, you cannot diagnose. Only tell the client what signs or symptoms you see. Do not name a specific condition. Ask the client to bring you a note from the physician, if possible, giving a diagnosis and communicating his/her opinion on whether or not bodywork is safe.

Whenever you have referred a client to another practitioner, it is wise to write the date, signs and symptoms, and what referral you gave in your notes, for two reasons: 1) the note will remind you to ask the client on their next visit to you if they did get checked, and 2) the note will serve as another legal limit of your liability because it shows that you recommended the client seek further care.

Speaking of liability, it is important that you know that you <u>might</u> be liable for damages if you do not refer a client to a physician when you observe or palpate signs or symptoms of illness. For instance, if your client reports acute lower right-sided abdominal pain and you do not refer the client to see a physician right away, and the client dies of an untreated ruptured appendix, then his/her family can sue you and, possibly, collect damages. Likewise, if you referred this client to a psychiatrist or dentist (in other words, practitioners that are not appropriate for the condition), and the client is harmed by not seeking appropriate care, you can be sued. If you are judged to be not at fault, you will still have the emotional, financial and time costs of your defense. For further clarification of these points, consult your State's massage/bodywork regulations, your professional association, and a lawyer who is knowledgable about health care liability issues in your State.

With this in mind, in terms of your legal protection, the SAFEST practitioners to refer to are the professionals who are licensed to diagnose and treat illnesses in your State. It is best to find out if chiropractors, naturopaths, nurse practitioners, or any other types of health professionals are licensed to diagnose and treat illnesses in your State. It is OK to refer to BOTH the licensed practitioners and alternative practitioners, and acknowledge the client's freedom and responsibility to choose.

GENERAL CONDITIONS TO REFER TO PHYSICIANS AND/OR OTHER HEALING PRACTITIONERS

Although each chapter of this book lists, by system, the specifics of when to refer a client, the following is a brief, general list for you to use as a beginning point.

- acute pain (sharp and localized; deep or superficial)
- fatigue and muscle weakness
- inflammation

- lumps and skin changes
- unexplained rashes
- edema
- unexplained mood changes
- infections
- changes in appetite, elimination, or sleep patterns
- bleeding or unexplained bruising
- nausea, vomiting, diarrhea
- fever or unusual coldness

EVALUATING THERAPEUTIC OUTCOMES

A *therapeutic outcome* is the effect your bodywork has on the client. Evaluation means determining the value. How valuable is your bodywork? You will not know unless you determine the value, or effectiveness of your work. How can you do this? The primary way is to compare the assessment information you obtained before the bodywork started with the assessment information you obtain at the end of the work. This might include pain, anxiety, range of motion, muscle tension, or any other subjective or objective parameter that you assessed.

The most clear and most widely respected evaluations come from using objective information, that is, information you can see, touch or measure in some way. The more clearly you evaluate, the more clearly you and the client will learn the effects of the bodywork. If you can not see or touch the changes, you can help the client evaluate and communicate it to you through the use of a rating scale. My perspective, after 15 years of practicing professional bodywork, is that consistently evaluating my therapeutic outcomes is the most efficient way for me to continually learn from my practice.

SAMPLE CASE PRESENTATION

The following sample case presentation illustrates all the components of Chapter 1: history, observation/palpation, client goal, indications, contraindications, application, referral, and evaluation of therapeutic outcome.

2/23/96: The client is a 45 year-old woman whose MD suggested massage therapy for neck and shoulder muscle spasm relief.

Health history: 2 serious motor vehicle crashes, 10 years apart, and a boating accident one year ago. Injuries included multiple fractures: both feet, both fibulae, pelvis, right hip, and spine at L4, L5, T11 and T12. Client required 8 months of rehab before returning to work after the boating accident. Now working full-time with moderate neck and shoulder pain 3-4x wkly.

Observation/Palpation: No visible deformities. Posture symmetrical at head, shoulders & hips. Gait normal. Range of motion decreased in shoulders and neck. Skin clear. Tenderness in erectors beside C1-5, T11, T12. Client states, "I have concrete blocks for shoulders," rates neck pain at 6 and lower back pain at 5 on 0-10 scale.

Client goal: Reduce tightness and tenderness in neck and shoulders.

Indications: Effleurage, petrissage, myofascial release, friction, ice to reduce spasm.

Contraindications: Excessive force to previously fractured areas.

Application: Light, superficial palpation to neck and back. Myofascial stretching and rocking motion to lumbar area. Scalp massage. Friction and ice to tender areas. Effleurage to extremities.

Referral: A. Chang, acupuncturist, for assistance with pain.

Outcome: Client voiced decreased pain (neck 3; low back 4). Range of motion increased in neck and shoulders.

CASE PRESENTATIONS

4/15/96: Client is 43 year old female.

Health history: sinus headaches, allergies, neck pains, shoulder pain, backaches, chronic fatigue, high cholesterol, digestive problems, arthritis, foot pain and numbness, rheumatoid arthritis x 10 yrs, fibromyalgia and Sjogren's syndrome x 4 yrs.

Current medicines: flexeril, trazadone, and multivitamin. Often consumes caffeine, diet drinks and fast food. No regular exercise. Today she reports no active joint pain or inflammation, however, says muscles feel stiff and tight.

Client goal: relaxation and reduce muscle tension. This is her first massage.

Assessment: muscles very tight & many knots.

Application: long, slow effleurage with moderate pressure; gentle ROM to neck & upper extremities; slow gentle passive stretching to low back.

Referral: yoga or swimming for regular exercise and dietician or nutritionist.

Outcome: stated "I'm very relaxed. I'll definitely try this again." Follow-up phone call 2 days later: client reported she slept well the night of the massage & felt increased energy the next day, plus decreased muscle stiffness.

4/15/96: Client is 17 year old female with ulcerative colitis for 4 months & depression for 6 months. Says MD told her colitis is from stress. Was hospitalized for 4 days last week for both problems. Takes antidepressant pills. No pain in abdomen since she left the hospital. This is first massage.

Client goal: Relax.

Assessment: Tender spots in trapezius, upper and lower back, hamstrings and calves. Right (R) shoulder lower than left (L), head is pulled forward, L hip higher than R, pelvis tilted back. Gait slightly unbalanced. Pain in R deltoid & pectoralis and in L pectoralis & trapezius with active ROM. Initial pain ratings (scale of 0-10): Pects 4, traps 10, neck 3, back 5, calves 10. Nervous, high-pitched laughter and ticklish for first 10 min. of massage.

Application: Effleurage, petrissage, circular friction, vibration and acupressure to areas described above. Gentle passive stretching and ROM to upper extremities. Often invited her to pay attention to body sensations during massage, and notice what was happening.

Outcome: Slight improvement in gait and posture, final pain ratings: pects 0, traps 0, neck 0, low back 0, calves 2. Client looks calmer & says she feels great!

STUDY QUESTIONS:

Which parts of the above case presentations are subjective?
Which parts are objective?
What questions would you have asked that were not asked?
What bodywork techniques would you have done?
What referral(s)?
What other ways could the therapeutic outcome have been evaluated?
Each of these cases was written in a different format.
Which format did you like best?
How might you have changed the way the cases were written?

FURTHER RESOURCES

Check your State's massage therapy laws and regulations for its legal definition of massage therapy and for the lists of indications and contraindications that apply to your practice. At the time of this writing, 20 states, plus the District of Columbia, license or certify massage therapists. Others are in the process of setting state licensing standards. An example of a detailed list of indications and contraindications can be obtained by contacting the Oregon State Board of Massage Technicians at 503-731-4064.

Hirshberg, C. & Barasch, M.I. (1995). Remarkable recovery: What extraordinary healings tell us about getting well and staying well. Institute of Noetic Sciences: 1-800-383-1586.

REFERENCES

Healthy people 2000: National health promotion and disease prevention objectives. Washington, D.C.: Dept. of Health and Human Services, Sept. 1990. DHHS publication 91-50212.
Annual summary of births, marriages, divorces and deaths: United States, 1994. Monthly Vital Statistics Report, Vol. 43, No. 13,
Disability Etiquette. The Rehabilitation Institute of Chicago, 345 E. Superior St., Chicago, IL 60611, phone (312) 908-6044.
Thomas, C.L. (1989). Taber's cyclopedic medical dictionary (16th ed.). Philadelphia: F.A. Davis Co.
Words With Dignity. Paraquad, 311 North Lindbergh Blvd., St. Louis, MO 63141, phone (314) 567-1558 voice, TTY 314-567-5222, fax 314-567-1559.

CHAPTER REVIEW

1. Define the following:

pathology _____

assessment _____

health history _____

subjective _____

objective _____

indication _____

contraindication _____

referral _____

therapeutic outcome _____

disease _____

disability _____

aging _____

2. Written assessment notes are important because:

a. _____

b. _____

3. A written health history is important because:

a. _____

b. _____

4. The components of assessment are:

a. _____

b. _____

c. _____

5. Four important questions to ask on a health history are:

a. _____

b. _____

c. _____

d. _____

6. Three important questions to ask before bodywork begins are:

a. _____

b. _____

c. _____

7. In assessing pain, the four areas to focus your questions around are:

a. _____

b. _____

c. _____

d. _____

8. An example of a LOCAL contraindication is: _____

_____

9. An example of a SYSTEMIC contraindication is: _____

_____

10. What three things are important to write in the client file when you have made a referral?
    a. _____
    b. _____
    c. _____

11. Maslow's theory says that people are most healthy and whole when they have been able
    to _____

12. The Holistic Health theory says that people are intricate beings that include the facets
    _____ , and what affects one facet_____

13. Why is it important that bodyworkers know the basic signs and symptoms of aging?

    _____

    _____

    _____

CHAPTER REVIEW ANSWERS

1. *Pathology*: the study of the nature of diseases and the structural and functional changes produced by them.

   Assessment: the collection and interpretation of information provided by the client, any referring health professionals, and your own observation.

   Health history: a record of past health events, including past illnesses, accidents, and surgeries.

   Subjective: information known only by the person experiencing it, e.g. pain. (symptom)

   Objective: something that can be seen, touched, and measured by an observer, e.g. a wart. (sign)

   Indication: any persuasive reason to do the action under consideration.

   Contraindication: any persuasive reason to avoid the action under consideration.

   Referral: a recommendation that the client seek the advice of another health care practitioner.

   Therapeutic outcome: the effect your bodywork has on the client.

   Disease: a lack of ease; any group of symptoms distinct from normal health conditions; impaired performance of any vital function

   Disability: limited function in any aspect of the body/mind.

   Aging: becoming older; maturing

2. a) it is very hard to remember personal details about each client over time, and a written record makes recall easier, b) being able to look back over time helps you see the progress (or lack of) that the client has made.

3. a) writing about oneself helps the client be more conscious of the components of his/her health; b) if your practice is ever reviewed in a court of law, your liability is limited to the information you were given by the client.

4. a) health history, b) observation, and c) palpation

5. a) what are the client's past surgeries, illnesses and accidents, b) what is their current problem or concern, c) are they under a physician's care, and if so, d) what condition is being treated, what is the therapy, medication or supplementation being received?

6. a) What do you want from this massage? b) What increases or decreases your problem? c) What have you been doing about the problem?

7. a) location, b) duration, c) intensity and d) quality

8. (name a specific area of the body)

9. (the whole body)

10. a) date, b) signs and symptoms, c) what referral you gave

11. meet their needs

12. body, mind, spirit, emotion; affects all

13. to be sensitive and supportive to older clients (and to yourself, as you age).

Chapter 2, Part 1

STRESS, STRESSORS, AND THE BODY/MIND

STRESSORS CREATE STRESS

The term *stress* means disequilibrium, strain or tension in a structure, system, or organism. A *stressor* is any factor that causes stress. Stressors usually require a person to adapt in some way. The most common stressors are changes in one's environment. Examples include: moving to a new home, starting a new job, entering school, leaving school, starting a new relationship, ending a relationship, any illness in yourself or people you care about, pressure from someone else who wants you to change, holidays, birthdays, and even changes in the weather.

It is generally believed that biological organisms, including people, require some stress in order to maintain well-being. There are many signs and symptoms of stress such as: rushing, excitement, being focused, overly-focused, forgetfulness, restlessness, etc. What are the signs and symptoms that tell you there is strain, disequilibrium or tension in your life?

> *Tip*: As an exercise in your wellness awareness, use the Holmes-Rahe scale (see page 36) to get a sense of how many stressors you have had in the past 12 months.

Although some stress is inevitable, research has shown that as stress accumulates, the person becomes increasingly susceptible to physical, mental, emotional and spiritual problems such as outbursts, accidents, illnesses and exhaustion. Long-term, or chronic, stress is particularly damaging if it is not interrupted with periods of rest, relaxation and nurturance. That is because the body's chemical and mechanical changes that are normal and helpful for short-term crisis become damaging when they occur constantly over time.

CELLULAR CHANGES IN RESPONSE TO STRESS

Cells respond to stress by changing their size, shape and function. When cells can adapt to the stress, they can continue to function normally. When they can not, cell injury results, reducing the ability to function. If the cell injury is reversible, the cells will return to normal when the stressor is removed. If it is irreversible, the cell will die and the problem may spread. A basic listing of the types of cell injuries is important, since most contraindications for bodywork are based on this information.

Holmes and Rahe Life Challenge Scale

Name _____ Date _____

     Review the last year and the events that happened to you. Beside each event, indicate the number of times it happened to you during the past 12 months only. Multiply the number times the mean value. A total score of 150-199 indicates mild challenge; 200-299 indicates moderate challenge; 300+ indicates major challenge.

Life event	Mean value		Challenge
Death of spouse _____	___ x100	=	_____
Divorce _____	___ x73	=	_____
Marital separation _____	___ x65	=	_____
Jail term _____	___ x63	=	_____
Death of a close family member _____	___ x63	=	_____
Personal injury or illness _____	___ x53	=	_____
Marriage _____	___ x50	=	_____
Fired from a job _____	___ x47	=	_____
Marital reconciliation _____	___ x45	=	_____
Retirement _____	___ x45	=	_____
Change in health of a family member _____	___ x44	=	_____
Pregnancy _____	___ x40	=	_____
Sex difficulties _____	___ x39	=	_____
Gain of a new family member _____	___ x39	=	_____
Business readjustment _____	___ x39	=	_____
Change in financial status _____	___ x44	=	_____
Death of a close friend _____	___ x37	=	_____
Change to different line of work _____	___ x36	=	_____
Change in number of arguments with spouse _____	___ x35	=	_____
Mortgage over $10,000 _____	___ x31	=	_____
Foreclosure of mortgage or loan _____	___ x30	=	_____
Change in responsibilities at work_____	___ x29	=	_____
Son or daughter leaving home _____	___ x29	=	_____
Trouble with in-laws_____	___ x29	=	_____
Outstanding personal achievement_____	___ x28	=	_____
Spouse begins or quits a job _____	___ x26	=	_____
Begin or finish school _____	___ x26	=	_____
Change in living conditions _____	___ x25	=	_____
Revision of personal habits _____	___ x24	=	_____
Trouble with boss _____	___ x23	=	_____
Change in work hours or conditions _____	___ x20	=	_____
Change of residence _____	___ x20	=	_____
Change of schools _____	___ x20	=	_____
Change of recreation_____	___ x19	=	_____
Change in church activities _____	___ x18	=	_____
Change in social activities _____	___ x18	=	_____
Mortgage or loan less than $10,000 _____	___ x17	=	_____
Change in sleeping habits _____	___ x16	=	_____
Change in number of family get-togethers _____	___ x15	=	_____
Change in eating habits _____	___ x15	=	_____
Vacation _____	___ x13	=	_____
Major holiday celebration _____	___ x12	=	_____
Minor violations of the law _____	___ x11	=	_____
		Total	_____

1. *Hypoxia*: significant reduction in a cell's oxygen supply. Can be caused by blood vessel obstruction, anemia or impaired respiration.

2. *Chemicals*: exposure to excessive amounts of normal internal chemicals can injure cells, as well as exposure to external, or "foreign" chemicals.

3. *Physical trauma*: temperature extremes, pressure changes, radiation, and electricity, are among the physical forces that can injure cells.

4. *Pathogens*: micro and macro organisms can injure cells, including viruses, bacteria, parasites and fungi.

5. *Immune system hypersensitivity:* Antigens are substances that induce the formation of antibodies. They can come from either inside the body, as in autoimmune diseases, or from outside the body, as in allergies.

6. *Mutations*: changes in a cell's chromosome pattern. Mutations can be inherited or can occur during life due to the effects of pathogens, radiation, etc.

7. *Abnormal nutrient levels*: lack of nutrients is a major cause of cell damage. Excessive nutrients can also injure the body, e.g., obesity and cardiovascular disease.

8. *Structural changes* in plasma membrane, cytoplasm, organelles and inclusions: when the plasma membrane is altered, the cell walls become more permeable, allowing abnormal chemicals to enter the cell. This can increase or decrease the cytoplasm content, leading to abnormal swelling or shrinking of the cell. When the organelles and inclusions are altered, the cell sometimes ruptures, self-destructs, or is otherwise unable to function.

BODY/MIND CHANGES IN RESPONSE TO STRESS

In response to stress, all systems of the body/mind are required to adapt. These adaptations, or changes, take place through the autonomic nervous system, which consists of two distinct sub-systems: the *sympathetic* and the *parasympathetic* nervous systems.

The *sympathetic* system is activated for energy production. It is commonly called the "fight or flight" response. Sympathetic activation provides bursts of energy when stress stimulates activity.

The *parasympathetic* system is activated by periods of rest and nurturance. During these periods, energy is conserved and energy reserves are replenished. Commonly called the "relaxation response," parasympathetic activation slows the heartbeat, decreases body temperature, increases the secretion of most of the glands, and increases digestion and elimination. It brings the body/mind back to its normal balance after sympathetic activation.

SELYE'S GENERAL ADAPTATION SYNDROME (GAS)

Hans Selye developed a model, called the General Adaptation Syndrome, to explain how people mobilize energy when they feel threatened by an actual or perceived harm (sympathetic activity). It is a very general model, but its three stages appear to be consistent no matter if the perceived threat is coming from a physical, mental, emotional or spiritual source.

The three stages are: 1) *alarm* (the *"fight or flight"* response), which is the body's initial reaction to the perceived stressor; 2) *resistance reaction*, which allows the person to continue fighting or fleeing long after the alarm phase is over, and 3) *exhaustion*, which occurs if the person becomes depleted before they get rest, relaxation and/or nurturance.

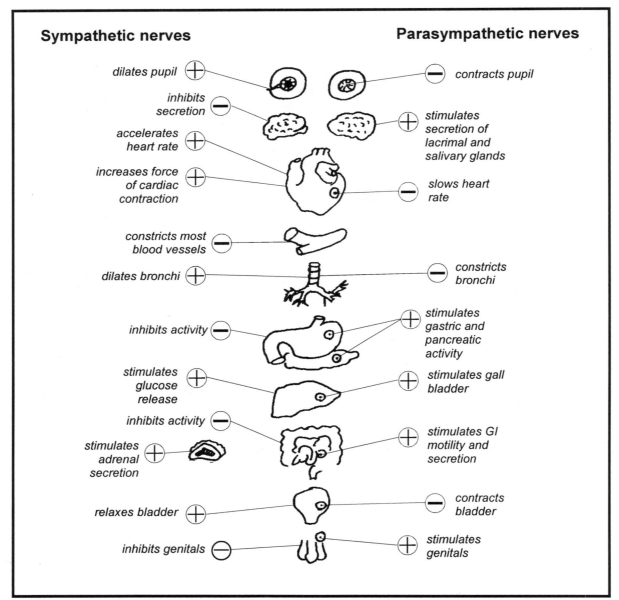

Illustration 1   Autonomic Nervous System

During *alarm* (stage 1), the body recognizes the stressor and the hypothalamus acts on the anterior pituitary gland to cause the release of adrenocorticotropic hormone, which stimulates the adrenal cortex to secrete glucocorticoid and the adrenal medulla releases epinephrine and norepinephrine. These hormones produce the energy we need to fight or flee the stressor. In this stage, the heart rate increases, blood sugar rises, pupils dilate, and digestion slows, with blood being sent away from the gut to the large skeletal muscles. (See illustration 1.)

During *resistance* (stage 2), the body begins to repair the effects of the alarm stage, and those acute symptoms diminish or disappear altogether. If, however, the stress continues without an adequate rest period, resistance will not be able to maintain the defense, and *exhaustion* (stage 3) occurs. When exhaustion continues without relief, any of a variety of disorders can begin to take shape, affecting all of the physical systems and the mental, emotional and spiritual facets.

Our body/minds are equipped to tell us when we have had enough sympathetic activation and it is time to let up. Initial signs and symptoms include: irritability, sweating, anxiety, high-pitched laughter or voice, teeth grinding, diarrhea, indigestion, nausea, fatigue, constipation, trembling, dizziness, emotional swings, forgetfulness, dryness in mouth or throat, increased heart rate, increased blood pressure, heart pounding, insomnia, nightmares, appetite changes, and hypervigilance. Unfortunately, these important messages are often misunderstood or ignored long enough for chronic illness patterns to develop and become the norm.

With long-term stress, muscles stay tight, restricting movement and reducing blood flow to cells, thus reducing oxygen and nourishment going in and out of tissues. Cortisol is released, causing fluid retention, hypertension (elevated blood pressure), muscle weakness, decreased immune responses, decreased blood glucose levels, and altered protein and fat metabolism. Long-term stress also causes decreased resiliency, including weakened connective tissue that is more apt to be injured, more emotional sensitivity, a predisposition to osteoporosis, ulcers, and headaches, and less confidence in (or awareness of) one's spiritual connection to life.

Techniques that may activate the parasympathetic response include: providing a safe, respect-ful, pleasant environment with low levels of temperature, light, sound, and smell stimuli, repetitive sound and touch rhythms at or below 60 beats per minute, slow, deep breaths, rocking, and acupressure.

In most bodywork scenarios, the client's sympathetic system is active as s/he arrives, meets the practitioner, and begins to receive massage. The bodyworker helps the client shift into a parasympathetic, or energy conservation state. However, in pre-event sports massage, the bodyworker stimulates sympathetic activation so that energy is produced and the client is ready for action. Compression, friction and tapotement are examples of techniques that stimulate the sympathetic response.

A considerable amount of research is being undertaken to better understand the mind/body connection. If you are interested in more information, refer to the headings Neuropeptides; Psychoneuroimmunology; and Endorphins in your search.

Chapter 2, Part 2

Mental and Emotional Conditions

The mental and emotional facets of wellness are discussed together because the American health culture interrelates them closely. The following are some abilities that mentally and emotionally healthy adults demonstrate:

- expressing thoughts and feelings in affirmative ways
- setting healthy boundaries for oneself
- a sense of humor
- loving and caring for oneself
- giving and accepting love and affection
- adapting and adjusting to change
- handling different degrees of anxiety, disappointment and anger
- accepting responsibility for one's decisions, feelings and actions
- controlling impulses until they can be fulfilled appropriately
- dealing with reality in a helpful way
- accepting and adapting to losses
- relating to others in ways that are helpful

In general, American psychological health professionals consider mental/emotional health to be based on self-respect and self-worth. However, we all have, at some time, felt low in self-respect and/or doubted our self-worth, so, there is more to mental/emotional health than that. For instance, even when we are feeling good about ourselves, it is much more difficult to stay mentally and emotionally balanced when we are dealing with serious losses, such as having an acute or chronic illness, a personal crisis, an environmental catastrophe, etc. Even having experiences we define as basically "good" can be stressful, and multiple stressors happening together can be overwhelming. Confusion, depression, anxiety, and agitation are common responses to having multiple stressors present in one's life.

The difference between mental and emotional health and illness behaviors is often a matter of degree. Signs and symptoms of mental/emotional illness differ from healthy reactions because they are more severe, intense and disabling. In general terms, *mental/emotional illness* is defined by behavior which is inappropriate to the life situation, as judged by the individual and/or by society. Mental/emotional illness can be temporary, occurring because of an overwhelming life event, or it can be long-term (chronic). In addition, certain types of mental/emotional illnesses are thought to result from imbalances in brain chemicals. At this time, it is not known how much these chemical imbalances are due to genetics, how much to life events, and how much to nutrition, environmental pollution, or other factors yet to be discovered.

Sometimes a person is aware that s/he is behaving inappropriately, and sometimes s/he is not aware of it. As a health care professional, it is important that you set and maintain clear and comfortable boundaries with your clients, in order to keep yourself emotionally, mentally, physically and spiritually safe, and to give your client an honest reflection in which to see him/herself, if they can. When you feel uncomfortable with a client's behavior, say so. Use your professional code of ethics as a reference, if you need to.

Signs and symptoms such as fatigue, apathy, anorexia, insomnia, headaches, and general all-over-the-body pain may be resulting from physical, mental, emotional or spiritual illness, or a combination. When you see severe, intense or disabling signs or symptoms manifesting in the mental/emotional facets of your client's health, it is your responsibility to recommend s/he see a health professional who is trained to help with the problem, just the same as you would refer clients with severe, intense or disabling problems manifesting in the physical facet of their health. The purpose of the rest of this chapter is to help you recognize deviations from health so you can understand, support and refer your clients appropriately.

DEFENSE MECHANISMS

The term *"defense mechanism"* means a mental process (often unconscious) that helps us deal with situations that are painful or that we feel anxious about. The short term use of defense mechanisms is *functional*. In other words, it helps us function in life without too many negative consequences. Defense mechanisms give us time to sort out information and process our thoughts and feelings. However, using defense mechanisms as an automatic way of life, over the long term, is *dysfunctional*, which means it does not help us function in life and gives many negative consequences.

The following are the names and descriptions of the major defense mechanisms:

Aggression is striking out at someone or something to get rid of pain or to defend oneself and is generally stimulated by frustration, which is a form of anger. An example of functional aggression might be to work extremely hard after a failure. An example of dysfunctional aggression might be to strike out at your child.

Denial is refusing to believe the truth about a situation, event or person. It can range from temporary to complete withdrawal from the world. An example of functional denial might be to ignore that you have not washed your dishes after supper when you are tired. An example of dysfunctional denial might be to pretend that you do not have an illness that needs attention.

Depression is feeling sad, pessimistic, dejected or discouraged. Symptoms vary in intensity and can include feeling hopeless, helpless, vulnerable, tired, angry, and low in self-esteem. In addition, depression is often accompanied by trouble concentrating, increased or decreased appetite, increased or decreased sleep, decreased sexual desire, and suicidal thoughts. An example of functional depression might be feeling sad after the death of a friend. An example of dysfunctional depression might be feeling pessimistic, or negative, about everything that presents itself in your life.

Projection is attributing one's own undesirable traits to someone else. This is a very common defense mechanism. An example of functional projection might be when children accuse their parents of being mean when they are feeling angry and mean, and they have not learned yet how to be responsible for their feelings. An example of dysfunctional projection might be when person A accuses person B of lying or cheating, without any objective basis, when, in fact, person A lies or cheats but does not acknowledge it. Dysfunctional projection often occurs with traits that are being repressed.

Repression is putting one's feelings or thoughts out of one's mind because they are unpleasant or painful. This can be temporary until the person is less overwhelmed and can sort through his or her feelings, or it can be extreme, where the person no longer can remember the event or the feelings. An example of functional repression might be to put the thoughts of a car wreck out of your mind while recovering from the fractures you sustained in it. An example of dysfunctional repression might be to refuse to think or talk about that experience so much that it eventually is pushed out of conscious memory.

Regression is behaving in ways that are less mature than the person is normally capable of. An example of functional regression might be to eat some chocolate to soothe myself when I am unusually stressed, after choosing to not eat it for the past 3 months. An example of dysfunctional regression might be to become dependent on our closest friend to spend time with us every day in a caretaking manner.

Rationalization is trying to justify what happens by blaming it on circumstances. When person A rationalizes, she explains her behaviors or motives as acceptable in order to reduce her anxiety. She is basically saying, "I'm capable, but it was impossible this time" or "I'm doing what's best for person B" when in reality the acts were meant for person A's own good. An example of functional rationalization might be to justify being 5 minutes late on being stuck in traffic. An example of dysfunctional rationalization might be to justify being 30 minutes late on picking up roses for the bodyworker.

Dissociation means separation from union, or detachment. This can be temporary and functional, as in separating one's attention from their arm while they get a flu shot, or it can be dysfunctional, as in separating one's awareness from one's body so completely that one is not even aware one is doing it. An example of dysfunctional dissociation might be to be unaware that your jaw, neck and shoulder muscles are clamped into spasm and your stomach is upset.

Hypervigilance means being overly concerned and overly attentive to one's inner state or outer environment. Again, this can be temporary and functional, as in watching for traffic when you cross a street. Or it can be dysfunctional, as in being constantly on the alert for any movement from any source within your vision. Hypervigilance often accompanies anxiety and is particularly common among people who have been either accidentally or intentionally hurt.

SPECIFIC MENTAL/EMOTIONAL ILLNESSES

When working with clients who have a diagnosed mental/emotional illness, it is best to be working in *collaboration* with the client's physician or mental health professional. If this is not possible, then at least ask the client to bring you an acknowledgment from their physician or mental health professional that they are in treatment for their mental illness and that they are aware the client is receiving bodywork. If neither of these options are possible, then document in the client's record that you have recommended that they seek help from a mental health professional or physician with the date(s) that you give the referral(s).

Depression is considered a mental illness if it lasts more than two months. Called chronic depression, it affects approximately 10% of the American adult population with women identifying symptoms more often than men. Chronic depression is often associated with physical illness, lack of physical activity, lack of sunlight, and drug or alcohol abuse. Bodywork is generally indicated for clients with chronic depression, and techniques that stimulate the client's sympathetic nervous system and stimulate the client to be more aware of his/her thoughts, feelings and physical sensations are especially helpful. Refer clients whose depression interferes with their functions in daily life to a psychologist, psychiatrist, social worker, physician or spiritual counselor.

Depression is a leading contributor to *suicide*, being present in 80% of suicide attempts. Sometimes suicide occurs during an acute phase of mental illness, but more often people who commit or attempt suicide are people who have not been diagnosed as mentally ill. Across all ages and races, American men complete a significantly higher number of suicides than women do. The suicide rate in males over age 75 is two to three times the rate of men at any other age, and approximately 10 times the rate in women at any age. (Source: U.S. National Center for Health Statistics, <u>Vital Statistics of the United States</u>, annual, 1992).

If a client brings up the subject of suicide, or mentions feeling uninterested in continuing to live, do not attempt to "hush up" their feelings. On the contrary, if you feel comfortable doing it, allow the client to talk about their feelings while you listen patiently and with care. Communicate that you understand what the client is saying and that it sounds like things are very difficult, painful or overwhelming right now. You can also tell the client that you would like to help, and ask what might help him or her feel better. Only agree to do what the client asks if it is a safe and reasonable choice.

Bodywork is generally indicated for people who feel suicidal. However, it is extremely important to report any suicide attempts or threats to the client's family, significant other, physician or therapist, with the client's permission. If you think a client is suicidal, ask him/her if s/he has someone to talk to. If s/he does not, refer him/her to a counselor or the Suicide Hotline. If s/he tells you or if you believe s/he has planned a suicide for the near future, you can call 911 (in the U.S.) and ask for an intervention.

Seasonal Affective Disorder (SADD) is depression related to a certain season of the year, especially winter. Symptoms usually begin during adulthood and include daytime drowsiness, fatigue, and diminished concentration. Women report symptoms four times as often as men do. The etiology is unknown, however, symptoms are reduced by exposure to bright light, especially during the early morning. Bodywork is indicated in the same way it is for depression.

Attention deficit disorder (ADD) is most commonly considered a children's disorder, but recently more and more adults are identifying symptoms, as well. The disorder is characterized by inattention, impulsivity, difficulty organizing and completing work, omissions or misrepresentations in communications, and sometimes hyperactivity and/or aggression. A variety of names have been applied to this disorder: hyperkinetic syndrome; hyperactive child syndrome; minimal brain damage; minimal brain dysfunction; minimal cerebral dysfunction. The etiology is unknown. Bodywork is indicated but may need to be modified to fit the client's attention span and/or need for movement.

Bipolar affective disorder is a condition with severe mood swings that range from mania (an exaggerated emotional high) to depression. This is also known as manic/depression. The manic state produces feelings of euphoria, restlessness, talkativeness, racing thoughts and grandiosity, and there is a decreased desire for sleep and food and often an increased tendency to do risky behaviors. In the depressive state, there is a loss of self-esteem and feelings of depression as already described. Bipolar affective disorder is more common in women than in men and usually starts between the ages of 20 and 35. The cause is not known, but it may have a genetic cause or may stem from emotional abuse or both. It is also sometimes associated with diabetes or stroke. Bodywork is generally indicated for bipolar affective disorder but is complicated due to the client's wide mood swings. Clients exhibiting mania generally need calm, gentle, soothing strokes and techniques, although you may want to start with more fast-paced, active techniques to start at the client's rhythm and gradually slow down as the session progresses. Techniques for working with depressed clients were mentioned earlier.

Anxiety is defined as a feeling of great apprehension, uneasiness and agitation, and can range from simple restlessness and irritability to an extreme feeling of powerlessness and panic. *Acute anxiety* is also known as a *panic attack.* In this situation, the feelings are very strong and accelerate quickly. The panic may be accompanied by a racing heartbeat, difficulty breathing, shaking, hot or cold sensations, phobias, and even feeling that one is about to die. Supportive attention and/or touch may or may not be useful to a person having acute anxiety (panic attack). Massage is contraindicated and, in some cases, agitates the person further. Refer this client immediately to medical or psychological help. *Chronic anxiety* is more generalized, less intense, and persists in varying degrees for a month or more. There may be insomnia, uneasiness, agitation, appetite changes, concentration problems and fatigue. Physically, there can be sweating, numbness in hands and feet, dry mouth, frequent urination, trembling and headaches. Bodywork is indicated for chronic anxiety and can be an important tool to help the client learn to relax and manage their symptoms.

Post Traumatic Stress Disorder (PTSD) comes from having a traumatic experience of any kind (e.g., combat, natural disaster, assault, rape, witnessing a murder, etc.). Generally, the person initially dissociates to repress the body/mind memories of the traumatic experience and then has anxiety, hypervigilance and sleep problems that alternate with emotional or physical numbness. There may also be unexplained rage, guilt, depression, phobias and suicidal thoughts. As memories surface, many persons use drugs or alcohol to repress the pain or terror as much as possible. Bodywork is indicated for persons with PTSD unless the client is behaving in an irrational and uncontrolled manner, and then immediate referral is indicated (also see *Abuse*, page 48).

Obsessive/Compulsive Disorder (OCD) consists of two different dimensions. *Obsession* is having uncontrollable thoughts over and over again. For example, a person might continually and uncontrollably think "My hands are dirty, this chair is dirty, this food is impure, etc." *Compulsion* is having an uncontrollable urge to act upon the obsessive thought. For example, if the person is obsessed with the idea that he or she is going to get sick, then they might also feel an uncontrollable urge to wash their hands or disinfect furniture before they sit on it, etc. Bodywork is generally indicated for OCD, however, it can be complicated by the client's compulsions.

Schizophrenia is an inability to distinguish reality from fantasy. The person generally dissociates, or separates, distinct mental processes, resulting in a decreased ability to think, plan and relate normally. They may hear or see things that others do not hear or see (hallucinations). Sometimes people who are schizophrenic can be violent to themselves or others. If you are working with a client who is having auditory or visual hallucinations, it is generally best to gently discontinue the work, acknowledge that you do not hear or see what the client does, and ask whether the client has had this experience before. If so, have they told anyone else? If, in your assessment, there are signs of dissociation occurring, it is important to take time to assess this symptom before proceeding. Like any sign or symptom of illness, dissociation can vary widely in its intensity.

Your decision to continue working or not (and which techniques you choose to use if you continue) is based on your education, experience and degree of comfort with the degree of dissociation present. When in doubt, gently end the work, offer to sit with the client, and listen. Recommend that the client talk to a person trained to help them, whether that is a psychologist, a shaman, a minister, etc. If the client seems unable to leave safely, offer to call someone to accompany the client home. Bodywork is indicated to persons under treatment for schizophrenia but is contraindicated to clients while they are out of touch (dissociated) with reality.

Paranoia involves feelings of persecution that are unsupported by actual evidence and results in unreasonable fears that someone or something is going to do them harm. Otherwise, emotional responses and social behaviors may appear normal. Paranoia can be complicated by the person's projection of their unacceptable feelings onto others in order to avoid conscious awareness of them. Bodywork is contraindicated during acute paranoid episodes, but is indicated for persons with chronic paranoia if they are in active treatment.

Multiple Personality Disorder (MPD) is a fairly rare condition in which the person exhibits two or more distinct personalities. Generally, each personality is unaware of the others and has its own identity or name, its own age, its own likes and dislikes, and, in some cases, its own distinct illnesses that the other personality(s) do not have. The person may also have consciously or unconsciously chosen to dissociate, or separate, whole segments of his or her personality, and make them no longer a part of the Self. Bodywork is indicated for persons with multiple personality disorder with some extra instructions: 1) If the client's personality changes during the session, it is appropriate that you stop working, introduce yourself again, explain what work you have to offer, do another health history and assessment, and ask this personality for consent, just as you did when the client first arrived. Obviously, this will be unusual and may be difficult to do. 2) A follow-up phone call, to check on the client a few hours after the bodywork will help you and the client determine if the session was helpful or upsetting. If upsetting, do not give more sessions unless the client is in active therapy and you have talked with the therapist (with the client's consent), so that you can tailor your work to what is appropriate to the client's needs.

Dementia is a broad, global impairment of intellectual function that usually is progressive and interferes with activities of daily living (ADLs). Most commonly, the onset of symptoms is slow, over month or years, as occurs in Alzheimer's disease or alcoholism. In some cases, onset is rapid (acute), over hours or days, as in drug overdose, brain tumors and infections of the brain. Symptoms include short-term memory loss, impaired abstract thinking, poor judgment, depression, agitation, insomnia, paranoia, impaired motor control, and sometimes impaired speaking ability. Disorientation to place and time occurs earlier, usually, than disorientation to recognizing oneself and familiar other people. Medical treatment is often curative for acute dementia, if initiated early enough. Medical treatment for slowly developing dementia is not usually curative and reduces symptoms minimally.

Bodywork is systemically contraindicated in cases of acute dementia, and a friend or family member should be called, if possible, to accompany the client to see a physician for assessment. Bodywork is indicated for people who have been assessed and diagnosed with slow-onset dementias unless contraindicated by the presence of another condition. Work may need to be modified to fit the client's energy level or shortened attention span. When working with people with short-term memory loss, be willing to repeat instructions or basic details of the visit several times, if necessary; the client may ask you to work on an area that you have already worked on, or there may be a sudden change in the client's attitude, and you might be asked to stop working. Do not take these things personally. Make each touch as complete as possible, since the session could end at any time. Keep conversation very simple, concrete (rather than abstract), and calming. Questions such as "Is there anything you want to say now?" are more helpful than "How was this session?" Provide physical cues and gently guide the person with your hands when s/he does not understand instructions.

A *somatoform disorder* occurs when the person is trying to resolve some mental or emotional conflict, but they are not able to do it directly so they unconsciously create physical signs or symptoms of illness. There are four main types of this disorder:

- *Somatization* is when the person feels physically ill but has no diagnosable disease. For example, the person has chronic nausea and vomiting and has seen many physicians for advice, but none have found physical evidence of a cause.

- *Conversion* is when the person has a hysterical reaction to an emotional event or trauma and physical symptoms emerge such as blindness or paralysis.
- *Psychogenic pain* occurs when a person feels pain but there is no diagnosable reason for the pain. For example, a person feels chronic sharp, shooting pains in their thighs and has seen many physicians, but none have found evidence of a cause.
- *Hypochondriasis* is when a person has a heightened awareness of their body and an abnormal fear of disease. For example, a person is aware of every ache, twinge, or adaptation their body makes and, generally, diagnoses themselves with one illness after another based on their awareness of what they believe are symptoms.

Many theories propose direct, predictable links between a person's mental, emotional, and/or spiritual facets and their physical body. One such theory has been proposed by Stanley Keleman, and another is proposed by Caroline Myss. To date, there is little scientific research to prove or disprove such theories. However, many books, tapes, and workshops are available to help people explore the possibilities of these important theories and their applications in personal and professional life (see *Further Resources*, page 52).

DRUG AND ALCOHOL ABUSE

Bodywork is contraindicated for any client who is intoxicated by drugs or alcohol. Can you imagine why this is? There are three primary reasons. First, a person who is intoxicated is, to some degree, numb or out of touch with their body, plus their mental awareness is clouded. Stimulants such as cocaine and amphetamines cause hyperactivity, irritability, muscle tension, aggression and sometimes hallucinations. Depressants such as alcohol and marijuana cause sedation, sluggish reflexes, decreased thinking and problem solving abilities and sometimes panic or paranoia. These effects decrease a person's ability to be responsible for themselves in giving you the assessment information you need for safe work. Second, the intoxicated person is usually not conscious of personal boundaries–yours or theirs–and, again, is unlikely to be responsible. Third, since bodywork can increase circulation, it can mobilize the drug or alcohol that is lying in the tissues so that it circulates to the brain and increases intoxication.

Bodywork can be helpful (indicated) for persons in drug or alcohol detox because it can help the person relax and be in touch with his or her body. However, depending on where the person is in their detox process, the bodywork can complicate or intensify the detoxification process. For instance, bodywork can contribute to increased emotional lability at a time when the person is not ready to deal with that, or conversely, really help the person contain (or ground) themselves. Bodywork may increase the circulating drug and its toxic effects, or conversely, help the body remove the drug. So, the timing of the bodywork is very important, and it should be included as part of the collaborative treatment plan with the therapist's or physician's awareness.

MENTAL/EMOTIONAL/PHYSICAL/SPIRITUAL ABUSE

Abuse is not a illness, per se, but it can greatly influence health. Abuse is defined as anything that hurts oneself or others, and it affects people mentally, emotionally, spiritually and physically. At its core, the intent of all abuse is the same: to dominate, humiliate, and gain control of a person. There are different kinds of abuse and different degrees, ranging from an unkind remark to an actual murder. The following terms are often used to identify abuse: belittle, ridicule, insult, offend, berate, criticize, attack, dishonor, neglect, exploit, harass, mistreat, molest, violate, batter, rape, torment, and persecute.

No matter how it occurs, abuse reduces a person's sense of worth, self-esteem, and empowerment. The severity of abuse's effects on a person seems to depend on its frequency, whether someone was able to validate the person's worth and help him/her cope at the time, and his/her own inner resources, or defense mechanisms. Generally, the older a person is at the time of the abuse, the more inner resources s/he has.

Contrary to the scary stories of strangers doing us harm, most abusers are our families and friends. This causes mixed emotions because, in addition to feeling the abuse, the person feels a measure of trust was there and now it is broken. In addition, the person who was abused often feels guilty, wondering if somehow s/he is at fault. Since bodywork requires trust and close physical presence, it is understandable that survivors of abuse often have difficulty receiving bodywork.

Sexual and physical attacks injure the body, and the body remembers its experiences. *State Dependent Memory* is a term for memories that are stored in the body as well as the mind. Body memories are not verbal. They are sensations of tastes, smells, sights, textures, pressures, postures, emotions, physical actions, and all the combined physiology of the person at the time the experience happened.

State dependent memory functions in all life experiences. However, during trauma, this mechanism locks in all the factors that coincide with the experience, and when the person has another set of circumstances where several sensations match with the trauma experience, the person experiences a flashback or relives the event as if it was occurring now. Flashbacks can last from a moment to several hours. When the flashback occurs, the person dissociates from the present.

The touch, pressure, position, or movements of either the client or bodyworker can trigger flashbacks to painful memories for the client. The areas of the mouth, throat, neck, chest, abdomen, buttocks, and inner thighs seem to most often be vulnerable. However, any touching or movement of any part of the body can trigger a flashback.

In addition, people who were abused before they became highly verbal (which generally happens about the age of four), seem to have especially difficult times trying to identify and put words to their body memories. In the place of words, they may have vague feelings of uneasiness or dissociation.

It is important that bodyworkers understand how to recognize and be supportive of clients who are experiencing flashbacks during the session. Generally, when a flashback occurs, the job of the bodyworker is to bring the client back to the present as quickly as possible. If the client feels overwhelmed by his/her experience, s/he may choose to stop. Many times, however, if you suggest that s/he sit up or simply open his/her eyes and looks around for a few moments, the client will choose to continue. If you are comfortable continuing, you can offer to work on a different body area. If the client is extremely upset or dissociated, assist him/her to get up, draped well with the sheet, and sit in a chair or walk around the room until s/he feels ready to dress again. In these cases, refer the client to a mental/emotional health professional with expertise in helping survivors of abuse.

A less obvious response to bodywork that also signals distress is dissociation, discussed on page 30. Clues that a client is dissociating include shallow breathing, holding the breath, and unusual muscle tension accompanied by a feeling that the client is somehow "not there" under your hands. Some bodyworkers report feeling "spacey" or disconnected, themselves, when the client is dissociating. If you notice these signs, you may want to gently ask the client what s/he is feeling or if there is anything going on that s/he wants to tell you about.

However, unless specifically requested by the client, it is not the bodyworker's job to remind the client to remain aware of his or her feelings. Being present in one's body is a double-edged sword for survivors of abuse. Each client has a right to use whatever coping mechanisms s/he wants. If the client is not ready to be more aware, s/he may withdraw from intrusive instructions or reminders. Conversely, if the client is aware of his/her discomfort with touch, and s/he trusts that you accept her/him, s/he may need you to work on his/her hands or feet for months before s/he is ready for other touch. It is not unusual for clients to need up to a year's experience with massage before they can have their unclothed backs or legs touched.

It is also not appropriate for a bodyworker to suggest to a client that s/he has been abused or that the client needs to deal with his or her experience in any way. The decision to deal actively with a painful history requires enormous commitment, time, and energy by the client. The bodyworker's job is to honor, respect, value, support, accept, appreciate, and recognize the client for who they are. Listening and acknowledging what the client says is enormously important. In this way, the client leads and the therapist follows.

Sexual abuse is "any unwanted or inappropriate sexual contact, either verbal or physical, between two or more people, that is intended as an act of control, power, rage, violence and intimidation, with sex as a weapon." (Benjamin, 1995.) Sexual abuse can range from seductive behavior to sexual intercourse and includes sexual harassment, incest, date rape, spouse rape, gang rape, and rape by a stranger. Sexual abuse can also take the form of ritual or cult abuse.

Sexual abuse is particularly devastating to people because it usually happens to people who are unable to defend themselves, because it is often accompanied by other types of mental, emotional, and physical abuse, and because it happens to so many people. Researchers estimate that, in the U.S., one woman in three and one man in six has been sexually abused before the age of 18. That is equivalent to 50 million Americans, or one in five.

According to Judith Herman, there are three stages of recovery from sexual abuse. These stages help us have a clear way to think about the recovery process, but, in reality, people often move back and forth between stages and can experience more than one stage at once. The three stages are: 1) Establishing safety. During this first stage, the person is learning how to take control of their body/mind. 2) Remembrance and mourning. The person is grieving the abuse and the losses associated with it. This is a deeply painful process. 3) Reconnection. The person begins to look toward the future. S/he remembers the abuse but begins to focus on other parts of life and building confidence.

A sensitive and respectful bodywork environment creates an opportunity for survivors of any type of abuse to begin to feel safe with emotions and physical sensations and to begin to rebuild personal boundaries. By being in charge of the session, the survivor gains another piece of control of his/her life and physical body. Touch that is neutral or pleasurable, and not sexual, provides internal foundations for a new experience, which, in turn, helps the client reconnect dissociated facets of his/her Self. Professional help and support from family or friends is often needed. Referral to an abuse recovery specialist (counselor, psychotherapist, etc.) can help the client integrate his/her memories and insights.

As a final note, clients who have been abused may not be able to adequately protect themselves when a bodyworker errs. Treatment mistakes can occur when the bodyworker presses too deeply or inadvertently violates one of the client's boundaries. Because survivors often have trouble knowing what they are really comfortable with, or voicing their boundaries, they may not be able to let the bodyworker know if he or she is using too much pressure or causing some other discomfort. Conversely, clients may sometimes ask for pressure or other bodywork that is not appropriate. It is important that the bodyworker be able to recognize these situations and respond knowledgeably, with patience, gentleness, and respect. The bodyworker may have to say "I'm sorry, I'm already working on this area as deeply as I feel it is safe to work," or "I do not feel that technique would be best for you right now."

If you have an interest in working with clients who are survivors of abuse or who experience mental/emotional illnesses, it is important that you get further education about the physiology and psychology of these conditions and the challenges your clients face. Advanced bodywork education is available nationally to help you learn appropriate bodywork techniques before you specialize in any of these areas.

MEDICATIONS RELATED TO MENTAL/EMOTIONAL ILLNESS

Persons with certain types of mental/emotional illnesses have been found to have imbalances in some of their brain chemicals. As stated earlier, it is not known how much these chemical imbalances are due to genetics, how much to life events, and how much to nutrition and environmental pollution. Hyperactivity/ attention deficit disorder, bipolar disorder, schizophrenia, seasonal affective disorder, and chronic depression are just a few illnesses thought to involve brain chemical imbalances.

Medication is often very helpful for people with brain chemical imbalances. The bodyworker should not judge clients who take medication for these disorders nor make statements that suggest the person is at fault, in any way, for their illness or wrong for their use of medications. The choice to take medications is a very personal one and is based on many factors. Unless the bodyworker is also a pharmacist, RN, MD or DO, he or she is not usually informed enough to advise a client on the appropriateness of their medication choices.

However, if a client is following his or her treatment plan, exercising regularly, and receiving bodywork regularly, s/he can often gradually reduce his/her dose and, in some cases, eventually stop taking the medication. It is very important that each client work closely with his/her prescribing health professional during that process. Bodyworkers can play an important part by noticing signs and symptoms of improvement, pointing them out to the client, and documenting them in the client's file.

CASE PRESENTATION

7/28/96 *Health history*: 32 yo female, complaining of headaches & neck/shoulder tension and pain. Sexual abuse survivor who's been in therapy x 3 yrs and is currently processing memories.

Assessment: Rates occipital pain at 3 on 0-5 scale. Hypertonic cervical and trapezius muscles. Skin and fascia felt extra tight. I noticed feeling a vague anxiety come and go in myself during the work, as well as feeling like I was walking through knee-deep mud. Sometimes I felt like I was touching a body, but the person wasn't in it.

Application: Gentle effleurage and petrissage to upper body, feet and lower legs. Focused on sending love, warmth and nurturance; checked with her often to see how she was doing.

Outcome: Neck pain rated at 1. Didn't have time to visit much with client after massage.

Post note: Client called about 2 hrs after session, crying. Said she didn't know why she was so upset. I acknowledged her feelings and explained that sometimes massage facilitates a release of emotions stored in the body. Recommended she call her therapist. I called client the next day & she said she was feeling much better. Is increasing her therapy and wants to continue massage to help her healing process.

STUDY QUESTIONS

Which part of the above case presentation was subjective?
Which parts was objective?
What questions would you have asked that were not asked?
What bodywork techniques would you have done?
What referral(s)?
What other ways could the therapeutic outcome have been evaluated?
How might you have changed the format or the way the cases were written?

FURTHER RESOURCES

Benjamin, Ben E., PhD and/or faculty, <u>Massage and bodywork with survivors of abuse.</u> Contact Dr. Benjamin at 508-369-3150 or 508-369-0514.

Ford, Clyde, DC, <u>Compassionate touch</u>, Simon and Shuster, 1993.

Herman, Judith L., <u>Trauma and recovery</u>, Harper Collins Publishers, Inc., 1992.

Katherine, Anne, <u>Boundaries: Where you end and I begin</u>, Fireside Parkside Books, 1993.

Keleman, S. (1985). <u>Emotional anatomy</u>. Berkeley, CA: Center Press.

Levin, Peter, PhD and Diana Poole Heller, <u>The body as healer: Transforming trauma</u>. Contact Kathy Allen at The Ergos Institute, 303-786-7544.

Myss, C. (1996). <u>Anatomy of the spirit: The seven stages of power and healing</u>. New York: Harmony Books.

Piantedosi, Sharon, RN, LMT, *Safe Touch® Seminars*. Contact Aleka Munroe at 603-749-4780.

Torrenzano, Suzanne, PhD, <u>Incest: Insults to the body-mind, bodywork with adult survivors</u>. Contact Suzanne Torrenzano at 21104 Crocus Terrace, Ashburn, VA 22011, 703-536-5012.

REFERENCES

Benjamin, B. E. (1995). Massage and bodywork with survivors of abuse, Parts I-V. <u>Massage Therapy Journal</u>, Summer 1995, Fall 1995, Winter 1996, Spring 1996, Summer 1996.

Bailey, K. (1992). Therapeutic massage with survivors of abuse. <u>Massage Therapy Journal</u>, Summer 1992, 79-85, 116, 118, 120, 122.

Kapit, W., Macey, R.I., & Meisami, E. (1987). <u>The physiology coloring book</u>. NY: Harper & Row.

Samuelson, P. (1994). <u>Pathophysiology for massage: The travel guide</u>. Overland Park, KS: Mid-America Handbooks, Inc.

Thomas, C.L. (1989). <u>Taber's cyclopedic medical dictionary</u> (16th ed.). Philadelphia: F.A. Davis Co.

<u>Vital Statistics of the United States</u>, (1992). U.S. National Center for Health Statistics.

CHAPTER REVIEW

1. Signs and symptoms of mental/emotional illness differ from healthy reactions because they are _____

2. Define the following terms:
   a. defense mechanism _____
   b. dysfunctional _____
   c. bipolar affective disorder _____
   d. acute anxiety _____
   e. obsession _____
   f. compulsion _____
   g. schizophrenia _____
   h. hypochondriasis _____

i. abuse _____

j. state dependent memory _____

k. hypoxia _____

l. pathogens _____

m. mutations _____

n. risk factors _____

o. stress _____

3. Bodyworkers can play an important role in the client's medication treatment by: _____

4. Depression is considered a mental illness if it lasts _____
   Chronic depression affects approximately ____% of the U.S. adult population.

5. (Circle one) People who commit or attempt suicide often <u>have/have not</u> been diagnosed as
   mentally ill.

6. Bodywork is indicated for persons with PTSD unless _____

7. (Circle one) Bodywork is <u>indicated/contraindicated</u> to clients while they are out of touch
   with reality.

8. Paranoia can be complicated by _____

9. (Circle one) Bodywork is <u>indicated/contraindicated</u> for any client who is intoxicated by
   drugs or alcohol.

10. (Circle one) Bodywork is <u>indicated/contraindicated</u> for persons in drug or alcohol detox.

11. When a flashback occurs, the bodyworker's job is to _____

12. Approximately one in every _____ clients may be a survivor of sexual abuse.

13. When working with survivors of abuse, treatment mistakes can occur when the
    bodyworker _____

14. List 4 common subjective responses to stress.
    a. _____
    b. _____
    c. _____
    d. _____

15. List 4 common objective responses to stress.
    a. _____
    b. _____
    c. _____
    d. _____

16. Cells respond to stress by changing their _____

17. The three stages of the GAS are: 1) _____,
    2)_____ and 3) _____

18. List 4 common results of long-term stress:
    a. _____
    b. _____
    c. _____
    d. _____

19. What is the function of the sympathetic nervous system? _____
    What is the function of the parasympathetic system? _____

ANSWERS TO CHAPTER REVIEW

1. more severe, intense and disabling

2. a. a mental process that helps us deal with situations that are painful or scary
   b. it does not help us function in life and gives many negative consequences
   c. severe mood swings ranging from mania to depression; also known as
      manic/depression
   d. panic attack; the feelings are very strong and accelerate quickly; can include a racing
      heartbeat, difficulty breathing, shaking, hot or cold feeling, phobias, and feeling that
      one is about to die
   e. having uncontrollable thoughts over and over
   f. having an uncontrollable urge to act upon the obsession
   g. inability to distinguish reality from fantasy
   h. a heightened awareness of ones body and an abnormal fear of disease
   i. anything that hurts oneself or others
   j. memories that are stored in the body as well as the mind
   k. significant reduction in a cell's oxygen supply
   l. organisms that can injure cells, including viruses, bacteria, parasites and fungi
   m. changes in cell chromosomes
   n. conditions that make a negative event more likely, but do not necessarily constitute the
      cause
   o. disequilibrium, strain or tension in a structure, system, or organism

3. noticing signs and symptoms of improvement, pointing them out to the client, and documenting them in the client's file

4. lasts more than two months; 10

5. have not

6. the client is behaving in an irrational and uncontrolled manner

7. contraindicated

8. the person's projection of their unacceptable feelings onto others

9. contraindicated

10. indicated

11. bring the client back to the present as quickly as possible

12. 5

13. presses too deeply or inadvertently violates one of the client's boundaries

14. anxiety, fatigue, nausea, irritability, insomnia, forgetfulness, dizziness, emotional swings, heart pounding, nightmares, appetite changes, hypervigilance

15. muscle weakness, muscle tension, joint stiffness, sweating dry mouth, increased incidence in accidents, stuttering, high-pitched voice, increased heart rate, teeth-grinding, diarrhea, constipation, trembling, increased blood pressure

16. size, shape, and function

17. 1) alarm ("fight or flight"), 2) resistance reaction, and 3) exhaustion

18. muscles stay tight, oxygen and nourishment are reduced to the tissues, cortisol is released, fluid retention, hypertension (elevated blood pressure), muscle weakness, decreased immune responses, decreased blood glucose levels, and altered protein and fat metabolism, decreased resiliency, weakened connective tissue, more emotional sensitivity, a predisposition to osteoporosis, ulcers, and headaches, and less confidence of one's spiritual connection to life

19. energy production or "fight or flight;" energy conservation

Chapter 3, Part 1

INTEGUMENTARY SYSTEM

ANATOMY AND PHYSIOLOGY REVIEW

The integumentary system consists of the hair, nails and skin, and each can reflect health or illness. Healthy hair is soft, shiny, resilient and secure. Hair loss should be minimal when massaging the scalp or body. Healthy nails are smooth. Vertical ridges can indicate nutritional difficulties, whereas horizontal ridges and/or clubbed nails can be signs of poor circulation. Hangnails, split skin around the nails and lips, and mouth sores are signs of prolonged stress or other pathology.

The skin, or *integument*, protects the body against heat, light, dehydration and microorganisms. It regulates body temperature through its sweat glands and blood vessels. It stores water, fat, and vitamin D. It serves as both an organ of elimination (through the sweat) and absorption. Nerve endings in the skin sense temperature changes, pressure, texture, and pain, sending the information to the spinal cord and brain. The oil glands provide a lubricant that keeps the skin soft and pliable. The skin continually and efficiently regenerates itself. It is the body's largest organ and weighs about six pounds. The skin is made of two layers: the outer layer (*epidermis*) and the inner layer (*dermis*) (see *Illustration 2*).

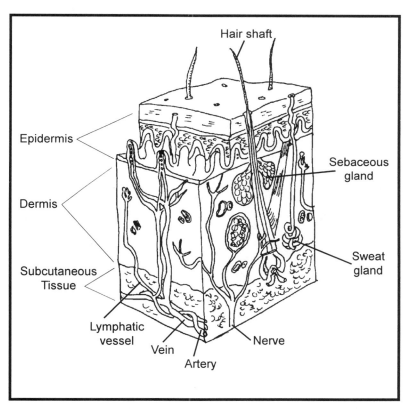

Illustration 2   Integument (Skin) Organization

The epidermis consists of layered epithelial cells. Basal cells in the bottom layer divide, forming new cells that gradually move up to the surface. Squamous cells at the surface die and become scale-like, providing the waterproof layer of the skin. The deepest part of the epidermis contains melanocytes which produce the melanin that gives the skin its color and protects it from the sun's ultraviolet rays. The epidermis is only about 0.07 to 0.12 mm deep in most areas. There are no blood vessels in the epidermis.

The dermis lies under the epidermis and contains blood and lymph vessels, nerve fibers, and connective and elastic fibers. Hair follicles, sweat (perspiration) glands, and oil (sebum) glands located below the dermis pass through it and connect to the epidermis through tiny openings called pores.

Beneath the dermis is the subcutaneous tissue, made up of fat and blood vessels. The hair follicles, sweat and oil glands are also located in the subcutaneous tissue. This fatty tissue connects the skin to underlying muscle, bone, or ligament tissues by means of fascia and can vary in depth from being only about 1/8" in thin, undernourished people, to 8" or more in very obese people.

ASSESSMENT: OBSERVATION AND PALPATION

Healthy skin is smooth, resilient and elastic, with rich, even coloring. Problems in the body are often indicated by changes is skin coloring. For instance, *cyanosis*, a blue color, is seen in the lips, nose, and nail beds when a person is not getting enough oxygen. This is different from bruises which can be blue, purple, red, yellow or a combination of those colors. Avoid giving any pressure or friction on bruised areas. Refer clients with cyanosis to physicians for diagnosis and treatment.

Jaundice, a yellow color, is present first in the sclera (whites) of the eyes and then in the whole body's skin when a person has liver disease. Bodywork is contraindicated for persons with jaundice until the client has consulted with his/her physician.

Erythema, a red color, is seen with fever, inflammation, and alcohol intake. If the redness is limited to a small area, such as around a scratch, cut or rash, only local massage is contraindicated. However, if you observe hot redness or red streaking on a client's body, refer him/her to a physician immediately.

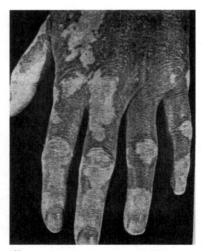

Pallor, a whitish look in the face and/or extremities, is present when a person is about to faint, go into shock, or die. Pallor is also present over the entire body when a person is anemic. A total absence of melanin (the skin pigment) may be present in a hereditary condition called *albinism*, or it may be absent in patches, signaling an autoimmune disease (*vitiligo,* see *Illustration 3*) in which the melanocytes are being destroyed. The significance of pallor must be evaluated in each case to determine if bodywork is contraindicated.

Illustration 3   Vitiligo

During bodywork, it is important to watch the skin carefully for its initial qualities and for its changes during the session and, with repeat clients, for changes over time. Bodyworkers often spend more time touching and observing a person's skin than anyone else, so our observations of skin are especially important.

Skin thickness can vary. Facial skin and the skin on the dorsal aspect of the forearms is often much thinner than other areas. The skin in the lumbar, upper arm, and buttocks areas is often thicker than other areas. However, variations within any particular area are signs of a problem. The skin often loses its elasticity and mobility over areas of dysfunction.

Another sign of a problem is when the skin is so dry that it stays peaked for a few moments after you pinch it. This sign is called *tenting*, and is a sign that the person is dehydrated. The best areas to check for tenting are the dorsal areas on the hands and forearms and on the sternum. Skin, blood vessels and connective tissues are more fragile than usual when the person is dehydrated.

When skin and underlying subcutaneous and muscle tissues are full of too much fluid, gentle pressure with your fingertips will cause dents. This is called *pitting edema* and is especially common in the feet, ankles and lower legs (see *Illustration 4*). Massage is always contraindicated in areas with pitting edema, because the added pressure can damage and even rupture fragile cell walls that are already being strained with too much fluid.

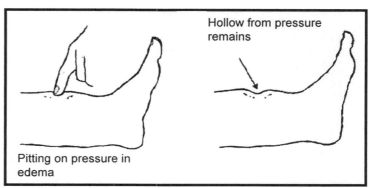

Illustration 4   Pitting Edema

A damp area of skin shows that the sympathetic nervous system is hyperactive in that area and has created what is called a *facilitated segment* (explained further in Chapter 5). Surface stroking with enough pressure to drag the skin will elicit a red response called *Sargent's line* over areas that are hyperactive, and deeper palpation will usually detect tenderness there. Lighter stroking will produce goose bumps, called the *pilomotor reflex*, over areas of hyperactivity.

IDENTIFICATION OF SKIN LESIONS

There is a broad range of *lesions*, or abnormal changes, in skin. The majority of skin lesions can be irritated by local bodywork, so it is best to avoid friction or petrissage directly on most skin lesions. If a lesion is inflamed or contagious through touch, then local bodywork is clearly contraindicated.

Skin lesions are described as "small" when they are less than 10 mm diameter, which is about the size of a pencil eraser. "Large" lesions are larger than 10 mm in diameter. *Primary skin lesions* develop on previously unaltered skin. The many different types are identified by the following terms and illustrations.

Macule

• Flat lesions: A non-elevated area of discoloration in the epidermis. Small flat lesions are called *macules,* and large flat lesions are called *patches.* Examples: freckles, flat nevi, vitiligo, petechiae, and measles. It is OK to massage macules and patches unless an infection is present..

Papule

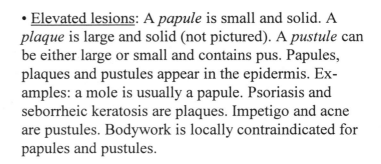

Pustule

• Elevated lesions: A *papule* is small and solid. A *plaque* is large and solid (not pictured). A *pustule* can be either large or small and contains pus. Papules, plaques and pustules appear in the epidermis. Examples: a mole is usually a papule. Psoriasis and seborrheic keratosis are plaques. Impetigo and acne are pustules. Bodywork is locally contraindicated for papules and pustules.

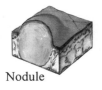

Nodule

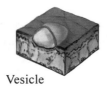

Vesicle

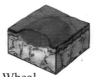

Wheal

Cyst

• Miscellaneous lesions: A *nodule* is a large, round, solid, flat or elevated mass that may extend under the dermis. A *vesicle* is a small, fluid-filled bubble in the epidermis. A *bulla* is a large, fluid-filled bubble in the epidermis (not pictured). A *wheal* is a small area of redness and swelling. A *cyst* is an encapsulated sac or pouch in the dermis or subcutaneous layer that contains fluid, semifluid or solid material and tensely elevates the skin. Examples: Fibromas and cancerous skin growths are nodules. A blister can be either a vesicle (if small) or a bulla (if large). Other examples of vesicles are herpes simplex, early chicken pox, and herpes zoster. Hives and mosquito bites are wheals. Bodywork is locally contraindicated for nodules, bullae, wheals, and cysts.

Secondary skin lesions are caused by an injury or by further deterioration in a primary skin lesion. Included are:

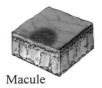

Crust or scab

Scale

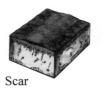

Scar

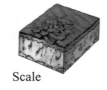

Keloid

• Elevated lesions: A *crust,* or *scab,* is an area made of dried drainage as often occurs with an abrasion or when vesicles, bullae, or pustules burst. Examples are impetigo, weeping dermatitis, and abrasions. *Scales* are collections of loose cells in the epidermis. They can be dry, greasy, silvery, or white. Examples are psoriasis, seborrheic dermatitis, eczema, and dry skin.

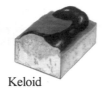

A *scar* is a collection of fibrous collagen tissue at the site of a healed lesion. A *keloid* is an elevated scar made of excessive collagen. Bodywork is locally contraindicated for crusts and scabs but usually appropriate for scales, scars and keloids.

• <u>Non-elevated lesions</u>: An *erosion* is a shallow depression where the epidermis has been partially destroyed. It is often moist but not bleeding. An *ulcer* is deeper and extends into the dermis. It may bleed. A *fissure* is any line-shaped ulcer. It looks like a crack in the skin and can be dry or moist. An *atrophic scar* is a scar with thinning of the epidermis which results in a depression in the skin. An example is a stretch mark. An *excoriation* is a superficial abrasion that may or may not be crusted. It is often caused by scratching an intensely itching area, e.g., insect bites, scabies or dermatitis. Bodywork is locally contraindicated for erosions, ulcers and fissures.

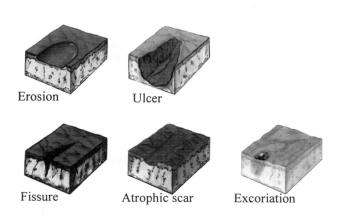

Erosion   Ulcer

Fissure   Atrophic scar   Excoriation

Combinations of primary and secondary lesions may co-exist. Those conditions can be described as maculopapular, vesiculopustular, papulovesicular, etc.

INFECTIOUS SKIN DISEASES

Infectious means capable of being transmitted and usually pertains to some type of infection that is caused by a *pathogen.* Pathogens are bacteria, viruses, fungi and parasites. The word infectious is synonymous with the word *contagious.* People whose immune systems are weakened due to stress, recent illness, and very young or very old age are especially susceptible to developing infections. In general, BODYWORK IS CONTRAINDICATED IN ANY AREA WITH AN INFECTION AND FOR ANY PERSON WITH A FEVER.

Bodywork is locally contraindicated to all areas of pain, heat, redness and swelling, which are the primary signs of inflammation and infection. Bodywork is also systemically contraindicated for anyone who has a *fever*. A fever is a 2° elevation of temperature for that person. Normal oral (by mouth) temperatures can range from 96.6° to 99.6°, depending on the person's general metabolism. During an infection, a moderate temperature elevation is actually beneficial to the work of the immune system. A very high fever is dangerous because it can cause convulsions, especially in children. Symptoms of fever are hot dry skin, flushed face, headache, aching all over, and sometimes nausea, chills or sweating. A physician should be contacted if a fever exceeds 102° or lasts longer than 24 hours. Bodywork is systemically contraindicated during fever because it could spread infection from one part of the body to another or from one person to another (including from client to bodyworker, from bodyworker to client, or from client to client). For more information on preventing infectious diseases, see Chapter 7.

BACTERIAL INFECTIONS

Impetigo is an acute, highly contagious skin infection common among children. It is caused by strep and staph organisms carried in the nose and passed to the skin. It most often appears on the face and hands. Erythema and oozing vesicles and pustules form. When these rupture, a yellow crust covers the lesion.

Cellulitis is usually not contagious unless your immune system is weak, however, massage is still contraindicated because the tissues are fragile. Cellulitis appears where a break in the skin has allowed bacteria to enter, causing a generalized infection in a large area. The area will appear red, swollen, and tender and is most often located in the extremities.

An *abscess* (or *boil*) is a deep pustule, usually caused by staph bacteria which is prevalent just about everywhere there are people, but which can cause serious infection when it has a chance to enter the body. Small, single skin abscesses are called *furuncles*. A group of furuncles is called a *carbuncle* and leaves scarring when it has healed. When an abscess forms in a hair follicle, it is called *folliculitis*. Acne is caused by interactions between bacteria, sebum (oil), and sex hormones and can be influenced by stress and/or food allergies. Cystic acne is produced by abscesses in the sebaceous (oil) glands.

Lyme disease is caused by the bacteria transmitted by the bite of deer ticks. An early symptom is an unusual "bull's eye" skin rash which sometimes has a small welt in the center. The outer red circle gradually expands and is surrounded by a lighter than usual area. Flu-like symptoms of chills, fever, headache, fatigue and musculoskeletal aches and pains may or may not accompany the rash, which appears from two days to five weeks after the tick bite.

VIRAL SKIN INFECTIONS

Cold sores, or *fever blisters*, on the outside of the mouth or lips are <u>contagious</u> and are caused by the herpes simplex I virus. This is a very common virus that is prevalent on most skin and mucous membranes, and which can live in the body for a long time without signs. When the person's immune system becomes weakened, the virus can suddenly become active.

Shingles are painful, red, swollen plaques and/or blisters that usually follow the path of a spinal nerve. Shingles usually occur in adults but rarely in children. Shingles are caused by the same herpes zoster virus that causes chicken pox. Shingles is highly contagious in its early stages, especially through the oozing of any blisters. After the lesions are gone, the person may still experience pain for months or even years, although s/he will no longer be contagious.

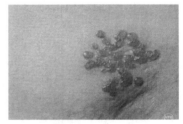

Illustration 21   Shingles

Warts are benign tumors of the keratin-producing cells, caused by viruses, and can occur in the epidermis or in the mucous membranes (such as genital warts). Warts are most common in children and young adults and can be spread by scratching. Warts are not usually serious or painful unless they form on the soles of the feet. These are called *plantar warts* and tend to grow inward.

FUNGAL SKIN INFECTIONS

All fungal infections are contagious through direct contact. Fungi thrive in warm, dark, moist environments, such as in the axillae, groin, genitals, vagina, beneath breasts, inside abdominal folds, between fingers and toes, and behind the ears. Anti-fungal medications are effective, but cleanliness and keeping the skin dry can also prevent and/or cure the problem. Most fungal infections are characterized by a foul odor or a yeasty smell.

Tinea is a very common fungus and is known by many names. *Ringworm, athlete's foot, jock itch,* and *toe/fingernail fungus* are all caused by varieties of tinea fungus and are all highly contagious. Tinea can be passed from pets to humans, from person to person, and/or from contaminated objects to humans. All are spread by scratching. The lesions are red patches that are itchy, scaly, sore, cracked, and/or blistered. If untreated, tinea can spread throughout the warm, moist, dark areas of the body. The tinea fungus that causes thick nails is usually contacted through working with the earth. It lives under the nails for years before its results become visible.

"Ringworm"

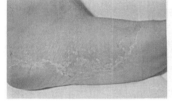

"Athlete's Foot"   "Nail Fungus"

Illustration 22	Examples of Tinea

Candida albicans is one of the common organisms found in the digestive tract (from mouth to anus), the vagina and the skin. It produces infection only when it becomes so prevalent that it crowds out other, more useful microorganisms. Candida can be likened to a weed in the garden. A few weeds are normal, but too many weeds crowd out the useful plants. Candida is a very common form of fungal infection. Diaper rashes are often caused by candida. Signs of Candida include: itching, swelling, pain, redness, and a yeasty smell. Sometimes pustules are also present.

PARASITIC INFESTATIONS

Parasites are organisms that live within, upon, or at the expense of another organism. *Lice* are tiny wingless insects that bite the skin and suck on human blood causing *pruritus*, or itching, and scratching. They are of medical importance because they are capable of transmitting epidemic typhus, trench fever, relapsing fever, and plague. Lice are spread by direct person-to-person contact and also by indirect contact, such as touching items onto which the lice have crawled. There are three main types of lice:

- *Head lice* are spread from person to person through shared combs, hats, and bed or massage linens. Head lice are usually not particularly dangerous, however, they bite the scalp and feed on the person's blood, causing the person to scratch a lot, and they deposit unsightly eggs along the hair shafts.

- *Pubic lice* are usually spread by erotic contact but can also be spread on bed and massage linens, as well. They are extremely small and may look like tiny pin dots. These lice also cause itching.

- *Body lice* can spread serious infections and have been responsible for typhus epidemics. These lice are most common among people who live in crowded quarters or who are unable to wash and change clothes regularly. They can be prevented by hygiene and are visible on white sheets.

Scabies is another contagious parasitic skin condition, caused by a microscopic insect called a mite. The female mite burrows into skin folds in the groin, under the breasts, or between fingers or toes. As she burrows, she lays eggs in the tunnels. As the eggs hatch, the mites spread and start the cycle over again. Intense itching, blisters, pustules, and grayish lines appear where the tunnels are. Scabies is easily transmitted by direct and indirect contact.

Ticks usually feed on the blood of animals but can attach and feed on humans, as well. Ticks often carry diseases such as typhus, Lyme disease, and Rocky Mountain spotted fever. Ticks are very easy to see and appear round and flat before they eat, and spherical, like a little balloon, after they eat.

ALLERGIC SKIN CONDITIONS

Allergic, or hypersensitivity reactions, are frequently manifested on the skin. These conditions are NOT contagious. Allergies all involve some amount of inflammation, and bodywork is locally contraindicated to the area.

Urticaria, or *hives*, are extremely itchy wheals that develop most often at pressure points like those under tight clothing but may appear anywhere on the skin or mucous membranes. Common causes for urticaria are stress and/or food allergies to wheat, nuts, berries, chocolate, and seafood.

Eczema (*contact dermatitis*) is a skin inflammation that can be either acute or chronic and involves erythema, papules, vesicles, pustules, scales, crusts and/or scabs. Eczema develops from skin contact with various plants, chemicals, latex and metals. Poison ivy, dyes used for hair or cloth, and the nickel in costume jewelry are examples of allergens that can cause eczema. Vesicles and bullae often develop after the tissue has become edematous. The area itches, and scratching causes the vesicles to burst and spread the antigen, or allergy-causing substance. Thin, dry skin and skin that has been damaged is more easily sensitized to contact dermatitis than healthy skin. Symptoms can develop within hours to days of contact. Stress can also sensitize a person.

Allergic drug reactions are very common and may appear as vesicles, itchy plaques, or erythema. People can be allergic to any food or drug taken internally and are most often allergic to food additives and pharmaceuticals. Some people are allergic to nuts and nut oils sufficient that the use of almond or other nut oils in bodywork can cause severe allergic drug reactions. Some allergic drug reactions are severe enough to cause anaphylactic shock and death. It is important to ask each client if they are allergic to anything. Many bodyworkers ask this on their health history, or intake form.

METABOLIC SKIN DISORDERS

Acne is the result of hormonal changes. The increased level of estrogen or testosterone stimulates all glandular activity, including the sweat and oil glands. When an oil gland becomes clogged with dirt or make-up, a little bump or whitehead is formed. Over time, this turns black, forming a blackhead. If bacteria enter the skin, pus forms, and a pimple or pustule results. Picking and squeezing opens the skin, allows more bacteria to enter, and spreads the bacteria to your hands. The most effective measures for controlling acne are thorough washing of the skin to remove excess oil and bacteria, avoiding heavy make-up, and avoiding foods to which the person may be hypersensitive, such as chocolate, dairy products, etc. Bodywork is locally contraindicated.

Sebaceous cysts form when a sebaceous, or oil, gland becomes blocked, forming a lump. If the cyst is painful or unsightly, it can be opened and drained using sterile technique. A sebaceous cyst that forms in the gluteal crease is called a *pilonidal cyst*, and often begins as an ingrown hair. Pilonidal cysts can be very painful and, if infected, can tunnel deeply. Surgery can remove the cyst and close the tissue. Bodywork is locally contraindicated.

Seborrheic dermatitis is known as *dandruff* in adults and as *cradle cap* in infants. This form of dermatitis can appear as either a dry or a greasy scaling on the scalp. The cause is excessive sebum (oil) secretion and can include the face, ears and eyebrows. Bodywork is not contraindicated.

Seborrheic keratosis is a raised, hard, waxy skin lesion that forms in the oil (sebaceous) glands of the sun exposed areas, such as the hairline or back. It occurs most often in persons over the age of 60. These lesions are harmless and begin with a yellow or tan color, darkening with time to brown or black. Their edges are often sharp or loose and can occasionally flake off during bathing or massage. There is no need for alarm if this occurs, however, the black lesions can be *pre-cancerous*, so observation for further changes is warranted. Bodywork is locally contraindicated for black lesions, but permissible for the others, however friction techniques should <u>not</u> be used on the lesions.

Psoriasis is a chronic, non-contagious skin disease in which the normal process of skin renewal goes awry, with skin cells being replaced every four days instead of every 28 and abnormal cells being shed in great numbers. Psoriasis may have a hereditary basis, but the exact etiology is unknown. The lesions may be itchy or sore and are pink or red patches with sharply defined edges usually covered with white or silvery scales. The most common areas affected by psoriasis are the extensor surfaces of the elbows and knees, but the trunk, arms, legs and scalp can also be affected. Periods of remission and exacerbation are common, with stress, infections, certain drugs, and lack of sunlight encouraging exacerbation. About 10% of persons with psoriasis also develop a related form of arthritis. Massage is NOT contraindicated unless the area is inflamed, tender, or the client asks you to avoid work on an area.

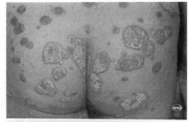
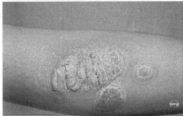

Illustration 23   Psoriasis

NEOPLASTIC SKIN CONDITIONS

A *neoplasm* is an abnormal tissue formation. In most cases, neoplastic growth serves no useful function and grows at the expense of the rest of the animal or person. Neoplastic growths are often called *tumors* and can be *benign, pre-cancerous,* or *malignant* (see Chapter 12). BODYWORK IS LOCALLY CONTRAINDICATED TO ALL ABNORMAL TISSUE FORMATIONS, regardless of whether you know if they are benign, pre-cancerous, or malignant.

Benign means causing no harm. Benign skin tumors usually grow slowly and do not spread or invade other tissues. An example of a benign skin tumor is a mole. *Pre-cancerous* means not yet (but at risk to become) cancerous.

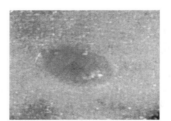

Small, smooth, shiny, pale or waxy lump.

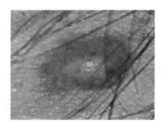

Firm red lump.

The word *"malignant"* is used as a synonym for the word "cancer." Malignant skin tumors grow rapidly, spread, or *metastasize*, to other areas of the body, and often have finger-like extensions that run into neighboring tissue. An example of a malignant skin tumor is the highly fatal malignant melanoma.

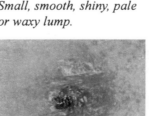

A lump that bleeds or develops a crust.

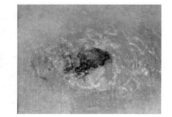

A flat, red spot that is rough, dry, or scaly.

Skin cancer is the most common form

Illustration 24   Examples of Skin Cancers

of cancer in humans. Most skin cancers appear on the sun-exposed surfaces of the head, neck, arms and back, however, skin cancer can occur anywhere. Fair-skinned people are particularly susceptible to skin cancer. Sun exposure and other forms of ultra-violet radiation, such as tanning beds, produce accumulative effects over a person's life-span. The radiation you have already been exposed to will continue to affect your skin cells and, accumulated with new exposure, may cause skin cancer to develop as you age.

BENIGN NEOPLASMS

A *nevus (mole)* is a benign skin tumor made of excessive melanin. A nevus looks like a pigmented macule, papule or nodule. Most people have several nevi. These are harmless unless they begin to change in size, shape or color (see *Malignant Melanoma* page 68).

A *skin tag (achrocordon)* is a small, soft, flesh-colored or pigmented skin growth that appears to hang from a small stem. Skin tags are located mainly in the neck, armpits and groin and are benign.

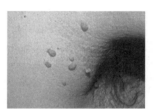

A *lipoma* is a large, soft, moveable nodule found primarily in the subcutaneous tissue of the trunk, forearms or neck. It usually can not be seen but can be easily palpated. Lipomas are very common and are formed mainly from adipose (fat) cells.

Illustration 25 "Skin Tags"

Angiomas are benign neoplasms of blood or lymph vessel and are most common in newborn infants where they are also called "port-wine stains" and "strawberry marks." Usually, these disappear sometime between a few months and a few years after birth. The "spider angioma" appears in adults and may accompany cirrhosis of the liver, pregnancy or use of oral contraceptives. Spider angiomas resemble a spider web with a small, pulsating center from which several blood vessels radiate.

Papillomas are benign tumors of the epithelial cells in the skin or mucous membranes. Included in this group are warts, condylomas, and polyps.

MALIGNANT (CANCEROUS) SKIN CONDITIONS

The most common warning sign of skin cancer is a change on the skin, especially a new growth or a sore that does not heal. Skin cancer has many different appearances (see below). Pain is NOT a sign of skin cancer. Skin cancers occur most often in people who have fair skin, light hair, and blue, green or gray eyes. However, anyone can develop skin cancer.

It is very important to avoid doing bodywork directly on any skin lesion that you think may be cancerous. Tell clients to see a physician if any skin change lasts for more than two weeks. With prompt treatment, over 95% of skin cancers are curable.

Basal cell carcinoma is the most common type of cancer, developing in approximately one in eight Americans. Basal cell is a slow-growing, usually non-metastasizing cancer and is caused by over-exposure to the sun in 95% of cases. Basal cell carcinoma can appear in many different forms:

- a persistent, non-healing open sore that bleeds, oozes, or crusts for 3 weeks or longer
- a reddish patch or irritated area, usually on the chest, shoulders, or limbs, that may or may not itch or hurt
- a smooth growth with an elevated, rolled whitish border and an indented center
- a shiny bump or nodule that is pearly or translucent and can be pink, red, white, tan, brown or black
- a scar-like area, white, yellow, or waxy, which often has poorly defined borders.

Basal cell carcinoma often develops on the face, ears, neck, scalp, shoulders, and back. In rare cases, it can develop on non-exposed areas. Basal cell tumors are easily treated by surgical removal, laser, or radiation therapies.

Squamous cell carcinoma is more serious than basal cell because it grows more rapidly, it infiltrates underlying tissues, and it sometimes metastasizes through the lymph channels. A squamous lesion appears as a small, reddish-brown plaque with a scaly surface and firm, elevated edges. Often the lesion may have a crater or ulcerated center. Squamous cell carcinoma can develop in any epithelium of the body, including skin and mucous membranes, and is often found on the head and neck and on areas where there has been previous sunburn damage. The cure rate is 75% to 80% when squamous cell carcinoma is identified early and is completely removed surgically and/or treated with radiation.

A lesion called *actinic keratosis* appears on the skin as a rough, red or brown scaly patch and is considered pre-cancerous because it sometimes develops into squamous cell carcinoma.

Malignant melanoma is the least common but the most dangerous skin cancer because it grows very fast and metastasizes early. The incidence rate of malignant melanoma is increasing dramatically. When people were born in 1930, the risk of developing it was one in 1500. Babies born in 1995 have a risk of one in 135. By the year 2000, the risk will be one in 90. Melanoma often develops as a new "mole" or from a mole that changes its size and color and becomes itchy or sore. The most common location of melanomas in women is on the legs. Clients with two or more of these signs in a lesion should be referred to a physician and encouraged to seek assessment as soon as possible.

Signs of malignant melanoma can be remembered with the acronym *ABCD* (see *Illustration*).

- *A* stands for *asymmetry*. If you drew a line down the middle of the lesion, the two sides would not match.
- *B* stands for *borders*. The borders are notched, scalloped, or indistinct.

- *C* stands for *color*. There will be two or more colors in the lesion, such as red and black, tan and blue, brown and white, etc.
- *D* stands for *diameter*. The lesion will be larger than the diameter of a pencil eraser.

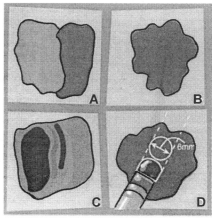

Surgical removal of melanoma often also takes the surrounding lymph nodes, to reduce metastasis. Prognosis depends on how early the lesion is identified, the depth of the lesion, and how completely the cancer is removed.

Illustration 26
ABCDs of Malignant Melanoma

MISCELLANEOUS SKIN CONDITIONS

Corns are cone-shaped areas of excessive keratin and are caused by pressure or friction. Corns are found mainly on or between the toes and may ache or be tender to the touch. If tender, bodywork is locally contraindicated.

Callouses are layers of thick keratinous tissue that have formed to protect the skin from friction. Bodywork is not contraindicated on callouses.

Decubitus ulcers, also called bedsores, are caused by a reduction in circulation to the area because of unrelieved pressure from sitting or lying too long in one position. Decubiti begin, initially, as small reddened areas that remain red for more than ten minutes after the pressure is relieved. As the person continues to remain in or return to the same position, the damage develops deeper and deeper, progressing into subcutaneous and, eventually, muscle and bone tissue. The areas that are most likely to develop decubiti are bony areas such as the heels, coccyx, sacrum, ischium, greater trochanters, elbows and occiput. Gentle massage around the area can increase circulation, however, massage, especially friction, is contraindicated directly on the decubitus lesion.

Pilonidal cysts are located in the sacro-coccygeal region, usually at the upper end of the gluteal cleft. These can develop into a fistula (an abnormal passageway) which can then easily become inflamed and/or infected. Bodywork is locally contraindicated.

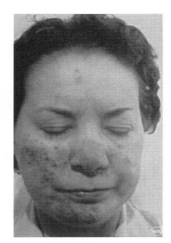

Rosacea is a chronic skin condition that produces dilation of the small facial blood vessels. The person may appear to have flushed cheeks or nose, papules, pustules, or eye inflammation. The skin may become chronically very dry. The etiology of rosacea is unknown, but stress, infections, hot and spicy foods, sunlight and physical exercise may aggravate it. In bodywork, locally avoid friction or deep tissue pressure.

Scleroderma is an autoimmune disorder that causes thick, red,

Illustration 27   Rosacea

leathery areas of inflammation and scar tissue on the skin and several organs. Frequently joint stiffness, muscle weakness, general skin thickening and finger swelling are present, as well as hypersensitivity to cold. Collagen deposits in the digestive tract and lungs can significantly affect the person's abilities to breathe and to absorb food. The disease is often fatal. Massage is NOT contraindicated but should be done in collaboration with the treating physician.

COMMON EFFECTS OF AGING ON THE INTEGUMENTARY SYSTEM

After age 50, the skin commonly becomes drier, secreting less oil and perspiration. The circulation to the skin also decreases and, in combination with more dryness, makes the skin more susceptible to injury, less elastic, and less able to regulate body temperature. The subcutaneous tissue also loses its elasticity. Finger and toenails become thicker and harder. Skin pigmentation becomes less even, and more benign and malignant lesions occur.

Chapter 3, Part 2

INFLAMMATION AND REPAIR

All living tissues (e.g., skin, muscle, bone, fascia, mucous membranes, etc.) react to allergens, injury, pathogens, and foreign substances by producing a protective response called *inflammation*. The cardiovascular, nervous, and immune systems work together to create inflammation and the repair that follows it. EVERY DISEASE OR ILLNESS ENDING IN "-ITIS" IS AN INFLAMMATION (e.g., arthritis, appendicitis, bronchitis, urethritis, etc.). Inflammation is easily confused with infection, however the additional presence of a pathogenic organism, or *pathogen*, is necessary to produce infection. It is very important for bodyworkers to understand physical inflammation and repair processes and recognize the signs and symptoms in order to avoid aggravating these conditions.

Stage one: *Acute inflammation*: Acute inflammation begins immediately after an irritation, injury, or foreign invasion (hereafter called a trauma) and lasts for 24-48 hours. A complex series of changes in blood vessels, white blood cells and chemicals takes place to send the body's nutritional and immune factors to assist in the injured area. There are four principal signs and symptoms of inflammation: *heat, redness, swelling, and pain*. Additionally, there may be some loss of tissue function.

The details of acute inflammation go like this: immediately after a trauma, the arterioles in the region vasodilate and the pre-capillary sphincters relax. This increases blood flow into the damaged tissues, causing heat and redness (*erythema*). The traumatized cells and certain immune system cells in the area release arachidonic acid, histamine and bradykinin. These chemicals irritate local nerve endings, causing pain, and send messages to the capillaries to open their pores to allow white blood cells (leukocytes) and protein-rich fluid (plasma) to flow into the traumatized area and produce swelling (*edema*).

Next, neutrophils and monocytes (two types of phagocytes) enter the area to engulf and digest any injured cells and/or bacteria that might be present. The phagocytes also produce chemicals that further increase the inflammatory response. As the process continues, the thickness, or viscosity, of the blood increases, which slows and stagnates the blood flow. While all this is happening, the repair process begins and continues until the traumatized area has returned to normal. Clotting chemicals, such as fibrinogen, are activated by any damaged blood vessels, and free radicals stimulate the inflammatory response but also may damage nearby healthy tissue.

Stage two: *Subacute inflammation*: Any inflammation that lasts longer than a few days is called subacute. The continued presence of a foreign body, like a splinter, can be one cause. Another can be that the person is functioning with a weakened immune system and it is taking longer than usual to finish the repair. A third possibility is that the person is continuing to irritate or re-injure the inflamed area. A fourth possibility is that there are pathogens present, creating infection, and they are overwhelming the body's immune response. Wound healing can only occur when the pathogens have been destroyed. If pathogens have created infection, there will be a thick yellow fluid (pus) that consists of dead and live bacteria, dead immune cells, and other debris.

Stage three: *Chronic inflammation*: When inflammation continues for more than a few weeks, the number of neutrophils decreases and the number of white blood cells increase, keeping the immune system working but not at its peak efficiency. In addition, an excessive amount of collagen fibers may be produced, causing scar tissue, or adhesions, to develop. This limits tissue mobility in the area. Chronically inflamed tissue often changes gradually from hot and swollen to cool and dense and is more easily re-injured. Chronic inflammatory conditions such as arthritis, asthma, eczema, and chronic bronchitis are often called inflammatory diseases.

Systemic signs and symptoms: In addition to the local signs and symptoms of inflammation, there may also be general, or systemic, signs and symptoms. These include fever, a high white blood cell count (leukocytosis), general discomfort (malaise), headache, loss of appetite, fatigue and general weakness. Usually signs and symptoms of systemic inflammation indicate a more serious situation than when the inflammation is localized to one area.

Tissue Repair: The first stage of repair is called *granulation*. Granulating tissue is soft, pink, and grainy, and has many new capillaries, fibroblasts and white blood cells. The fibroblasts are the key element in all wound healing. Ideally, granulation tissue is gradually replaced by normal cells that are identical to the cells that were present before the trauma. Sometimes, however, normal cells can not be regenerated and fibrous connective tissue is made in its place, resulting in *fibrosis, scarring,* or *adhesions*. This limits the area's ability to function and will be described further in Chapter 4.

Most tissue repairs are a combination of normal cells and fibrous cells. A goal in the healing process is to promote the growth of new cells and minimize scarring. All of the following factors are necessary for successful tissue repair.

- Immobilization and alignment. The cut or raw edges of the injured tissue must be lined up as closely as possible to the way they were before the trauma. Common examples of immobilization treatments are stitches and casts.

- Sterility. Pathogens must be removed from the trauma area by washing, by the body's immune system, and/or by antibiotics. Any break in the skin should be covered with clean or sterile material to prevent environmental pathogens from entering.

- Nutrition. Good nutrition, including protein, carbohydrates, vitamins, minerals, and fats are required for repair to occur.

- Blood supply. If circulation into or out of the traumatized area is reduced, healing will be delayed or prevented altogether.

- Contact inhibition. In cuts or any kind of broken skin, the body normally makes just enough new cells to cover the surface of the wound, then contact inhibition causes this production to stop. Cells that do not stop growing may form excessive scar tissue or tumor growth.

- Growth-stimulating chemicals. These are required in order for the body to make the new cells that are needed for repair.

- Regeneratability of tissue. Some types of tissue regenerate more easily than others. Damaged skeletal muscle, cardiac muscle, and nervous system tissues are particularly hard for the body to regenerate. Also, regeneratability of all tissues gradually decreases with advanced aging.

CASE PRESENTATION

4/14/96: 27 yo male; Goal: relaxation
History: Has had psoriasis "all his life." Having chronic low back and R hip discomfort. Takes no meds. Does not see an MD. Uses tanning beds to decrease skin problems.
Subjective: hip pain 3, low back 4 (0 - 10 scale)
Objective: Many raised, scaly and broken areas on trunk, arms, and legs from knee up; limited AROM in R hip, esp. adduction; shoulders slope anteriorly; tight pectoralis minors, R sartorius and quadriceps; breathing is shallow; didn't look at me when he spoke.
Application: PROM and a lot of stretching, since rubbing was uncomfortable for me; iliopsoas release technique to low back; petrissage to quads; trigger point work in pects minor; facilitated deep breathing and breath awareness
Referral: local MD for help with skin
Outcome: Said he felt "100% better;" hip 0 and low back 1/2;
Follow up call two days later: said he thinks oil helped his skin, it's less scaly now.

STUDY QUESTIONS

Which parts of the above case presentation was subjective?
Which parts were objective?
What questions would you have asked that were not asked?
What bodywork techniques would you have done?
What referral(s)?
What other ways could the therapeutic outcome have been evaluated?
How might you have changed the format or way the cases were written?

REFERENCES

Jarvis, C. (1992). Physical examination and health assessment. Philadelphia: W. B. Saunders Co. [Illustrations (pages 60-61,63,67) used with permission. *See page 76.]

Kapit, W. & Elson, L.M. (1977). The anatomy coloring book. NY: Harper & Row.

Kapit, W., Macey, R.I., & Meisami, E. (1987). The physiology coloring book. NY: Harper & Row.

Malasanos, L., Barkauskas, V., & Stoltenberg-Allen, K. (1990). Health assessment. St. Louis, MO: C.V. Mosby Co. [Photos *(Illus. 3, 21, 22, 23, 27)* used with permission.]

Mulvihill, M.L. (1995). Human diseases: A systemic approach (4th ed.) Norwalk, CT: Appleton & Lange.

National Cancer Institute, (1988). What you need to know about skin cancer. US Department of Health and Human Services, Public Health Service, National Institutes of Health, Publication No. 90-1564.

Newton, D. (1995). Pathology for massage therapists. Portland, OR: Simran Publications.

Thomas, C.L. (1989). Taber's cyclopedic medical dictionary (16th ed.). Philadelphia: F.A. Davis Co.

U.S. National Center for Health Statistics, Vital Statistics of the United States, annual, 1992.

CHAPTER REVIEW

1. The body's largest organ is the_____

2. The upper layer of the skin is the _____ and the lower layer is the _____

3. The _____ gives the skin its color and protects it from the sun's ultraviolet rays.

4. Beneath the dermis is the _____

5. Match the following skin colors:

   _____ cyanosis   a. red
   _____ pallor   b. yellow
   _____ jaundice   c. blue
   _____ erythema   d. white

6. Tenting is a sign that the person is _____

7. True/False: Massage is locally contraindicated for pitting edema.

8. Skin lesions are described as "small" when they are less than _____

9 Bodywork is locally contraindicated to all areas displaying _____, _____, and _____, which are the primary signs of inflammation and infection.

10. True/False: Bodywork is generally contraindicated for anyone who has a fever.

11. List 3 bacterial skin infections: _____

12. List 3 viral skin infections: _____

13. List 3 fungal skin infections: _____

14. _____ are organisms that live within, upon, or at the expense of another organism.

15. List 3 allergic skin conditions: _____

16. List 3 metabolic skin disorders: _____

17. List 3 benign neoplasms: _____

18. List 3 malignant neoplasms: _____

19. How long does acute inflammation usually last? _____

20. Chronically inflamed tissues gradually change from hot and swollen to _____

ANSWERS TO CHAPTER REVIEW

1. skin

2. epidermis; dermis

3. melanin

4. subcutaneous tissue

5. c, d, b, a

6. dehydrated

7. True

8. 10 mm diameter, or the size of a pencil eraser

9. pain, heat, redness, swelling

10. fever

11. impetigo, cellulitis, abscess/furuncle/carbuncle/boil, lyme

12. cold sore/fever blister/herpes, shingles, warts

13. tinea/ringworm, athlete's foot, jock itch, candida/yeast

14. parasites

15. urticaria/hives, eczema/contact dermatitis, drug reactions

16. acne, sebaceous cysts, seborrheic dermatitis/dandruff/cradle cap, seborrheic keratosis, psoriasis

17. nevus/mole, skin tag, lipoma, angioma

18. basal cell carcinoma, squamous cell carcinoma, and melanoma

19. 24-48 hours

20. cool and dense

*Illustration 22 "Ringworm" original source from Hurwitz S: Clinical Pediatric Dermatology: A Textbook of Skin Disorders of Childhood and Adolescence. Philadelphia, WB Saunders, 1981, p 283.

*Illustration 25 original source from Lookingbill DP, Marks JG: Principles of Dermatology. Philadelphia, WB Saunders, 1986, p 62.

CHAPTER 4

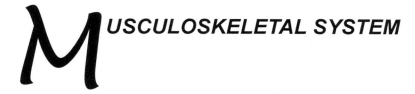

MUSCULOSKELETAL SYSTEM

ANATOMY AND PHYSIOLOGY REVIEW

The musculoskeletal system is made up of bone, muscle, and the *connective tissues*: fascia, joint cartilage, bursa, tendon and ligament. Muscles are groups of contractile fibers that can lengthen/relax or shorten/contract. Most muscles originate on one bone and insert on another so that the second bone is moved when the muscle is contracted. The ends of the muscles blend into the tendons and the tendons blend into the fibrous sheath (the periosteum) that covers the bones. The periosteum is continuous with the ligaments, which attach bone to bone, and with the inner coating of the hollow bones (the endosteum). The joint cartilage covers and cushions the bone ends. The *bursae* are sacs or cavities in the connective tissue, usually near a joint. Bursae are lined with synovial membrane and filled with synovial fluid that reduces friction between tendon and bone, tendon and ligament, or between other structures where friction is likely. For an excellent review of the anatomy and physiology of the musculoskeletal system, I recommend the following books: *Job's Body*, *Anatomy of Movement*, and/or *Functional Assessment in Massage Therapy*. All are listed in the references. What follows is a brief and simplified synopsis.

All of the connective tissues contain and are formed by a transparent fluid called *ground substance*. The ground substance is a liquid that surrounds all the body's cells and can vary from a watery sol-state to a viscous gel-state that is like raw egg whites or a solid state that is like gelatin. Ground substance is produced by the fibroblast cells and works constantly to maintain equilibrium between the body's tissues. The fibroblasts also produce *collagen* fibers, which are protein chains that give strength, elasticity and structure to skin, ligaments, tendons, cartilage, bone, blood vessels, and all the organs. Taken as a whole, connective tissue can be likened to fluid crystal.

Connective tissue exhibits a phenomenon called *thixotropy*, meaning that it becomes more fluid when it is moved and/or heated and more solid when it is cool or sits undisturbed. The movement, pressure, stretching, and friction that accompany bodywork can literally provide the heat and mechanical activity that restores some fluidity in the connective tissues. This in turn promotes healthy exchange of nutrients and cellular wastes.

Connective tissue forms a continuous net throughout the entire body by means of the fascia. Fascia is a fibrous membrane that unites the skin with the underlying tissue and covers, supports and separates the muscles. It resembles spiderwebs in that it is very thin but also very strong and elastic. Fascia has a tensile strength of over 2,000 pounds per square inch (Barnes, 1996).

Fibers in the fascia run in all directions, allowing it to be stretched by body movements. If you have ever cut up a chicken, you have probably seen the thin, white, translucent fascia connecting the skin to the fat and muscle. Fascia organizes the muscles into functional groups, wraps each individual muscle, and honeycombs the interior of the muscle bellies. The many compartments of fascia throughout the body help prevent the spread of infections, tumors and diseases by means of its structural and chemical nature, and the ground substance provides the fluid medium through which the white blood cells, antibodies, hormones, and other immune system elements circulate.

Most of the fascia is not living tissue. The only living part is the fibroblastic cells that make the collagen fibers. These fibers give connective tissue its strength but also create its most common degenerative problems. Trauma draws the fibers together to make scar or adhesion tissue. Inflammation and immobility also shrink fascia. As injuries and habit patterns develop, collagen molecules tend to bunch up and become thicker and more rigid. Fascial restrictions can exert enormous pressure on pain receptors, nerves and/or circulatory vessels.

Structures that were originally designed to function separately, such as two muscles lying side by side or a tendon within its sheath, can become "glued" together by fascial adhesions. When palpated, these areas can be felt as thick, lumpy masses at the muscle origins, insertions, or bellies. Using ice on injuries in the acute stage of inflammation reduces the number of fibers that migrate to the trauma area, thus reducing adhesions. Myofascial release techniques loosen fascial adhesions and encourage fibers to spread out and become elastic again.

Fascia can be torn or overstretched by overzealous, uninformed bodywork. It is important to warm and energize tissue before doing deep, demanding work. The attitude that intense pain is necessary to produce myofascial improvements must be questioned. Acute pain announces imminent tissue damage. Even in the absence of actual damage, acute pain creates a reflex neuromuscular contractile response which reverses the desired process of softening and lengthening (Juhan, 1987).

Along the sol to gel connective tissue continuum, bone is the most rigid form. To achieve this rigidity, the tissue is packed with crystallized minerals, principally calcium and phosphorus, but also traces of magnesium, sodium, carbonate, citrate, and fluoride. Living bone requires minerals to give it rigidity, and collagen fibrils to give it tensile strength and flexibility. It also requires a dense distribution of blood vessels and nerves. The dry, brittle bones you might have handled from dead bodies are only 75% of what makes up living bone. When bone is part of a living being, it is a lot like a stiff sponge, hard but still flexible, and full of body fluids, including ground substance, blood, and liquid fats (lipids).

The osteo<u>blasts</u> take calcium and phosphorus from the blood and imbed them into the bone matrix to make bone cells. The osteo<u>clasts</u> liberate the crystallized minerals and disperse them into the blood stream again, as needed, in an attempt to maintain the correct amounts of circulating minerals and the correct thickness of bone wall. When mineral levels in the blood and body fluids are low, the call for more minerals in the circulation over-rides the bones' call for minerals. That is why blood tests for mineral levels can appear normal when the person is actually mineral deficient. The process of bone building and bone resorption is continual throughout the human life-span and keeps the bones responsive to dietary, mechanical, chemical, and psychological factors. In addition, red and white blood cells and platelets are formed in the bone marrow. The femur has the largest amount of bone marrow.

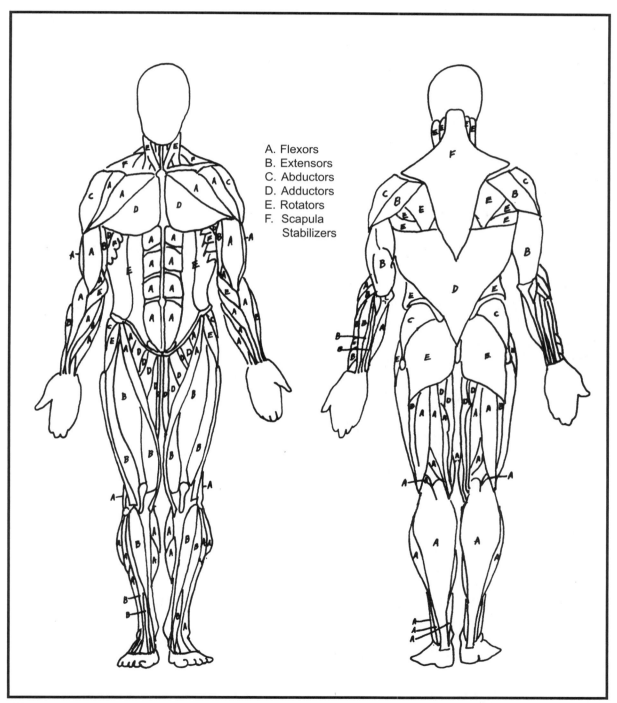

A. Flexors
B. Extensors
C. Abductors
D. Adductors
E. Rotators
F. Scapula
  Stabilizers

Illustration 28   Human muscle pattern

The extensive fascia and bone network provide a complex and flexible structure made up of connective cables and bony spacers. Many of us have been taught that the skeleton provides body structure like steel beams support a building. However, there is nothing inherently stackable, stable, or upright about the skeleton. The whole thing would slide to the floor if not for the complex muscle system that constantly contracts and relaxes to counterbalance the forces of gravity and movement.

Muscle tissue comprises the large majority of what is beneath our skin, making up 70-85% of the body's weight. The activities of the body's muscles consume the vast majority of all the food and oxygen we take in. There are three basic types of muscle tissue in the body: smooth muscle in the internal organs and blood vessels; striated muscle that moves the bones; and cardiac muscle that comprises and pumps the heart. In massage, we primarily focus on the striated (or skeletal) muscles, and so the rest of the information in this chapter relates to skeletal muscle.

There are over 600 separate muscle compartments in the human body, and normally no one compartment acts independently. In bodywork, we almost never find just one single muscle that is tense, but rather we find areas or patterns of tension. According to Juhan, we can "regard the body as having only one muscle, whose millions of fiber-like cells are distributed throughout the fascial network and are oriented in innumerable directions, creating innumerable lines of pull. This single muscle may contract or lengthen any number of fibers distributed in any number of compartments in order to change its consistency and shape" (1987).

Like connective tissue, skeletal muscle tissue displays a sol to gel range of consistency. The main difference is that muscle tissue can shift between these states almost instantaneously: it can soften and lengthen (relax) or shorten and harden (contract), depending on the needs of the moment. In states of dysfunction, it can also lock into place, preventing motion (contracture).

The skeletal muscles are often referred to as the voluntary muscles because they more or less respond to our minds' directions. However, in healthy skeletal muscle, relaxation is relative: we are never completely relaxed unless we are under deep general anesthesia. In fact, skeletal muscles need a certain amount of stimulation to maintain enough tone to hold the joints in place. Also, our motor skills are set up by our genetics and trained through daily repetition. With time and attention, we are free to re-train ourselves, but it is very difficult to respond suddenly in a different way than we have been trained.

Skeletal muscle must be used, or worked, frequently in order to stay healthy. If not, it will atrophy. When muscle tissue works, it requires much more food and oxygen than it does at rest. The normal contracting/relaxing, contracting/relaxing muscle work makes a pumping action that helps the food and oxygen circulate throughout the muscle tissue.

Muscles that are chronically tense are exerting a chronic pull against either a fixed structure or, more commonly, against another opposing muscle. At the same time, the sustained muscle contractions are squeezing the small arterioles and capillaries and reducing the amount of nourishment that can get to the muscle tissue, creating a vicious cycle in which the more there is tension, the less there is fuel delivered, which makes the work harder and harder until the tissue is exhausted and toxic wastes settle in. This lack of circulation is called *ischemia*, which means a local and temporary deficiency of blood supply due to obstruction of circulation. Chronically unrelieved ischemia creates a burning sensation, pain, diminished flexibility and eventual disuse.

Tendons normally feel elastic and mobile. Trauma and inflammation can cause adhesions which can glue tendons to the underlying bone or to the tendon's sheath, where one is present. Gentle, skilled bodywork is usually indicated and beneficial after the acute stage of inflammation is past.

Except for range of motion (ROM), the scope of practice for bodywork usually does not include unsupervised work directly on ligaments and joints. However, these structures can benefit from the bodywork done to adjacent tissues. Also, remember that ligament and cartilage tissue regenerate very slowly so healing from any trauma or inflammation will take much longer. During the healing process, these tissues need rest and as little mobility as the person can maintain.

Medications Related to Musculoskeletal Illnesses

When working with clients who are experiencing musculoskeletal pain, always ask what medications they are taking, including both pharmaceuticals and herbs. Medications that treat musculoskeletal problems usually can be categorized as either *anti-inflammatories, analgesics,* or *muscle relaxants*. When people take any of these, they may underestimate their discomforts so it is best to take that into account when you assess their level of pain and decide how deep you will work. If you choose to ask about medications on your health history form, you might want to list anti-inflammatories, analgesics, and muscle relaxants as specific types you want to be aware of.

NSAIDs (non-steroidal anti-inflammatory drugs) are primary drugs commonly used to treat musculoskeletal inflammations. Examples include: ibuprofen, Advil, Motrin, aspirin, Aleve, Clinoril, Indocin, Naprosyn, Nuprin, Relafen, etc. There is considerable variability among people in terms of effectiveness and tolerance of NSAIDs. The most common side effects are: stomach upset, nausea, indigestion, peptic ulcers, constipation, diarrhea, headache, dizziness, vision disorders, kidney necrosis, jaundice, liver toxicity, fluid retention, rash, itching, and ringing in the ears.

Cortisone, and products that include cortisone, are the other type of anti-inflammatory drugs. Cortisone is a synthetic steroid, closely related to the hormone cortisol, which is made by the adrenal glands in response to stress (see chapter 2). It relieves the symptoms of inflammation "like magic," but it does not cure the underlying problem, and repeated or long-term use has a high potential for the following side effects: glaucoma, cataracts, hypertension, psychic disorders, myopathy, osteoporosis, peptic ulcers, skin atrophy, increased intracranial pressure, carbohydrate intolerance, and potassium, calcium, and sodium imbalances. Cortisone can also mask infections and suppress the immune response. It should not be used when a person has bacterial, viral, or fungal infections and should not be used continuously or preventively.

Analgesics are pain relievers and are categorized as narcotics and non-narcotics. *Narcotics* are natural or synthetic forms of opium and are federally controlled due to the potential side effects of central nervous system depression and habituation. They include Buprenex, Darvocet, Darvon, Demerol, Dilaudid, Dolophine, Duragesic, Tylenol or Aspirin with co-deine, Lorcet, Lortab, Morphine, Nubain, Oxycontin, Percocet, Percodan, Roxanol, Stadol, Talwin, Tylox, Vicodin, etc. Common side effects include dizziness, drowsiness, allergic reactions, rash, stomach upset, nausea, constipation, and urinary retention. *Non-narcotic* analgesics include all of the NSAIDs, plus acetaminophen (Tylenol). Side effects of Tylenol include rash and kidney toxicity.

Muscle relaxants may include Valium, Flexeril, Equagesic, Lioresal, Norgesic Forte, Parafon Forte, Soma, valerian root, etc. Again, clients taking these drugs may underestimate their discomfort. Muscle relaxants work on all the skeletal muscles, not just an area of spasm, so you are apt to feel more "openness" in the tissue. Take this into account and proceed more gently than usual, particularly with range of motion (ROM). Common side effects of muscle relaxants are: liver toxicity, hepatitis, drowsiness, photosensitivity, allergic reactions, stomach upset, prolonged bleeding time, faster heartbeat, dizziness, dry mouth, blurred vision, weakness, headache, urinary retention, and rash.

For more information about the effects of medications, consult a pharmacist or one of the many books about medications available in local bookstores.

ASSESSMENT: OBSERVATION AND PALPATION

There are three main areas to consider during the musculoskeletal assessment:

- balance (is the posture leaning or crooked?),
- function (do all parts move efficiently?), and
- symmetry (does one side match the other?).

There are four main ways to assess, or get information about balance, function and symmetry. These are:

1) <u>Observe the client walking</u>. Watch what parts move, how they move, and what parts are not moving. The upper and lower body should move in rhythm and the arms should move freely, in sync with the legs. The pelvis should rock evenly from side to side. The toes should point directly forward with each step (see *Illustration 29*).

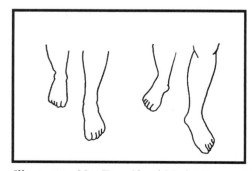

Illustration 29   Toes Should Point Forward

2) <u>Observe the client's standing and lying posture</u>. Postural asymmetry is often a result of hypertonic muscles, shortened connective tissue, and/or overstretched ligaments. It is less often a result of genetic deformity. The following are some key areas to observe when assessing postural symmetry:

- chin, sternal notch and navel should be in a direct line that falls evenly between the knees and feet
- shoulders should be level and neither rolled forward or back
- arms should have the same rotation
- elbows, wrists and fingers should be level with each other
- rib cage should be symmetrical
- waist curves should be even on both sides
- spine should be without lateral curves
- scapulae should be level with each other
- iliac crests should be level with each other
- greater trochanter, knees and ankles should be level
- legs should have the same slight rotation out of the hip
- patellae should be level and pointed slightly laterally
- knees should not hyperextend
- ankles should sit over the feet without rotating in or out
- feet should have even arches that are not exaggerated or flat; toes contact the floor

3) <u>Observe the client's active and/or passive range of motion (ROM)</u>. Active range of motion (AROM) is when <u>the client</u> moves his/her own joint(s) through each direction that is possible. Passive range of motion (PROM) is when <u>you</u> move the client's joints through each direction that is possible (see illustration). Pay attention to the client's remarks about location, quality, intensity, and duration of pain or discomfort during ROM and use these as important assessment information. Never do ROM past the point of pain. Listen for *crepitation* which is a grating, clicking, or crackling sound heard on joint movement usually due to roughness and irregularities on the articulating surfaces. Crepitation is a sign of wear and tear. However, it is not a local contraindication for massage unless inflammation is also present. Practice watching other students' active and passive movements to become familiar with normal ROM. Watch for ROM that is limited.

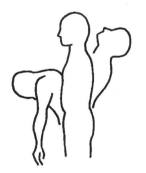 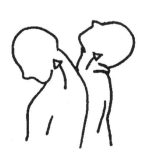 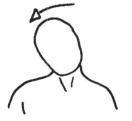 

Illustration 31   Joint Range of Motion

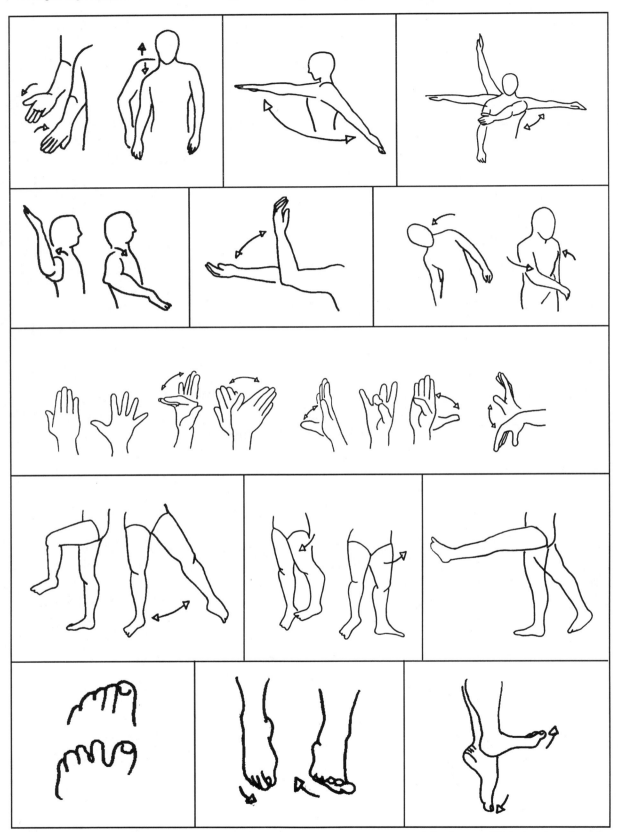

Illustration 32   Joint Range of Motion (continued)

During PROM, notice what you feel in the joint at the end of each movement. This is called the end-feel and will either be soft or hard. An example of a soft end-feel is where the joint motion has come to a stop, but the joint could give a little bit more with gentle pressure, e.g., normal wrist and finger joints. With hard end-feel, the joint has no give, e.g., the elbow. If you observe a hard end-feel in a joint that normally should be soft, this is a sign of *contracture*. Contracture is abnormal shortening of fascia, muscle, tendon and/or ligament tissue and occurs when a body area is paralyzed, as in stroke or spinal injury. In many cases, contracture can be prevented by doing ROM and massage every 6 hours (around the clock), however, that is a difficult schedule to maintain. Contracture is gradually progressive and causes permanent damage.

How to distinguish between muscle/tendon problems and joint/ligament problems.

Therapeutic massage and bodywork can only deal with soft tissue dysfunction. Joint dysfunction is not in the bodywork scope of practice unless there is specific training and supervision by a physician or physical therapist. Therefore, it is important to know how to distinguish between muscle/tendon problems and ligament/joint problems. The following methods are suggested for assessing conditions that are NOT acutely injured or inflamed:

  • If AROM produces pain and PROM does not, it is usually a sign of a muscle or tendon problem.
  • Pain on gentle traction is usually a muscle or tendon problem.
  • If both AROM and PROM produce pain, then it is usually a sign of a ligament or joint problem.
  • Pain on gentle compression is usually a ligament or joint problem.

When in doubt, always refer the problem to a physician. With experience, you will probably find that most muscle dysfunction, including trigger points and micro-scarring from previous injuries, occurs at the musculo-tendinous junction (where the muscles and tendons meet).

---

4) <u>Observe and palpate the neck, limbs, shoulders, hips and back</u>. Learn through practice how to identify different types of tissue by their feel under your hands and fingertips. Also learn to distinguish differences in contour, texture, tension, and mobility within the same tissue type. A common deviation from normal muscle tissue is *hypertonicity*, which is excessive muscle tone. Another deviation is *spasm*, which is a sudden, involuntary muscle contraction. Another possibility is fibrillation, where individual muscle bundles are spasming (but not the whole muscle), and feels like twitching or vibrating within a muscle. Muscles can feel also feel *flaccid*, or limp. This is called *hypotonicity* and represents an inability of the muscle to contract normally.

Practice palpation by starting with a gentle, light touch and gradually move in deeper. Notice how the tissue feels when you first touch it and how it changes as you work on it. Notice the tissue's color, temperature, mobility, the client's rhythms of respiration, and the client's reports of pain or numbness. Pay attention to the client's remarks about location, quality, intensity, and duration of pain or discomfort.

GENERAL MUSCULOSKELETAL CONDITIONS

The following are definitions and descriptions of general musculoskeletal findings. Information on more specific musculoskeletal disorders follows in the next section. As a general rule, refer clients with the following musculoskeletal findings to a physician for assessment and diagnosis:

- progressive or persistent pain
- misalignment of any extremity
- asymmetry of muscle contours
- pain with loss of function or strength
- numbness with loss of function or strength
- hard or firm lumps (also called masses)
- pallor or coolness in one extremity and not the other
- erythema or heat in one extremity and not the other
- asymmetry in the size of one extremity over the other
- fever, nausea, and lethargy
- signs and symptoms of infectious disease
- signs and symptoms of acute inflammation

The following are more specific descriptions of musculoskeletal problems that you may encounter, with more specific information about contraindications and referral.

SPECIFIC MUSCULOSKELETAL CONDITIONS

Ankylosing Spondylitis: This is an autoimmune disease that occurs most often in men between 20-40 years old. It causes connective tissue along the spine, hip, and knee joints to inflame and eventually become solid, restricting joint movement (ankylosis). The symptoms are similar to those seen in rheumatoid arthritis. A major symptom is pain at night that decreases with activity. The etiology is unknown. Bodywork is locally contraindicated unless the client has discussed it with a physician and s/he thinks it is safe.

Arthritis, Miscellaneous: There are many miscellaneous kinds of arthritis. Two of the most common are:

- *infective arthritis*, which occurs when a bacterial infection in the body spreads to a joint. It is treatable with antibiotics and rest, but can cause permanent joint destruction if left untreated. This condition is potentially contagious with contact. Bodywork is systemically contraindicated.

• *psoriasis arthritis,* which is joint inflammation that flares up when psoriasis flares up. It can progress to deformity, ankylosis, and joint destruction. Bodywork is locally contraindicated.

Arthritis, Osteo (OA) or Degenerative Joint Disease (DJD): This is the most common form of arthritis and affects 16 million Americans over age 45. OA/DJD is progressive and is associated primarily with the wear and tear of normal living, however, it can also occur as a result of trauma, infection, or congenital malformation. The spine, fingers, hips, and knees are most often affected. The articular cartilage gradually erodes, and new bone (called a spur) forms in its place. Inflammation at the joint may or may not be present. If present, it causes pain and stiffness and can increase or decrease in intensity. A grating or grinding sound (crepitation) often develops in the affected joints and the joints may tend to subluxate or even dislocate in some cases. Bodywork is usually indicated because it can increase circulation to the area and relax the muscles adjacent to the joint, which can reduce stiffness and joint pressure. BODYWORK IS LOCALLY CONTRAINDICATED TO ACUTELY INFLAMED AREAS. Appropriate bodywork on persons with OA/DJD in the vertebrae includes gentle effleurage on muscles near the spine but never includes instructing client to bend or twist past their comfort level, manipulations of the vertebrae, or tapotement over the spine.

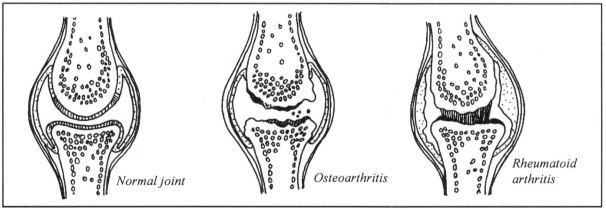

Illustration 33   Normal and Arthritic Joints

Arthritis, Rheumatoid (RA): This is an autoimmune disease where the body's immune system is attacking its own joint tissue. It often begins much earlier than osteoarthritis and can even occur in children. RA is progressively deforming and crippling, causing joints to inflame, cartilage and bone to degenerate, and joints to enlarge and fuse together (ankylosis). The small joints of the hands, wrist, elbow, ankles, and feet are most often affected. Rheumatoid arthritis can also affect the skin, heart, blood vessels, muscles and lungs. The person often experiences periods of remission and exacerbation. Bodywork is usually indicated because people who relax on a frequent, regular basis can often reduce the rate of the disease's progression. However, BODYWORK IS LOCALLY CONTRAINDICATED TO ACUTELY INFLAMED AREAS AND CAUTION IS ADVISED IN MOVEMENT ASSESSMENT AND THERAPY.

Bone cancers: Cancer can occur in bone or cartilage. *Osteomas* are benign tumors of the bone. There are few symptoms or signs other than being palpable as a hard and bony mass in a bone. *Osteosarcomas* are malignant bone tumors, occurring most often in the ends of the long bones in men between 10-25 years old. They can be treated successfully if diagnosed early. Cancers that originate in other tissues sometimes metastasize into bone tissue, as well. When cancer has metastasized to a bony area, deep constant pain is common, along with increased pain on movement and increased susceptibility to spontaneous fracture (also see *Chapter 12*). Bodywork is locally contraindicated in any areas of bone cancer.

Bursitis: This is inflammation of a bursa, or joint capsule, and is usually caused by injury, overuse or a systemic inflammatory disorder, such as gout. Sometimes the etiology is unknown; and sometimes bursitis can occur during acute arthritis. Bodywork is locally contraindicated during the acute inflammation stage, however, gentle work on the muscles proximal and distal to the area can be helpful. Rest, Ice, Compression, and Elevation (RICE) will help reduce symptoms and speed healing. After pain and swelling are gone, gentle bodywork within the client's comfort zone can help the tissue finish its repair.

Degenerative Disc Disease: This is also called osteoarthritis of the spine, and it affects many people over the age of 60. It is a deterioration or impairment of the fibrocartilaginous tissue between the vertebral bones. Excessive use, injury, and/or aging deteriorates the cartilage that covers the edges of the spinal vertebrae so the discs between the vertebrae become worn and the spaces between the bones narrow. Inflammation sets in. Bony spurs develop, which further rub into the discs. Symptoms include back stiffness and gradual loss of flexibility, pain and, if a disc ruptures, sudden severe pain (see *Herniated Disc*). Appropriate bodywork on persons with degenerative disc disease includes gentle effleurage on muscles near the spine, but contraindicates instructing a client to bend or twist past their comfort level, manipulations of the vertebrae, or tapotement over the spine.

Fibromyalgia: This is a condition that affects the muscles and connective tissue of the whole body, causing pain, tenderness, stiffness, and fatigue. Its etiology is unknown. It has a gradual onset, and it is worsened by stress and overuse. It is usually associated with insomnia, but researchers are unclear if the insomnia precedes the soft tissue pain or vice versa. Fibromyalgia is diagnosed by identifying symptoms that must have been present for at least three to five months including: pain (radiating and/or localized); chronic fatigue; morning stiffness; sensitivity to light, sound, cold and heat; joint swelling; numbness and tingling in the extremities; diarrhea and/or constipation; an irritable urinary tract; dry mouth and eyes; depression; headaches; and predictable tender points. Clients with fibromyalgia are often taking analgesic, anti-inflammatory, and/or anti-depressant medications. PMS, TMJ, carpal tunnel, sciatica, thoracic outlet syndrome, and dysfunctions in posture and respiration often accompany this illness. Bodywork is indicated within the client's comfort zone. Gentle cross-fiber friction over entire muscles seems to be very beneficial, as does stretching and effleurage (Stephens, 1996).

Fractures: Bone repair is much like the repair process described in Chapter 3, as follows: First, a blood clot forms. Next granulation tissue forms and provides a foundation for other tissues to build upon. Third, a callus forms between the broken ends, forming cartilage first and gradually filling bone cells and calcium into the area until the repair is complete. Bodywork is locally contraindicated on fractures until they are completely healed and the physician has either released the client from care or has written a prescription for the work.

Gout: This is a painful inflammation of the joints caused by excess uric acid in the blood. Combined with calcium, the uric acid forms deposits in the joints. It occurs most often in the big toe joint and occurs in men more often than women. Like other chronic joint inflammations, it can come and go. Its etiology is uncertain, but a diet high in red meat and/or alcohol seems to contribute to its occurrence. Dehydration can also cause a flare-up. It is readily treatable with diet and/or medication. Permanent damage can result if gout is untreated. Local bodywork is contraindicated during acute inflammation.

Herniated disk: Also known as "ruptured disk." This is a rupture of the soft disk between two spinal vertebrae, and it creates pressure on the adjacent nerve (see *Illustration* next page), which causes numbness, tingling, and/or pain radiating downward along the compressed nerve. The most common sites for a herniated disk are L4-5 and L5-S1. It can also occur between the cervical vertebrae. Men under the age of 45 are most commonly affected. In the neck, a herniated disk can cause severe pain, numbness, tingling and/or pain down one or both arms. In the back, it can cause pain, numbness, tingling and/or pain down the thigh and leg. Gentle massage is indicated to adjacent muscles, UNLESS THERE IS NUMBNESS OR SEVERE PAIN. In that case, avoid the area, refer the client to a physician, and massage only with the physician's approval.

Joint dislocation: This is the displacement of a bone from its joint and is caused by injury, congenital defect, or advanced arthritis. The signs are pain, swelling, and clearly visible misalignment. Shoulder dislocation usually involves an injury to the acromioclavicular joint. DO NOT work on persons with dislocations. Apply ice and refer the person for immediate medical assessment and treatment before further inflammation develops.

Joint replacement: This is a surgical procedure in which a diseased or damaged joint is removed and replaced with a mechanical joint, usually made of a special steel alloy. At this time, the most common replacements are of the hip and knee joints, but shoulder replacements are also occurring. These are major surgeries, because all of the connective tissues attaching to the joint are cut loose, the joint is literally cut off the body, the ends of the mechanical joint are cemented into the cut ends of the bones, and then the ligaments, tendons, and muscles are reattached. All these tissues, plus the neighboring fascia, blood and lymph vessels require great healing. During this healing process, and the person should rest and learn what has been cut and why movement may be limited for awhile. Very gentle massage can be beneficial during healing, after consultation with the surgeon. It is important that replaced hips are not adducted over the body's midline because that can put too much strain on the connective tissues that hold the joint in its socket. Other joints may have similar movement contraindications. After the joint is well-healed, massage and movement are indicated within the client's range of comfort.

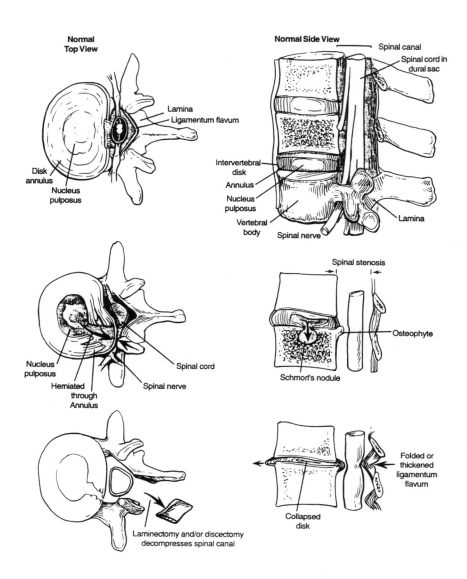

Illustration 34   Vertebral Disc Problems

Joint subluxation: This is a partial dislocation, where the antagonistic muscle is too tight or the ligaments are stretched causing a misalignment, but the bone is not entirely out of socket. This is particularly common in the hip joint and spinal vertebrae. There may be discomfort but not severe pain, swelling, or disfigurement. Massage is indicated to adjacent muscles if comfortable for the client. If not comfortable, avoid the area and refer the client to a physician.

Kyphosis: This is an exaggerated thoracic curve, also known as "hunchback." It is most often caused by arthritis or by the collapse of spinal vertebrae from osteoporosis. Bodywork is indicated if the condition is mild. If pain, functional limitation, or deformity are present, the client should discuss it with his/her physician first (see *Illustration 35*).

Lordosis: This is an exaggeration of the lumbar curve, also known as "swayback." It can be caused by excessive use of high heels, pregnancy, weak abdominal muscles, or obesity. Bodywork is indicated if the condition is mild. If pain, functional limitation or deformity are present, the client should discuss it with his/her physician first (see *Illustration 36*).

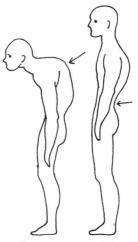

Illustrations 35-36
Kyphosis and Lordosis

Low back (lumbar) pain: This is the #1 most common problem that clients bring to bodyworkers. (It is the #2 most common pain that clients bring to physicians, with headache being #1.) There are many possible causes, including hypertonic erector spinae, spasm, tumors, arthritis, a herniated disc, vertebral subluxation, poor posture, and/or weak abdominal muscles. If the cause is poor posture, weak abdominal muscles, hypertonic erectors, or spasm, bodywork is indicated. If sharp or shooting pain is present, or if there is leg weakness or numbness present, bodywork is contraindicated until the client has consulted his/her physician for assessment (see illustration of vertebral problems).

Lupus: This is the shortened name for Systemic Lupus Erythematous (SLE), which is an autoimmune disorder that causes chronic inflammation affecting the skin, joints, kidneys, nervous system, and mucous membranes. The etiology is unknown. Lupus often causes redness on the cheeks and nose, called a butterfly rash. Women are affected more often than men. Lupus may begin with a fever, joint pain, and a general feeling of illness, and increase gradually over a period of years, with intermittent fevers and illness. Symptoms from any organ system may be present. Diagnosis can be made if four or more of the following symptoms are present: butterfly rash, red, scaling skin lesions, Raynaud's phenomenon, hair loss, photosensitivity, ulcerations in the mouth, nose or throat, arthritis without deformity, increased protein in the urine, and several different changes in the blood. Bodywork is usually indicated, but clients are advised to discuss it with their physician, first (also see *Raynaud's* in Chapter 6).

Muscular Dystrophy: This is a hereditary disorder, primarily affecting males, in which the skeletal muscles gradually atrophy. Muscular weakness in the pelvic and shoulder girdles begins soon after birth. Bodywork is systemically contraindicated without a physician's approval.

Myasthenia Gravis: This is an autoimmune disorder characterized by weakness, fatigue, and swelling in the face and extremities. It is progressive and has periods of remission and exacerbation. Bodywork is indicated, but if pain, functional limitation, or deformity are present, the client should discuss it with his/her physician first. Massage/bodywork results may vary and the practitioner should monitor changes closely.

Osgood-Schlatter disease: This is inflammation of the bone and cartilage with necrosis (death) of the tissue. It affects the tibial tuberosity (at the knee) and occurs most often in children from 10-15 years old. Bodywork is locally contraindicated.

Osteomyelitis: This is a bacterial infection of the bone that can be local or systemic. It causes deep pain, fever, bone destruction and necrosis (death). Bodywork is systemically contraindicated until a physician verifies that the infection is gone.

Osteoporosis: This is a gradual reduction of bone mass, most notably in the ribs, femur and spinal vertebrae, that is caused by the minerals and collagen being pulled out of the bones. This leaves small holes, or pores, in the bones, making them weak and susceptible to spontaneous fracture. People at highest risk are women over 60 years old of Asian and/or European descent. Osteoporosis can be prevented by building a strong calcium reserve before a woman is 24 years old, by maintaining adequate calcium intake after age 24, by getting regular weight-bearing exercise, and by getting at least 20 minutes of sunlight three times per week. If a client tells you s/he has osteoporosis, it is best to

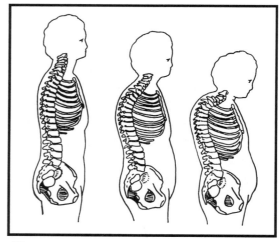

Illustration 37
Progressive Kyphotic Deformity of Osteoporosis

have a physician's approval for bodywork and then proceed with gentle pressure and movements, using extra caution over the anterior and posterior ribs and spine.

Paget's disease: This disease causes abnormal bone metabolism, with osteoclastic hyperactivity followed by an osteoblastic phase in which bone is replaced in an abnormal, misshapen way. The etiology is unknown, but it affects primarily older men and can be associated with congestive heart failure or some bone tumors. Signs and symptoms include: bone pain, general muscle weakness, and visible bone deformity. There may also be increased skull size, headache and central nervous system problems. Bodywork is locally contraindicated and the client should discuss it with his/her physician before proceeding.

Post-polio syndrome: This is a general muscular weakness that develops gradually many years after a person has recovered from acute poliomyelitis. Unlike acute polio, it is not infectious and is characterized by progressively hypotonic (flaccid) muscles, degenerating motor neurons, and decreasing motor function. The muscles in the legs are most often affected, initially. Bodywork is indicated and can help invigorate and tonify the tissues.

Sciatica: This is inflammation of the sciatic nerve, most often caused by compression from arthritis, a herniated disk, spinal misalignment, poor posture, prolonged periods of sitting, or muscle spasm. Some cases are caused by infectious, metabolic or toxic disorders, or the pain may be referred to the sciatic nerve from another source. Sciatica can begin abruptly or gradually and is characterized by a sharp shooting pain running down the posterior thigh. Pain in the anterior, medial or lateral leg is probably not sciatica. Movement of the leg generally intensifies the pain. Sometimes numbness or tingling are also present. Bodywork is indicated if the cause is myofascial or postural, after a physician has assessed the condition to rule put other causes (also see Chapter 5: *Nerve Compression*).

Scoliosis: This is a lateral curve in the spine that causes the vertebrae to rotate (see illustration), starts in the teenage years, and occurs more often in girls. The etiology can be from a variety of things, including a difference in leg length, a congenital deformity, abnormal pelvic tilt, infection, postural habits, diseased vertebrae or hip, rickets, and muscular paralysis. Scoliosis is usually mild, but in severe forms it can become progressive and deforming. Bodywork is indicated unless pain, functional limitation or deformity are present. In those cases, the client should discuss it with his/her physician first, and the bodyworker should proceed gently.

Sjogren's Syndrome: This is an autoimmune disorder that results from chronic dysfunction of the exocrine glands (glands whose secretions reach an epithelial surface either directly or through a duct) and is characterized by dryness of the eyes, mouth, urethra, vagina, and other areas covered by mucous membranes. It is frequently associated with rheumatoid arthritis, lupus erythematosus, and scleroderma, and often affects women between the ages of 40 and 60. Bodywork is indicated for general relaxation and body awareness.

Sprain: This is excessive stretching and/or tearing of ligament tissue and adjacent fascia. It is most often caused by falls, twisting, or motor vehicle accidents. The symptoms are those of acute inflammation with severe pain. The lower extremities are the most common locations of sprain, however, any area close to a joint can be affected. Sprains take longer to heal than strains because there is less blood flow to ligament tissue. Sprains are graded 1 to 3. A first-degree sprain is mild and usually heals in about two weeks if not re-injured. A second-degree sprain involves more tearing of the ligament fibers and can require up to two months to heal. A third-degree sprain is a complete rupture of the ligament and requires surgical repair. For first- and second- degree sprains, Rest, Ice, Compression, and Elevation (RICE) will help reduce symptoms and speed healing. Bodywork is contraindicated during the acute inflammation stage. After swelling is gone, gentle bodywork (with a physician's prescription) can help the tissue finish its repair.

Strain: This is excessive stretching and/or tearing of a muscle or tendon and its adjacent fascia. It is caused by overuse or by sudden use without warm-up. Strains most often occur at the site of previous injury and at the musculotendinous junction, although they can also occur at the place where the tendon attaches to the bone or in the muscle belly. Strains are graded 1 to 3. A first-degree strain produces mild inflammation and usually is repaired rapidly. A second-degree strain involves moderate inflammation and damage. A third-degree strain involves marked inflammation and tearing of more than half of a muscle's fibers. It may require surgical repair. Bodywork is locally contraindicated during the acute inflammation stage. Rest, Ice, Compression and Elevation (RICE) will help reduce symptoms and speed healing. After swelling is gone, gentle bodywork within the client's comfort zone can help the tissue finish its repair. Post-swelling work on grade 3 strains requires a physician's prescription.

Tendinitis: This is inflammation of a tendon and is usually caused by injury, overuse, or a systemic inflammatory disorder such as rheumatoid arthritis. Tendinitis can also occur when an adjacent joint is inflamed. Bodywork is locally contraindicated during the acute inflammation stage, however, gentle work on the muscles superior and inferior to the area can be helpful. Rest, Ice, Compression, and Elevation (RICE) will help reduce symptoms and speed healing. After swelling is gone, gentle bodywork within the client's comfort zone can help the tissue finish its repair.

TMJ (Temporo Mandibular Joint Dysfunction): This is a hypertonicity in the jaw muscles, caused by misalignment of the jaw bone, which can be caused by mental/emotional tension, teeth grinding, or injury. The muscle that is most often sore is the masseter, although the temporalis may also ache. Teeth pain, dizziness and/or ringing in the ears is common. Bodywork is indicated unless an acute inflammation is present, however, the client should see his/her dentist or general physician for assessment before seeking relief through bodywork.

Torticollis: This is also known as "wry neck," and is a shortening of the sternocleidomastoid muscles on one side only, from any cause. It causes the head to be flexed to one side and slightly rotated and is usually a permanent condition. Bodywork is indicated to the involved muscles if no acute inflammation is present, however, the client should see his/her physician for assessment before receiving bodywork.

Trigger Point: This is an area of hyperirritability in a tissue that is tender when compressed. If it is sufficiently irritable, it may refer pain, tenderness, autonomic phenomena and/or distortion of proprioception to other areas (Travell & Simons, 1983). Myofascial trigger points are the most common, usually occur within a taut band of skeletal muscle, and respond well to certain massage/bodywork techniques. Other types of trigger points include cutaneous, fascial, ligamentous and periosteal.

Whiplash: This is an imprecise term for injury to the cervical vertebrae and adjacent soft tissues. It usually involves strain and also sometimes a sprain. It is most often caused by a sudden stop or a rear-end collision in a motor vehicle. Clients who have experienced a sudden stop or rear-end collision should see a physician immediately for assessment and should not receive bodywork until they have done so. Bodywork is locally contraindicated during the acute stage of inflammation, but work on the mid to low back may be very helpful during this time, as that area often becomes hypertonic from trying to splint, or keep the neck immobile.

ENDANGERMENT SITES

Endangerment sites are areas that are not well protected by muscle or connective tissue, with nerves and/or blood vessels lying close to the surface. Deep sustained pressure to these areas can damage the nerves and vessels. In addition, the kidney area is included because heavy pounding is contraindicated in that area. A list of areas commonly considered endangerment sites includes (see *Illustration* next page):

1. <u>Anterior triangle of the neck</u>: includes the carotid artery, jugular vein, and vagus nerve located deep to the sternocleidomastoid

2. <u>Posterior triangle of the neck</u>: brachial plexus, brachiocephalic artery and vein (superior to the clavicle) and subclavian arteries and vein

3. <u>Axillae</u>: brachial artery, axillary vein and artery, cephalic vein, brachial plexus

4. Medial epicondyle of the humerus: ulnar nerve

5. Lateral epicondyle of the humerus: radial nerve

6. Sternal notch and anterior throat: vagus nerve, nerves and vessels to the thyroid gland

7. Umbilicus: descending aorta and abdominal aorta

8. Twelfth rib, dorsal side: kidney

9. Sciatic notch: sciatic nerve

10. Inguinal triangle: external iliac artery, femoral artery, great saphenous vein, femoral vein, femoral nerve

11. Popliteal fossa: popliteal artery and vein, tibial nerve

12. Additional: deep effleurage in the arms or legs in a direction away from the heart is contraindicated because it can weaken or damage the valves in the veins.

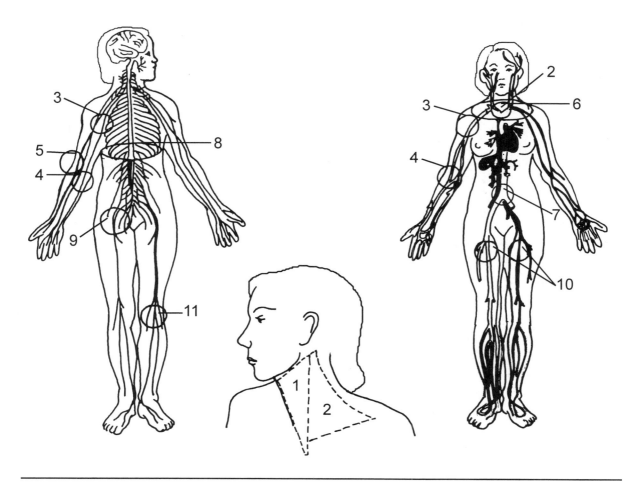

COMMON EFFECTS OF AGING ON THE MUSCULOSKELETAL SYSTEM

After age 65, the vertebral ligaments progressively become more calcified, causing kyphosis and scoliosis postural distortions. Joints progressively become more calcified, causing more joint stiffness and decreased ROM. Bones lose calcium and become less dense and more brittle. Muscles become weaker, more hypotonic, and progressively atrophy. (This may be caused by less activity and exercise, rather than by aging.) Overall endurance and stamina decrease. Intervertebral discs compress and vertebrae demineralize, causing a decrease in height in women of about 2-3" between the ages of 25 and 75.

EFFECTS OF EXERCISE

A key ingredient to a healthy musculoskeletal system is physical activity. When people are physically active their muscles and bones stay strong, their joints and connective tissues stay flexible, and their balance and coordination are maintained. Inadequate levels of physical activity are associated with increased risk for osteoporosis, heart disease, hypertension, non-insulin dependent diabetes, colon cancer, depression, and anxiety.

A recent review of research has concluded that "every US adult should accumulate 30 minutes or more of moderate intensity physical activity on most, preferably all, days of the week" (Pate, et al., 1995). Moderate physical activity is defined as the equivalent of a brisk walk at 3 to 4 mph, and can include work, play, or physical fitness types of activities. As a bodyworker, clients will ask you for advice about physical activity and health maintenance. It is important that you familiarize yourself with additional information in this area.

CASE PRESENTATIONS

Each of these cases reflects a real client and his/her bodywork session. Each was written in a slightly different way, reflecting the individual style of the massage therapist.

5/6/96: 34 yr old female presenting with R shoulder pain & stiffness

Health history: Asthma, migraine & sinus headache, R rotator cuff repair '90, gallbladder surgery '95. Married w/ 4 kids. Exercises 3-5x/wk. Job requires lifting & pushing with arms.

Assessment: Decreased R shoulder flexion, extension and abduction, knots palpated in all 4 R rotator muscles, extending into shoulder blade.

Goal & intervention: Increase AROM; decrease pain & stiffness of R shoulder. Swedish techniques + strain/counter-strain.

Evaluation: Increased AROM & decrease in pain & stiffness.

Follow-up instructions: Continue therapeutic massage, good body mechanics & ROM exercises previously prescribed by MD.

11/11/96: 63 yr old woman presenting with neck pain

History: arthritis in fingers and lumbar spine; dislocated R shoulder 20 yrs ago (fixed with
   pins & screws); L sciatica
        Gets massage 2-4x/month.

S: pain, tension, & stiffness in neck & shoulders; L leg numb

O: very limited AROM in R shoulder; shoulders drawn forward; traps extremely tight.

Goal: increase relaxation & neck mobility, decrease neck pain

A: effleurage, petrissage & deep friction on neck, shoulders & back; trigger point work on
   neck, traps & lumbar areas; gentle petrissage on legs; deep petrissage & trigger point
   work on gluts; No PROM on R shoulder

Outcome: increased mobility in neck, increased relaxation, decreased pain in traps & lumbar area

---

3/25/97: 73 yo woman presenting with pain from fibromyalgia

History: fibromyalgia & arthritis the past few yrs; lumbar injury 6 yrs ago with dislocated
   lumbar disc. Sees MD, chiropractor, & neurologist regularly. Planning to get cortisone
   injections in tender points this week.

S: Pain ratings on 0-10 scale: R shoulder 8, neck 5, upper back 5, lower back 9, L hip 8, R hip 6

O: posture slightly stooped; grimaced when she removed her jacket; edema in L ankle & foot

G: reduce muscular pain; wants bodyworker to locate tender points today, so she can direct
   cortisone injections; relax

A: applied warm moist heat to lumbar area; trigger point work on tender points in shoulders,
   hips and lower back. Recorded location of points on diagram for her use; PROM to joints

TO: decreased pain: R shoulder 6; neck 3; upper back 3; lower back 6; L hip 7; R hip 5. Said
   she loved the work!

STUDY QUESTIONS:
        What questions would you have asked that were not asked?
        What bodywork techniques would you have done?
        What referral(s)?
        What other ways could the therapeutic outcome have been evaluated?
        How might you have changed the format, or way the cases were written?
        What were the indications for massage/bodywork?
        What were the contraindications?

FURTHER RESOURCES

Journal of Soft Tissue Manipulation, 324 Oakdale Avenue, Ottawa, Canada K1YOE4, 613-722-8588.

Massage Magazine, 1315 W. Mallon, Spokane WA 99201, 1-800-533-4263.

Massage Therapy Journal, 820 Davis St., Suite 100, Evanston IL 60201-4444, 1-708-864-0123.

REFERENCES

Barnes, J. F. (1996). Myofascial release: The new therapy for fibromyalgia. Nurse's Touch, 2(2), 14, 20, 21, 24.

Calais-Germain, B. (1993). Anatomy of movement. Seattle, WA: Eastland Press, Inc.

Fritz, S. (1995). Mosby's fundamentals of therapeutic massage. St. Louis: Mosby Lifeline.

Jarvis, C. (1992). Physical examination and health assessment. Philadelphia: W. B. Saunders Co.

Juhan, D. (1987). Job's body: A handbook for bodywork. Barrytown, NY: Station Hill Press.

Kapit, W. & Elson, L.M. (1977). The anatomy coloring book. NY: Harper & Row.

Kapit, W., Macey, R.I., & Meisami, E. (1987). The physiology coloring book. NY: Harper & Row.

Lowe, Whitney W. (1995). Functional assessment in massage therapy. Corvallis, OR: Pacific Orthopedic Massage.

Malasanos, L., Barkauskas, V., & Stoltenberg-Allen, K. (1990). Health assessment. St. Louis, MO: C.V. Mosby Co.

Mulvihill, M.L. (1995). Human diseases: A systemic approach (4th ed.) Norwalk, CT: Appleton & Lange.

Newton, D. (1995). Pathology for massage therapists. Portland, OR: Simran Publications.

Pate, R. R., Pratt, M., Blair, S. N., Haskell, W. L., Macera, C. A., Bouchard, C., Buchner, D., Ettinger, W., Heath, G. W., King, A. C., Kriska, A., Leon, A. S., Marcus, B. H., Morris, J., Paffenbarger, R. S., Patrick, K., Pollock, M. L., Rippe, J. M., Sallis, J., & Wilmore, J. H. (1995). Physical activity and public health: A recommendation from the Centers for Disease Control and Prevention and the American College of Sports Medicine, JAMA, 273(5), 402-407.

Ribeiro, C. & Bourdelais, M. (1996). Prevention and rehabilitation of shoulder injuries. Massage Therapy Journal, 35(3), 87-88.

Sameulson, P. (1994). Pathophysiology for massage: The travel guide. Overland Park, KS: Mid-America Handbooks, Inc.

Stephens, R. R. (1996). Massage therapy for fibromyalgia. Massage Therapy Journal, 35(3), 76-80.

Thomas, C.L. (1989). Taber's cyclopedic medical dictionary (16th ed.). Philadelphia: F.A. Davis Co.

Travell, J. and Simons, D. (1983; 1992). Myofascial pain and dysfunction: The trigger point manual, Volumes 1 and 2. Baltimore, MD: Williams and Wilkins.

Zerinsky, S. S. (1987). Introduction to pathology for the massage practitioner. (S. Weinstein & J. E. Thompson, eds.) The Swedish Institute.

CHAPTER REVIEW

1. All of the connective tissues contain a transparent fluid called _____ that is the basis for their production.

2. _____ are protein chains that give strength, elasticity and structure to skin, ligaments, tendons, cartilage, bone, blood vessels, and all the organs.

3. _____ is a fibrous membrane that unites the skin with the underlying tissue and covers, supports, and separates the muscles.

4. Living bone requires _____ to give it rigidity and _____ to give its tensile strength and flexibility.

5. In massage, we primarily focus on the _____ muscles.

6. Chronically tense muscles cause a lack of circulation called _____, which means a local and temporary deficiency of blood supply due to obstruction of circulation.

7. The scope of practice for bodywork usually does not include unsupervised work directly on _____ and _____. However, these structures can benefit from the bodywork done to adjacent tissues.

8. The 3 main areas to consider during the musculoskeletal assessment are:

   _____

9. The 4 main ways to assess, or get information about the musculoskeletal system are to observe the client's: _____

   _____

   _____

   _____

TRUE/FALSE

10. _____ If AROM produces pain and PROM does not, it is usually a sign of a muscle or tendon problem.

11. _____ Pain on gentle traction is usually a muscle or tendon problem.

12. _____ If both AROM and PROM produce pain, then it is usually a sign of a ligament or joint problem.

13. _____ Pain on gentle compression is usually a ligament or joint problem.

14. _____ is the name for excessive muscle tone.

15. Refer the following musculoskeletal findings to a physician:

   _____

   _____

   _____

   _____

   _____

   _____

16. _____ is the most common form of arthritis and is associated primarily with the wear & tear of normal living.

17. _____ is an autoimmune disease where the body's immune system attacks its own joint tissue; it is also progressively deforming and crippling.

18. _____ is a painful inflammation of the joints caused by excess uric acid in the blood and often occurs in the big toe joint.

19. _____ is a gradual reduction of bone mass caused by the minerals and collagen being pulled out of the bones.

20. _____ can be prevented by building a strong calcium reserve before age 24, by maintaining adequate calcium intake after age 24, by getting regular weight-bearing exercise, and by getting at least 20 minutes of sunlight three times/week.

21. _____ is an autoimmune disease that causes connective tissue along the spine, hip, and knee joints to inflame and eventually become solid.

22. _____ is an autoimmune disorder that causes chronic blood vessel inflammation and affects many other body tissues, including the joints.

23. _____ is a lateral curve in the spine that causes the vertebrae to rotate.

24. _____ is an exaggerated thoracic curve; "hunchback."

25. _____ is a bulge or rupture of the soft disc between two spinal vertebrae.

26. _____ is the displacement of a bone from its joint.

27. _____ is excessive stretching or tearing of a muscle or tendon caused by overuse or by sudden use without warm-up.

28. _____ is excessive stretching or tearing of ligament tissue caused by wrenching or twisting motion.

29. _____ is also known as "wry neck," and is a shortening of the sternocleido-mastoid muscles on one side only.

30. _____ are areas that are not well protected by muscle or connective tissue, with nerves and/or blood vessels lying close to the surface.

31. _____ is a key ingredient to a healthy musculoskeletal system.

ANSWERS TO CHAPTER REVIEW

1. *ground substance*

2. collagen fibers

3. fascia

4. minerals; collagen fibers

5. striated or skeletal

6. ischemia

7. ligaments & joints

8. balance, function & symmetry

9. 1) walk; 2) standing and lying posture; 3) AROM & PROM; 4) palpation, or the way the tissues feel

10. T

11. T

12. T

13. T

14. hypertonicity

15. progressive or persistent pain
    misalignment of any extremity
    asymmetry of muscle contours
    pain with loss of function or strength
    numbness with loss of function or strength
    hard or firm lumps (also called masses)
    pallor or coolness in one extremity and not the other
    erythema or heat in one extremity and not the other
    asymmetry in the size of one extremity over the other
    fever, nausea, and lethargy
    signs and symptoms of infectious disease
    signs and symptoms of acute inflammation

16. osteoarthritis (OA) or degenerative joint disease (DJD)

17. rheumatoid arthritis (RA)

18. gout

19. osteoporosis

20. osteoporosis

21. ankylosing spondylitis

22. lupus (SLE)

23. scoliosis

24. kyphosis

25. herniated, ruptured or slipped disc

26. dislocation

27. strain

28. sprain

29. torticollis

30. endangerment sites

31. physical activity

Chapter 5

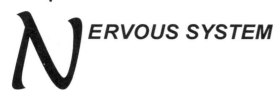

NERVOUS SYSTEM

ANATOMY AND PHYSIOLOGY REVIEW

The nervous system is the body's communication system, and its functions are to receive stimuli from the internal and external environments, organize that information, and provide responses. It consists of two main divisions: the *central nervous system (CNS)* and the *peripheral nervous system (PNS)*. The CNS can be compared to a central information processing station and consists of the brain and spinal cord and their coverings called meninges. The PNS is like the lines that carry nerve impulses to the CNS and then back out again, to the muscles, glands, skin and other organs. The PNS consists of the cranial and spinal nerves and their ganglions.

The PNS is divided into the *autonomic nervous system (ANS)* and the *somatic nervous system (SNS)*. The ANS is divided into the *sympathetic* and *parasympathetic* systems, which control the fight or flight and relaxation responses of the smooth muscles in the organs, the cardiac muscle, and the glands (see Chapter 2 for a more detailed review). The SNS consists of the nerves of the joints and skeletal muscles. A description follows.

Afferent nerves carry stimuli from the senses to the spinal cord and brain (CNS). Afferent nerves are also called *sensory nerves*, because they carry sensory information (sensations), such as position, rate of movement, pain, temperature, pressure, contraction, tension, and stretch of tissues. *Efferent nerves* carry stimuli from the brain and spinal cord to the muscles. Efferent nerves are also called *motor nerves*, because they cause motion/movement in the body. One way to remember which nerves are which is to remember that "A" comes before "E," and the afferent nerves first carry stimuli from the senses to the spinal cord and brain before the efferent nerves can carry the message from the CNS back to the muscles and other peripheral tissues (see *Illustration 39*).

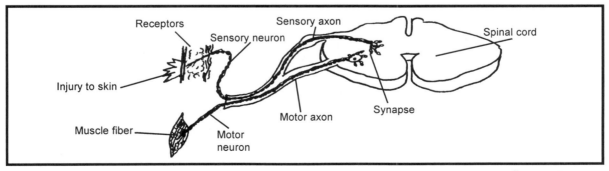

Illustration 39   Reflex Arc Pattern

The effects of bodywork on the nervous system are largely reflexive, that is, based on the body's reflexes. A *reflex* is a specific, purposeful and predictable involuntary neuromuscular response to a stimulus. Stimuli that produces a reflex can transfer either in the brain or the spinal cord. The drawing on the previous page is of a simple arc. Many reflexes are more complex.

From a European/American perspective, many of these neuro-muscular responses can be understood by *scientific laws*. A scientific law is a statement that is uniformly true for a whole class of natural occurrences. Below are brief descriptions of some of these laws.

Scientific Laws of the Nervous System

All-or-None Law: In cardiac and skeletal muscle and in nerves, any stimulus capable of producing a response produces the maximum response contraction. This law implies that bodywork techniques do not have to be extremely intense to produce the maximum response.

Bell's Law: Anterior spinal cord nerve roots are motor, and posterior spinal cord nerve roots are sensory. This law implies that a back massage along each side of the spine stimulates sensory, not motor, responses.

Law of Facilitation: When an impulse has passed through a certain set of neurons to the exclusion of others, it will tend to take the same course on future passes, and each time it travels this path there will be less resistance. This law implies that once a pain or other sensory pattern is established, minor stimuli that would normally cause no response are able to stimulate the nerve, muscle, or organ tissue to be contracted or hyperactive.

Hilton's Law: Any nerve trunk that serves a joint also serves the muscles of the joint and the skin over that muscle's insertions. This law implies two things: 1) it is difficult to determine if pain is from a joint, the muscles around the joint, or the skin over the joint, and 2) stimulation of other skin, muscle, or joint also affects these other parts.

Law of Specificity of Nervous Energy: Excitation of a receptor always results in the same sensation, regardless of the nature of the stimulus. This law implies that no matter what technique is used, if a receptor is activated, the receptor always sends the same sensation.

Law of Symmetry: If a stimulation is sufficient to provoke a strong response on one side of the body, the other side will have a similar neuromuscular response. This law implies that a bilateral effect can be stimulated, even if bodywork is only being done on one side. This is especially helpful when direct work on one side is contraindicated, such as in the case of a fracture.

References for the above information: Fritz, S. (1995), <u>Mosby's Fundamentals of Therapeutic Massage</u>, and Thomas, C. L., ed. (1989), <u>Taber's Cyclopedic Medical Dictionary</u>.

Proprioceptors are sensory receptors in the muscles and connective tissues that give the person kinesthetic information about position, movement, pressure, tension, stretch, and balance. Proprioceptors include: muscle spindles, located mainly in the muscle bellies that respond to stretches; tendon and joint receptors that respond to movement and strain; pacinian corpuscles, located in subcutaneous tissue, pancreas, penis, clitoris and nipple that respond to deep or heavy pressure; and labyrinthine receptors, located in the inner ear that respond to the body's equilibrium (or balance) in space.

NERVE COMPRESSION

Nerve compression is also called nerve impingement or a pinched nerve. Tissues that can cause pressure on a nerve are: taut skin, shrunken fascia, hypertonic and/or spasmed muscles, shortened ligaments, and misaligned joints. Pressure on nerves results in pain or tingling. If the pressure is unrelieved, it can progress to numbness of a sensory nerve or to paralysis of a motor nerve.

When nerve compression occurs, it is often at one of the major nerve plexuses. Compression in the cervical plexus can cause headaches, neck pain, and dyspnea (breathing difficulty). Vertebral misalignment, shortened connective tissue at the cranial base, hypertonic suboccipitals and/or sternocleidomastoid muscles are often the cause of cervical plexus compression.

Compression in the *brachial plexus* can cause unilateral or bilateral pain, tingling, numbness, or paralysis in the shoulder, chest, arm, wrist, and hand. Vertebral misalignment, shortened connective tissue in the upper thoracic or the axillae areas, hypertonic scalenes, pectoralis minor, and/or subclavian muscles are often the cause of brachial plexus compression.

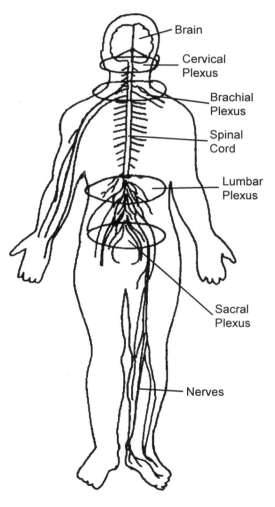

Illustration 40   Major Nerve Plexuses

Compression in the *lumbar plexus* can cause localized or radiating lumbar, lower abdominal, genital, thigh, and/or medial lower leg pain, tingling, numbness or paralysis. Vertebral misalignment, shortened connective tissue in the lumbar area, and hypertonic quadratus lumborum and psoas muscles are often the cause of lumbar plexus compression.

Compression in the *sacral plexus* can cause localized or radiating pain in the buttock, pelvis, leg and/or foot. Sciatica is one example. Vertebral misalignment, shortened connective tissue, and hypertonic piriformis and/or gluteal muscles are often the cause of sacral plexus compression.

Bodywork can be beneficial by stimulating nerves to reflexively change muscle tone, by mechanically lengthening and softening tight muscle and connective tissues, by positional stimuli, and by interrupting the pain-spasm cycle.

ASSESSMENT: OBSERVATION AND PALPATION

There are five main areas to consider during the neurological assessment:

- pain,
- tingling or numbness,
- balance,
- paralysis or involuntary movements, and
- changes in sensory or mental abilities.

There are four main ways to assess, or get information about the nervous system. These are:

- ask the client to describe to you any problems they have in the above five areas;
- observe the client's posture, gait, and movement;
- observe the client's speech, hearing, and other sensing abilities, and
- palpate for reflexes and tactile sensation.

The assessment of pain has already been discussed in Chapter 1, however, this chapter will discuss pain in more depth. Although pain does not always mean neurological problems, there are certain descriptions of pain that call for specific assessment because neurologic structures might be involved. For instance, pain described as burning, shooting, or electrical in nature may indicate neurogenic pain due to stretching or compression of a nerve trunk or root.

Paresthesia (a sensation of pins and needles) is usually caused by compression somewhere along the nerve path and is usually felt after the compression has been released. The duration of the compression affects how long afterwards the paresthesia is felt. For instance, compressing the peroneal nerve by crossing your leg for five minutes will probably result in paresthesia of less than one minute after the compression is released. However, when a nerve is compressed all day, such as in brachial plexus compression, the paresthesia might not occur until after you have rolled onto your side in bed, and have relaxed for several hours. In this case, the person may wake up in the middle of the night with his/her arms "asleep" (also see *Nerve Compression* page 105).

Tingling is a prickling or stinging sensation that is most often caused by cold temperatures, nerve injury, or decreased circulation (ischemia). *Numbness* is a lack of sensation (pain, pressure, temperature, texture, etc.) in any part of the body and often occurs after tingling from the further progression of cold temperatures, nerve injury, or decreased circulation.

Numbness can be caused by some block or interruption in the afferent route to the brain.

PAIN

When assessing pain, it is best to organize your questions around the following four areas:

- location,
- duration,
- intensity, and
- quality.

To assess the location, ask the client to show you where he/she hurts. To assess duration, ask when the client first noticed the pain, and whether the pain is steady or comes and goes. To assess intensity, ask the client to rate the pain on a scale, e.g., mild, moderate, severe, or 0-5 with 0 being no pain and 5 being the worst pain imaginable. Then ask the client what increases and decreases the pain. To assess quality, ask the client to describe how the pain feels (sharp, dull, aching, burning, stabbing, constant, intermittent, squeezing, cramping, etc.).

The location of pain can be further identified as *localized* (pain confined to its source), *projected* (pain perceived in the distal tissue served by a compressed nerve, e.g., paresthesia), *radiating* (pain that diffuses out and around its site of origin or travels along a nerve), and *referred* (pain that is felt in an area distant from the site of its origin).

Referred pain occurs when there is an exceptionally large amount of sensory input from an area and the brain receives a flood of information. The brain relays its response back to the spinal cord where the efferent messages are spilled into the muscular or connective tissue areas that are enervated by the same spinal cord segment as the original source of pain. Visceral (organ) pain is a common source of referred pain and stimulates pain and/or the reflex contraction of skeletal muscles innervated by the same spinal cord segment. For example, the cardiac pain of a heart attack is often also felt as left arm and neck

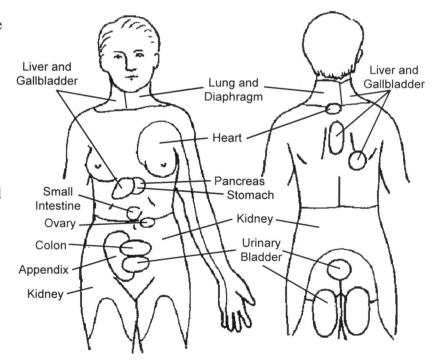

Illustration 41   Common sites of referred pain.

pain (see *Illustration 41*). Clients experiencing acute, persistent, or progressively worsening pain in any area shown should be immediately referred to a physician for assessment and diagnosis. However, these sites are not always exactly the same in everyone, in fact, unusual sites are fairly common. The safest procedure is to REFER ALL CLIENTS WITH ACUTE, PERSISTENT, OR PROGRESSIVE PAIN.

Myofascial *trigger points* are another example of referred pain. When a muscle develops an area of hyperirritability, and that area is also stressed, the brain sends a flood of information back to that segment of the spinal cord, and the message can spill over into the efferent innervation of another area. For instance, a trigger point in the neck can cause pain in the temporal areas. For more information about myofascial trigger points, see books by Travell and Simons listed in the Further Resource section at the end of this chapter.

The International Association for the Study of Pain defines pain as the sensory and emotional experience associated with actual or potential tissue damage. An estimated 700 million work days, at a cost of over $60 billion, are lost annually in the U.S. due to chronic pain (Taber's, 1989). The experience of pain is influenced by constantly changing, dynamic, and interacting factors from every facet of the body/mind. Thus, the pain that is perceived at one time will, most likely, be perceived differently at another point in time. There are many different kinds of pain. The four that are most common are: *acute, chronic, intractable*, and *phantom*.

Acute pain activates the sympathetic nervous system, is short in duration, and is experienced as sharp or cutting. The intensity usually ranges from 6-10 on a 0-10 scale. Acute pain is usually easily relieved once its cause is corrected. It is often associated with acute inflammation of tissue, or involvement of a posterior spinal nerve root. It is clearly localized, warns the person of actual or impending tissue damage, and prompts the person to rest and/or attend to the problem. However, persistent acute pain can interfere with the healing and recovery process by causing a series of reflexes that prevent optimum functioning of the heart, lungs, and other essential body systems.

Common signs of acute pain are: increased heart rate and blood pressure, dilation of the pupils, sweating on the palms, increased breathing rate/hyperventilation, restlessness, irritability, and anxiety. Bodywork is systemically contraindicated until the client's condition has been assessed by a physician and the cause has been identified. Clients who have acute pain are advised to discuss bodywork as a treatment option with their physicians before choosing it. If bodywork is chosen, it can be beneficial to the client for systemic relaxation and biofeedback, but bodywork is locally contraindicated for the area in pain.

Chronic pain persists beyond the usual or expected course of an acute pain, or after the expected time for an injury to heal. It often has a vague or subtle onset and serves no known purpose. It is diffuse and generalized with the character and quality changing from time to time. The intensity usually ranges from 1-5 on a 0-10 scale. Common signs of chronic pain are: appetite and/or sleep disturbances, irritability, constipation, restricted movements, decreased pain tolerance, social withdrawal, and depression. Bodywork is systemically indicated for persons with chronic pain but is locally indicated only within the client's comfort zone. Clients who have chronic pain are advised to discuss the bodywork with their physicians.

Intractable pain feels acute but is not easily relieved and persists despite treatment. It often occurs as a result of cancer, mental illness or neurological disorder. Bodywork is contraindicated until a physician has assessed and diagnosed the cause, and then it may be beneficial.

Phantom pain feels like it is occurring in a part of the body that has been amputated, as if the part were still present. One explanation for phantom pain is that the sensory nerves that were cut may be activated at their distal ends and sending signals to the CNS that are interpreted as occurring beyond that point. Bodywork is beneficial, both systemically and locally.

The Gate Control Theory of Pain (also called Afferent Inhibition)

This theory was proposed in 1965 by Melzack and Wall and has been used extensively as a base for pain research. It is widely accepted as a possible explanation but has not been conclusively proven or disproven. It is known that pain signals travel on two types of sensory nerves, large-diameter nerves and small-diameter nerves. The hypothesis is that there is a "gate" mechanism at the spinal cord through which pain signals must pass to reach the brain. The signals traveling on the small-diameter nerves, such as the aching pain signals, seem to be prevented from reaching the brain when the larger sensory nerves that carry friction and the sharp signals are stimulated (see *Illustrations 42 and 43*). This may be because the larger nerves carry a faster signal which arrives at the gate first and blocks the smaller nerve signals. Examples of this theory are that rubbing, massaging, or shaking an area of aching pain seems to suppress it. The gate control theory is one of the proposed Western explanations of the action of acupuncture.

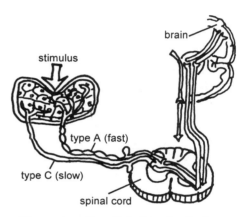

Illustration 42   Pain Impulse Pathways

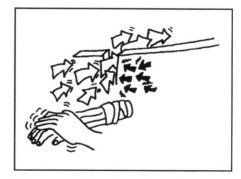

Illustration 43   Gate Control Theory

Pain Medications

Analgesics are substances that give temporary relief from pain without causing a loss of consciousness. There are two major types of analgesics: narcotics and non-narcotics. The most commonly used non-narcotics are acetaminophen and NSAIDs (non-steroidal anti-inflammatory drugs) such as ibuprofen. In addition to reducing pain, the NSAIDs also reduce fever and inflammation. Narcotic medications are prescribed only for severe pain that is not relieved by non-narcotics, because these are gradually addictive. Narcotics are natural or manufactured forms of opium, such as Codeine, propoxyphene (Darvon), meperidine (Demerol), and morphine. An intermediate step between non-narcotics and narcotics are drugs that are a combination of the two, such as Tylenol with Codeine, or Darvocet.

Most pain medications have the potential of creating undesirable side effects including dry mouth, constipation, nausea, drowsiness, and dependence (narcotics); increased bleeding time and ringing in the ears (aspirin); and stomach upset and irritation (NSAIDs). Acetaminophen (Tylenol) has fewest side effects but should be avoided in persons with kidney or liver disorders. Stomach irritation and nausea side effects are reduced when the drugs are taken with food. Pain medications should not be taken more often than prescribed, and bodyworkers are advised to work with the awareness that pain medications can dull a person's sensory awareness. For more information about the effects of pain medications, consult a pharmacist or one of the many books, available in local bookstores, about medications.

GENERAL NERVOUS SYSTEM CONDITIONS

The following are definitions and descriptions of general neurological findings. Information on more specific neurological disorders follows in the next section. As a general rule, refer clients with the following neurological findings to a physician for assessment and diagnosis:

- acute pain
- pain that is persistent or progressively worsening
- pupils of unequal size
- seizures
- changes in mental ability
- changes in sensory ability
- abnormal reflexes
- headache with fever and neck rigidity
- headache that is persistent or progressively worsening
- headache followed by vomiting
- involuntary movements
- numbness
- paralysis
- inability to maintain balance

SPECIFIC NERVOUS SYSTEM CONDITIONS

ALS (Amyotrophic Lateral Sclerosis): This is a progressive degenerative disease that causes destruction of motor neurons in the brain and spinal cord, which then causes gradual weakening, atrophy and hyperreflexia of skeletal muscles. It is also called Lou Gehrig's disease. There is no known cure, and ALS is eventually fatal, but some people have remained active for 10 to 20 years. Bodywork is beneficial if it is given with respect to the person's wishes, energy level, and range of comfort.

Alzheimer's Disease: This is a progressive degenerative disease of the cerebral cortex which causes mental and emotional abilities to gradually waste away. It affects approximately 5% of the U.S. population over age 65, usually begins after the age of 50, has no known cure, and is usually fatal in 8-10 years. Bodywork is beneficial if it is given with respect to the person's wishes, attention span, energy level, and range of comfort. These areas can be difficult to assess in confused persons. Astute observation of verbal and non-verbal communication is required, as well as informed consent of the responsible guardian if the client is not mentally competent to give consent.

Bell's Palsy: This is a unilateral facial paralysis of sudden onset. The etiology is unknown but is thought to involve swelling of the seventh (facial) nerve due to immune or viral disease, resulting in compression and ischemia of the nerve where it leaves the skull. It usually resolves in several months, with 20% to 90% likelihood of complete recovery. Bodywork is locally contraindicated, and clients are advised to consult with their physician for assessment and diagnosis.

Brain Cancer: This can cause intense headaches and changes in motor, mental and emotional function, including confusion, agitation, mood swings, changes in personality, seizures, loss of balance or coordination, and loss of bodily functions. Bodywork is NOT contraindicated to the head unless there are palpable masses present, however, it is best to work with the physician's approval. If cancer is present in another part of the body, or if the person is undergoing chemotherapy or radiation, other precautions and contraindications may be warranted (see *Chapter 12*).

Brain Injuries: There are three basic types of brain injuries. In all cases, bodywork is systemically contraindicated until a physician has determined that the client's condition is stable and able to tolerate the stimulation. There are three main types of brain injuries: compression, concussion and hemorrhage.

- *Compression*: squeezing from tumor, increased fluids or swelling of brain tissue; patient can progress into seizure, coma or death.
- *Concussion*: a blow to the head or a fall on the end of the spine shakes the brain against the skull; causes dizziness, paralysis, or unconsciousness, with or without vomiting or headache, and usually resolves within 48 hours.
- *Hemorrhage*: bleeding into the brain tissue, as a result of a severe blow to the head, a skull fracture, or the spontaneous rupture of an artery or arteriole (also called *stroke* or *CVA*); signs are confusion, unconsciousness and, if severe, death.

Carpal Tunnel Syndrome (CTS): This is a chronic compression of the median nerve at the point where it goes through the carpal tunnel of the wrist. It is most often caused by repetitive motion, with inflammation in the tendon sheath causing the compression. Symptoms are pain, tingling, numbness, and/or weakness in the affected thumb, wrist, and hand. The compression may have other causes, such as a tumor, so it is best to advise clients to consult a physician for assessment and diagnsis before choosing bodywork as their treatment option. Trigger points in the forearm and/or shoulder girdle can mimic carpal tunnel syndrome.

Cerebral Palsy: This is a bilateral, symmetrical, non-progressive paralysis and/or involuntary movements that are a result of either developmental defects in the brain or from injury at birth. Bodywork is systemically indicated, with the physician's advice if the client is currently receiving treatment.

Headaches: These may be due to trigger points, diseases of the sinuses, teeth, eyes, ears, nose or throat; acute infections; injury to the head; tumors; mental/emotional stressors; metabolic conditions; endocrine disorders; allergies; exposure to toxic chemicals, or from unknown causes. Clients with persistent or progressively worsening headaches must be referred to a physician for assessment and diagnosis. Of the many types of headaches, there are four main types you will encounter in bodywork practice:

- *Cluster headache*: This is a cluster (or series) of headaches over the span of a few days. The etiology is unknown, but it is more common in men and is aggravated by alcohol, overwork, and emotional stress. The onset is abrupt and characterized by intense throbbing pain behind one nostril and/or eye. The eye and nose may water and the skin in the area may become red. These occur most often at night and rarely last longer than 2 hours, but may recur 2-3 times per night. Bodywork is beneficial, but clients are advised to consult with their physician for assessment and diagnosis.

- *Migraine headache*: The etiology is unknown, but theories suggest that changes in the blood vessels and blood flow to the brain are triggered by food allergies, menstrual cycle, emotional stress, and/or environmental stimuli such as bright lights or strong odors. In the first stage, the cerebral arteries constrict causing visual or auditory auras (warning signals). In the second stage, the arteries dilate causing the feeling of stabbing, throbbing, or pressure. This stage can last from a few hours to several days, and pain is aggravated by emotional and environmental stimuli. Usually pain is felt only on one side of the head, reaches its peak in one to two hours, and then gradually lessens. Although it is common for the migraine to resolve completely within six hours, patterns are individual, and the migraine may last for days or even a week. Migraines can also be accompanied by visual disturbances or digestive upset. Sometimes bodywork can prevent a migraine if it is given during the warning signal (aura) stage, and it is given within the person's particular energy level and range of comfort at that time. Soothing approaches are usually more beneficial than stimulating approaches. Light, sound, odor, and movement sensitivities may be more acute than usual.

- *Sinus headache:* These are caused by inflammation or infection of the nasal sinuses, and are characterized by pain and pressure in the sinus areas, which increases when the person leans far forward. Sinus headaches begin gradually and can last for days or weeks until the infection or inflammation is resolved.

- *Tension headache*: Nine out of ten headaches are tension related. Tension head-

muscles and often include trigger points (see Travell & Simons, 1983). Adults between 20 and 40 are most likely to be affected. Pain is usually bilateral and occurs most frequently in the temporal, frontal and occipital areas. The onset is gradual but if not relieved it may last for several days, months, or even years. Poor posture with prolonged neck flexion, depression, fatigue, emotional upset, and injuries causing misalignment of the cervical vertebrae can all cause tension headaches. Bodywork is very beneficial, both locally and systemically.

Meningitis: This is an infection of the meninges (the membranes around the brain) and can be viral or bacterial. The symptoms are headache, fever, and neck rigidity. Treatment requires hospitalization and intravenous antibiotics. Bodywork is systemically contraindicated until a physician has determined that the client's condition is able to tolerate stimulation.

MS (Multiple Sclerosis): This is a progressive degeneration of the myelin sheath around the nerves, especially in the brain, spinal cord and eyes. Its onset can be sudden or gradual, and the primary symptoms are weakness or numbness in one or both limbs, with hyperactive reflexes, unsteady gait, visual disturbances, dizziness, nausea, depression, and irritability commonly associated. MS commonly begins between ages 20 and 40 and affects about 6-14 persons per 100,000 in the southern U.S. and 30-80 persons per 100,000 in the northern U.S. MS can take either a steadily progressing path or a remission/exacerbation path. Some persons die a few months after disease onset and others are still working after 25 years. There is no known cure. Bodywork is beneficial, but clients are advised to consult first with their physician.

Paralysis: This is the temporary or permanent loss of sensation or voluntary motion. It is divided into two groups: *spastic paralysis* that is due to a lesion in the part of a motor neuron that is in the brain, and *flaccid paralysis* that is due to a lesion in the part of a motor neuron that runs to a muscle. In spastic paralysis, muscle tone is increased and there is no atrophy except that from disuse. Reflexes may be abnormal or increased. In flaccid paralysis, reflexes are reduced or lost, and muscles lose tone and atrophy (wither away). Acute or chronic compression of the spinal cord or of a nerve is one of the main causes of paralysis. Another common cause is *stroke*, or cerebrovascular accident (*CVA*), which damages the brain and motor neurons there. Other causes are: polio, prolonged voluntary movement that exhausts the nerve centers, and brain or spinal cord lesions. Bodywork must be modified to fit the type of paralysis, using a knowledge of the individual client's physiology, and is best accomplished in collaboration with the client and his/her health care team.

Parkinson's Disease: This is a progressive degenerative disease of the nervous system which causes hand tremors during rest, weakness, stooped posture, shuffling gait, severe muscle rigidity, drooling, and a decrease in facial expressions. It affects about 1% of the U.S. population over age 65, and men more often than women. Its etiology is unknown, it has no known cure, and it is usually fatal after about 10 years. Bodywork is beneficial but extra attention should be given to respect to the person's wishes, energy level, and range of comfort.

Peripheral Neuropathy: This is a general term meaning disease of the peripheral nerves (sensory or motor). Its symptoms are tingling, pain, numbness and/or weakness in the extremities, and it can be caused by anything that reduces the blood or nerve impulse flow to the tissues, such as diabetes, trauma, narrowed arteries, chemical poisoning, compression, etc. Bodywork is beneficial locally and systemically, but clients are advised to consult with their physician for assessment and diagnosis.

Polio: This is a shortened name for poliomyelitis, which is a viral infection that attacks the motor neurons. Polio is communicable, and can be transmitted through contact with oral, respiratory, and fecal secretions. It is preventable by immunization, and is one of the vaccinations required for children in the U.S. Polio causes muscle weakness, atrophy, and sometimes paralysis. Bodywork is indicated only after a physician has determined that the client's condition is no longer infectious.

Rabies: This is a viral infection that attacks the brain and spinal cord. It is most often transmitted by an animal bite, but is preventable by vaccination. Rabies causes progressive mental confusion, convulsions, and paralysis that ends in death if not treated in its early stages. Bodywork is systemically contraindicated until a physician has determined that the client's condition is able to tolerate nerve stimulation.

Sciatica: This is inflammation of the sciatic nerve, most often caused by compression from arthritis, a herniated disc, spinal misalignment, poor posture, or prolonged periods of sitting. Some cases are caused by infectious, metabolic or toxic disorders, pregnancy, tumor, or constipation with hard feces. The pain may also be referred to the sciatic nerve from another source. Sciatica can begin abruptly or gradually, and is characterized by a sharp shooting pain running down the posterior thigh. Movement of the leg generally intensifies the pain. Sometimes numbness or tingling are also present. Symptoms often grow worse at night and on the approach of stormy weather. Bodywork is indicated if the cause is muscular, after a physician has assessed and diagnosed the condition (also see Chapter 4).

Seizures: These occur when the brain experiences abnormal electrical activity, similar to an electrical storm in the brain. Seizures are thought to be caused by certain drugs, kidney failure, chemical poisoning, toxemia in pregnancy, brain tumor, and epilepsy. They temporarily alter the person's brain function, so that s/he experiences motor, sensory, and/or mental symptoms. The location of the unusual electrical activity determines the kind of seizure and the person's signs and symptoms. There are basically four types of seizures:

- A *simple partial seizure* occurs in the brain's cortex and causes stiffening or jerking of an arm or leg on one side of the body. The person does not lose consciousness unless the seizure progresses to a generalized tonic-clonic type.
- A *complex partial seizure* occurs in the brain's temporal lobe, and, although symptoms vary between people, each person's symptoms are fairly consistent for him/her. Generally, people have a warning sign (aura) that precedes the seizure. Examples of auras include: seeing spots, tingling in the extremities, and ringing in the ears. The seizure symptoms can include: staring, not responding, confusion, unusual mouth motions, aimlessness, or a drunk appearance. These may last one

to three minutes, and the person often does not remember these behaviors.

- A *generalized tonic-clonic seizure* affects the entire brain, and usually gives no warning. The person may cry out as s/he loses consciousness and falls. Next the whole body stiffens and the muscles alternately spasm and relax, causing jerking or thrashing motions. Breathing may also be irregular and facial color may pale or blush. There may be loss of bowel or bladder control. These seizures may last from one to three minutes, and as the person begins to regain consciousness, s/he is often confused, sleepy, and has headache. Again, the person probably will not remember the seizure.
- An *absence seizure* has no identifiable focus in the brain and lasts about one to ten seconds. There is no aura, the person only momentarily loses consciousness, and does not fall. Often there will be a blank stare, eye blinking, or facial twitching. Some people have hundreds of these seizures daily.

Some people wear a Medic-Alert bracelet to let you know that they sometimes have seizures. Other people do not. Seizures can happen anytime, anywhere. If a client seizures in your presence, protect him/her from injury and turn him/her onto his/her side. Loosen any clothing that is around the neck. Do not put anything in the person's mouth. There is no danger that s/he will swallow his/her tongue as we were taught years ago. After the seizure, talk to the person and relate what happened. Offer to call someone to drive him/her home. Be sure that the person can safely resume activities before leaving him/her alone. Bodywork is systemically contraindicated during a seizure, but is beneficial for persons with a history of seizures, with their physician's advice if they are currently receiving treatment.

Shingles: This is a viral infection that affects one or more nerves, causing intense pain and red blisters that follow the nerve's path. It usually affects only one side of the body. The blisters' fluid contains the virus, and the virus can be transmitted by contact with this fluid. Shingles occur in adults and are caused by herpes zoster which is the same virus that causes chicken pox in children. Bodywork is systemically contraindicated while the person has blisters, and locally contraindicated after that until the person can be touched without feeling pain.

Spinal Cord Injuries: There are three types of spinal injuries:

- *Compression*: squeezing of cord, most often caused by tumor or vertebral fracture; results in numbness or paralysis below site. Bodywork is beneficial after the diagnosis has been made and the client's condition is no longer considered acute (also see *Paralysis* page 113).
- *Contusion*: a bruise, causing swelling and pressure on cord, which can cause compression until swelling subsides. Bodywork is locally contraindicated until a physician has determined that the client's condition is able to tolerate the stimulation.
- *Laceration*: a cut or tear in the spinal cord; symptoms include paralysis, loss of sensation and altered reflexes below the level of the injury. Bodywork is beneficial after a physician has determined that the client's condition is able to tolerate the stimulation.

Tetanus: This is a deadly infection caused by bacteria that lives in soil and thrives in the absence of oxygen. Puncture wounds are most susceptible to tetanus infection because they are deep and close quickly at the top, reducing contact with air. It attacks the motor neurons and causes painful muscle spasms that progress to death by asphyxiation. Since it affects the jaw muscles first, it is also known as lockjaw. Tetanus is preventable by receiving a vaccination every 10 years. It is treatable, if caught early enough, by a vaccine and massive doses of antibiotics. Bodywork is systemically contraindicated until a physician has determined that the client's condition is able to tolerate nerve stimulation.

Thoracic Outlet Syndrome: This is a chronic compression of the subclavian artery and/or nerves in or near the brachial plexus, caused by hypertonic pectoralis minor or scalene muscles, aneurysm, tumor, or rib protrusion against the clavicle. Symptoms are tingling, numbness, pain, and/or weakness in the chest or upper extremities. It often occurs after swimming, weight lifting, backpacking, and other activities involving shoulder rotational stress while the muscles are contracted to perform weight-moving. Bodywork is indicated if the cause is muscular, after a physician has assessed and diagnosed the condition. A focus on relaxing and lengthening the anterior muscles of the neck and shoulder is often beneficial. A retraining program to develop muscle strength and balance in the pectoral girdle is recommended (Ribeiro and Bourdelais, 1996).

Tourette's Syndrome: This is a disease of unknown etiology that begins in childhood and may continue through life. It affects boys three times more often than girls and is estimated to affect 1 to 5 people per 10,000. Symptoms include lack of muscle coordination, involuntary movements, tics, and incoherent vocalizations that may resemble grunts, barks, or obscenities. Clients are advised to consult with their physician when choosing bodywork therapies.

Trigeminal Neuralgia: This is pain along the trigeminal nerve in the face. It is usually an intense, intermittent stabbing or burning pain and is aggravated by touch, chewing, or temperature change. Bodywork is locally contraindicated, and clients are advised to consult with their physician for assessment and diagnosis.

MISCELLANEOUS TERMS DESCRIBING NERVOUS SYSTEM CONDITIONS

Dyskinesia: This is a general term meaning "defect in voluntary movement." The most common type is tardive dyskinesia, which is slow, rhythmical involuntary movements that can be generalized or localized in single muscle group. It occurs as an undesirable side effect of certain psychotropic drug therapies. Bodywork is beneficial for general relaxation purposes.

Dystonia: This is a general term meaning "impaired or disordered tonicity," especially muscle tonicity. It most often occurs as an undesirable side effect of certain psychotropic drug therapies, and includes abnormal facial grimacing and torticollis. Bodywork is beneficial for general relaxation purposes.

Insomnia: This is a general term meaning "disorders of initiating or maintaining sleep." The disorder may be primary or secondary to some other illness, condition, or circumstance.

Clients are advised to consult their physician for assessment and diagnosis of the cause. If the cause is mental/emotional stress, worry or muscular tension, bodywork is beneficial. Clients may also benefit from establishing a more regular sleep routine starting earlier in the evening, avoiding caffeine, and exercising early in the day, preferably before the last meal.

COMMON EFFECTS OF AGING ON THE NERVOUS SYSTEM

After age 65, the surface of the brain and the inner brain cells begin to atrophy, influencing behavioral changes, reducing emotional intensity, changing self-image, slowing adaptability, and narrowing interests. Sensory nerve transmission begins to slow, causing a slower reaction time and reducing sensitivity to light touch and pain. Spinal cord synapses begin to degenerate causing a reduction in overall coordination of neuromuscular, circulatory, and glandular functions, and an increase in susceptibility to shock, slower motor nerve transmission, and sensitivity to heat and cold. Kinesthetic and vestibular sensations are reduced, causing less awareness of position and increasing likelihood of falls. Sleep patterns change, making falling to sleep more difficult, reducing Stage IV and REM sleep, increasing time spent in bed, but causing the person to wake up earlier than previously.

CASE PRESENTATIONS

08/09/96: 70 yo female presenting with pain and stiffness in neck and R shoulder, weakness in R arm and hand

History: Lyme disease that has resulted in permanent neuropathy, shooting or stabbing pain in various parts of the body, rashes that itch, muscle cramps, tingling and numbness in extremities, and occasional mental confusion. Also had rotator cuff surgery 10 months ago in the R shoulder and has had 1 lumbar and 2 cervical surgeries to repair ruptured discs. Has arthritis in hands and knees and varicose veins in R leg.

Objective: Rash on lower R abdomen and L ankle. No open sores or broken skin. Hypertonicity in rhomboids and traps. Limited AROM in R shoulder and neck.

Goals: reduce pain and increase AROM

Interventions: relaxation massage to back, neck, and limbs; avoid rashes and varicose veins; gentle PROM to neck and shoulders.

Outcome: said she felt less tense and more invigorated immediately after the session. On follow-up 3 days later, said she still felt invigorated. She had talked to her MD about it, and he encouraged her to get more massages.

5/6/96: 69 yo woman in poor health; neck and shoulder pain

History: degenerative arthritis in hip and spine; Parkinson's, diabetic neuropathy; R hip replacement; general weakness since being confined to bed. Under MD's care, and he gave approval for bodywork. Taking many medications. Receives help with meal prep, bathing, and housekeeping. Can only do minimal exercise in bed and stand with assistance.

S: dull pain, tension, stiffness in neck; tight shoulders; poor circulation in feet and legs, pain, weakness and stiffness in R hip; pain in spine; amazingly positive attitude.

O: hand tremor at rest; few facial expressions; coldness and reddish/brown discoloration in lower legs and feet; hypertonic traps and cervicals.

Goals: increase relaxation, mobility in neck, and lower extremity circulation; decrease pain and tension in neck and shoulders

Treatment: light effleurage and petrissage to neck and shoulders, legs and feet. Avoided R hip. Light palmar friction to warm feet. Worked slowly and did a lot of listening.

Outcome: moderate increase in neck mobility; significant increase in relaxation; moderate decrease in neck and shoulder pain. Client plans to continue twice weekly.

STUDY QUESTIONS

What questions would you have asked that were not asked?

What bodywork techniques would you have done?

What referral(s)?

What other ways could the therapeutic outcome have been evaluated?

How might you have changed the format or way the cases were written?

What were the indications for massage/bodywork?

What were the contraindications?

FURTHER RESOURCES

Travell, J. and Simons, D. (1983; 1992). Myofascial pain and dysfunction: The trigger point manual, Volumes 1 and 2. Baltimore, MD: Williams and Wilkins.

REFERENCES

Fritz, S. (1995). Mosby's fundamentals of therapeutic massage, St. Louis, MO: Mosby Lifeline

Jarvis, C. (1992). Physical examination and health assessment. Philadelphia: W. B. Saunders Co.

Juhan, D. (1987). Job's body: A handbook for bodywork.. Barrytown, NY: Station Hill Press

Kapit, W. and Elson, L.M. (1977). The anatomy coloring book. NY: Harper and Row.

Kapit, W., Macey, R.I., and Meisami, E. (1987). The physiology coloring book. NY: Harper and Row.

Lowe, Whitney W. (1995). Functional assessment in massage therapy. Corvallis, OR: Pacific Orthopedic Massage.

Malasanos, L., Barkauskas, V., and Stoltenberg-Allen, K. (1990). Health assessment. St. Louis, MO: C.V. Mosby Co.

Mulvihill, M.L. (1995). Human diseases: A systemic approach (4th ed.) Norwalk, CT: Appleton and Lange.

Newton, D. (1995). Pathology for massage therapists. Portland, OR: Simran Publications.

Ribeiro, C. and Bourdelais, M. (1996). Prevention and rehabilitation of shoulder injuries. Massage Therapy Journal, 35(3), 87-88.

Sameulson, P. (1994). Pathophysiology for massage: The travel guide. Overland Park, KS: Mid-America Handbooks, Inc.

Stephens, R. R. (1996). Massage therapy for fibromyalgia. Massage Therapy Journal, 35(3), 76-80.

Taber's cyclopedic medical dictionary, 16th ed. (1989). (C. L. Thomas, ed.) Philadelphia: F.A. Davis Co.

Zerinsky, S. S. (1987). Introduction to pathology for the massage practitioner. (S. Weinstein and J. E. Thompson, eds.) The Swedish Institute.

CHAPTER REVIEW

1. The nervous system consists of two main divisions:
   a. _____ b. _____

2. The autonomic nervous system (ANS) consists of two parts _____ and
   _____

3. The somatic nervous system (SNS) consists of nerves in the: _____

4. Afferent nerves are also called _____ nerves and carry stimuli from
   _____ to _____.

5. Efferent nerves are also called _____ nerves and carry stimuli from
   _____ to _____.

6. _____ are sensory receptors in the muscles and connective tissues that
   give the person kinesthetic information about position, movement, pressure, tension, balance.

7. Pain that diffuses out and around its site of origin is called _____

8. Pain that is felt in an area distant from the site of its origin is called _____

9. As a rule, refer clients with the following neurological findings to a physician for
   assessment and diagnosis: _____
   _____
   _____
   _____
   _____

10. The four most common kinds of pain are _____
    _____, _____, and _____

11. Common signs of acute pain are: _____
    _____

12. TRUE/FALSE: Bodywork is systemically indicated for persons with acute pain.

13. Common signs of chronic pain are: _____

_____

14. TRUE/FALSE: Bodywork is systemically indicated for persons with chronic pain.

15. When rubbing, massaging, or shaking an area of sharp pain seems to suppress the pain, this is an example of _____

16. _____ is the temporary or permanent loss of sensation or voluntary motion.

17. Pressure on nerves results in _____, which, if unrelieved, can progress to _____ of a sensory nerve or to _____ of a motor nerve.

18. Bodywork can be beneficial to nerve compression that is being caused by _____

_____

19. _____ is a progressive degenerative disease of the cerebral cortex, which causes mental and emotional abilities to gradually waste away.

20. What are the three basic types of brain injuries? _____

_____

21. What is a chronic compression of the median nerve? _____

_____

22. What are the four main types of headaches? _____

_____

23. What is a progressive degeneration of the myelin sheath? _____

24. What is a progressive degenerative disease of the nervous system which causes hand tremors, weakness, stooped posture, shuffling gait, severe muscle rigidity, and a decrease in facial expressions? _____

25. What are uncontrollable (involuntary) movements that can range from minor eye staring, muscle rigidity or twitching to total body stiffening and convulsions? _____

26. What is a viral infection that affects one or more nerves causing intense pain and red blisters that follow the nerve's path? _____

25. What is a chronic compression of the subclavian artery and/or nerves in or near the brachial plexus? _____

28. TRUE/FALSE: After age 65, sensory nerve transmission begins to slow, causing a slower reaction time and reducing sensitivity to light touch and pain.

ANSWERS TO CHAPTER REVIEW

1. central nervous system (CNS)/peripheral nervous system (PNS)

2. sympathetic and parasympathetic

3. joints and skeletal muscles

4. sensory; the senses; brain and spinal cord

5. motor; the brain and spinal cord; muscles

6. proprioceptors

7. radiating

8. referred

9. acute pain
    pain that is persistent or progressively worsening
    pupils of unequal size
    seizures
    changes in mental ability
    changes in sensory ability
    abnormal reflexes
    headache with fever and neck rigidity
    headache that is persistent or progressively worsening
    headache followed by vomiting
    involuntary movements
    numbness
    paralysis
    inability to maintain balance

10. acute, chronic, intractable, and phantom

11. increased heart rate and blood pressure, dilation of the pupils, sweating on the palms, increased breathing rate/hyperventilation, restlessness, and anxiety

12. FALSE

13. appetite and/or sleep disturbances, irritability, constipation, restricted movements, decreased pain tolerance, social withdrawal, and depression

14. TRUE

15. gate control theory

16. paralysis

17. pain or tingling; numbness; paralysis

18. hypertonic skeletal muscles and shrunken fascia

19. Alzheimer's

20. compression, concussion, hemorrhage

21. carpal tunnel syndrome

22. cluster, migraine, sinus, tension

23. multiple sclerosis (MS)

24. Parkinson's disease

25. seizures

26. shingles

27. thoracic outlet syndrome

28. TRUE

Chapter 6

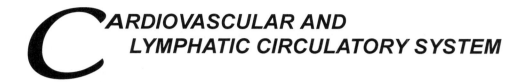

CARDIOVASCULAR AND LYMPHATIC CIRCULATORY SYSTEM

ANATOMY AND PHYSIOLOGY REVIEW

The circulatory system consists of the heart, blood, and blood vessels (cardiovascular system) and the lymph, lymph nodes and vessels (lymphatic system). Its functions are to:

- transport oxygen, nutrients, and the components needed for inflammation and repair to the cells,
- transport waste products away from the cells,
- maintain hydrostatic pressure.

Increases in the circulation are among the most widely recognized physiologic effects of bodywork. Bodywork may influence the blood and lymph vessels by:

- direct mechanical action (pumping) on the vessel walls in which alternating pressure increases the movement of fluid;
- reflex action through the vasomotor nerves,
- neurochemical action through the release of vasodilators and vasoconstrictors.

CARDIOVASCULAR SYSTEM

The *heart* is a hollow, muscular organ that pumps the blood throughout the body. Its walls consist of three layers: a tough inner lining (endocardium), a serous outer lining (epicardium), and the heart (cardiac) muscle in between (myocardium). The heart is surrounded by a tough fibrous sac (pericardium). The heart has four chambers: the right and left upper chambers (atriums) and the right and left lower chambers (ventricles). The ventricles are thick-walled because they contract to pump the blood out. The atriums are thinner-walled and serve mainly as receiving chambers. The right side receives blood from the body via the veins and pumps it to the lungs for oxygenation. The left side receives blood from the lungs and pumps it to the body via the arteries. Each of the four chambers has a set of valves at the exit to prevent back-flow. A healthy adult heart rate averages between 60 to 80 beats/minute.

The *blood* circulates through the heart and blood vessels, carrying nourishment (carbohydrates, proteins, fats, and vitamins), electrolytes (minerals), hormones, antibodies, heat, and oxygen to the body's tissues and taking away waste matter and carbon dioxide. The blood consists of approximately 22% solids and 78% water and makes up about 7-8% of the body's weight. There are six main types of blood cells, and each has its own particular function. Blood in the arteries is bright red because it contains a lot of oxygen. Blood in the veins is purplish or blue because it has little oxygen and a lot of carbon dioxide.

The *blood vessels* are arteries, capillaries, and veins. *Arteries* carry oxygenated blood away from the heart. With one exception, arteries warm and nourish the body's tissues. The exception is the pulmonary artery, which carries blood to the lungs to pick up oxygen and release carbon dioxide. The walls of the arteries are normally thick and elastic because they withstand the highest pumping pressure as the blood leaves the heart. The largest artery is the aorta. The *capillaries* are microscopic vessels that connect the ends of the smallest arteries (arterioles) with the beginnings of the smallest veins (venules). All of the exchange of nutrients and wastes that pass between the body and the blood occurs in the capillaries because the walls are thin enough to let these exchanges occur. The *veins* carry deoxygenated blood from the body's tissues back to the heart. With one exception, veins carry blood to the lungs for oxygenation. The exception is the pulmonary vein, which carries oxygenated blood to the heart from the lungs. Veins differ from arteries in that they are larger in diameter, greater in number, have thinner walls, lower pressure, and periodically have valves inside to prevent back-flow of blood.

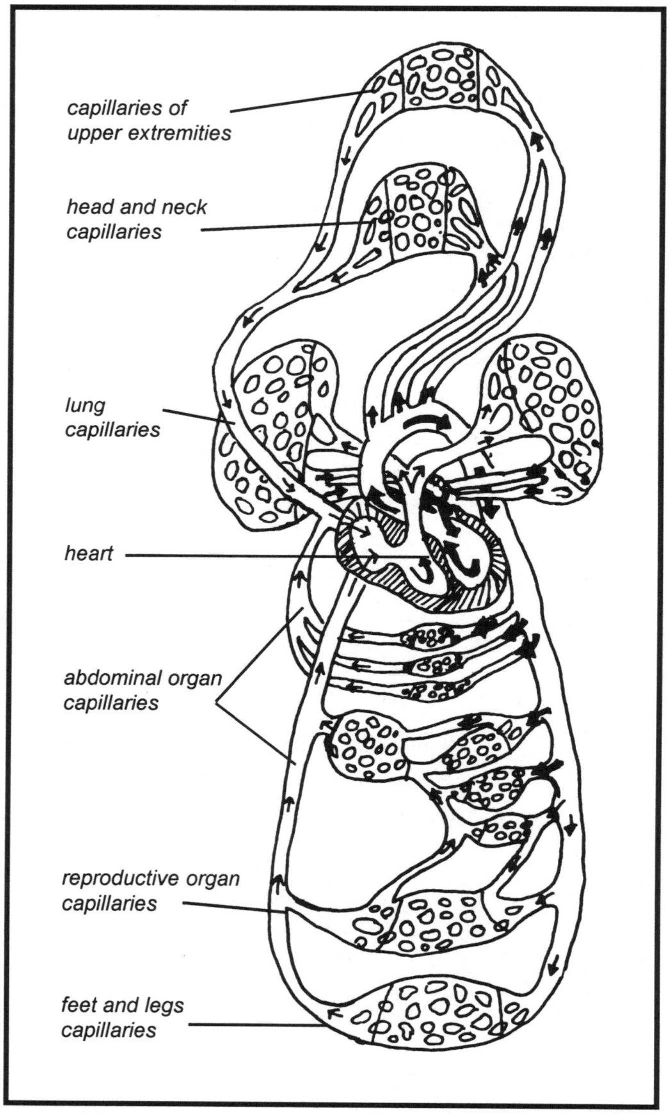
capillaries of
upper extremities
head and neck
capillaries
lung
capillaries
heart
abdominal organ
capillaries
reproductive organ
capillaries
feet and legs
capillaries

Illustration 44 Simplified view of the heart and blood vessels. Arrows indicate path of blood flow.

The term "*blood pressure*" means the pressure exerted by the blood on a blood vessel wall. This pressure is highest at the moment when the ventricles contract/pump, and lowest when the ventricles rest. Blood pressure is written as a fraction, such as 120/80. This is read or spoken as "120 over 80." A healthy adult blood pressure averages between 140 and 100 for the highest number (systolic), which is written on the top, and between 90 and 60 for the bottom (diastolic) number. Blood pressure varies with age, sex, altitude, muscular development, stress, and fatigue. It normally rises during activity or excitement and falls during rest or sleep.

The term *ischemia* means local, temporary deficiency of blood supply due to an obstruction of circulation. Common examples of ischemic areas include: muscles that are chronically hypertonic; tissues that have restrictive fascia around them; tissues distal to arterial obstruction.

When a tissue becomes active, it releases a number of metabolites which dilate local arterioles. This brings the active tissue more nourishment and washes away waste products. The smooth muscle inside the blood vessel walls are also controlled by sympathetic nerves. These nerves cause the vascular smooth muscle to contract. When the frequency of sympathetic impulses increases, blood vessel constriction is more intense; when the frequency is decreased, the muscle is more relaxed and blood vessels dilate (see *Illustration 45*).

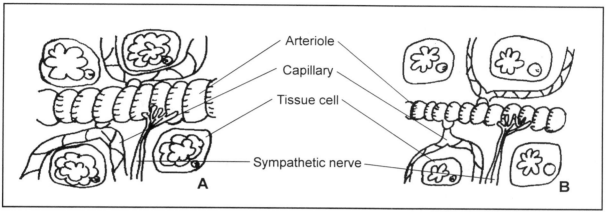

Illustration 45   Local Vasodilation (A) and Constriction (B)

Lymphatic System

Lymph is a clear, colorless alkaline fluid that varies in composition as it passes through different parts of the body. Lymph contains proteins, salts, glucose, fats, water, lymphocytes, and various body waste products, and is carried to the body's cells by the blood vessels.

Lymph is conveyed from the tissues to the bloodstream by *lymph vessels*. These are thin-walled tubes with paired valves, and are one-directional, resembling veins. The smallest lymph vessels are lymph capillaries, which are microscopic and made of a single layer of cells, each ending blindly in a rounded end. Lymph enters these capillaries from the body's cells through the thin lymph vessel walls and travels into larger and larger vessels until it empties into either the thoracic duct or the right lymph duct. Lymph from the head, neck, and right arm empty into the right duct and then into the right subclavian vein. Lymph from the rest of the body (the majority of the lymph) empties into the thoracic duct, which then empties into the left subclavian vein, near the clavicles (see illustration). In the abdomen, the lymph vessels absorb nutrition from the small intestine and carry it into the blood vessels for circulation to the body.

Lymph vessels flow to and through the *lymph nodes*, which are small, rounded bodies that vary in size from a pinhead to an olive, and may occur singly or in groups. The principal node groups are located in the neck, armpit, and groin (see *Illustration*). Lymph nodes produce lymphocytes and monocytes and filter the lymph, freeing it of foreign particles, especially bacteria. They can stop cancer cells from passing through, but, in turn, often become a metastatic site. The lymph nodes, spleen, tonsils, and thymus are all made primarily of lymphatic tissue.

Lymphocytes (a type of white blood cell) are important components of the immune system and are of two types: small B cells that originate in the bone marrow and produce antibodies that circulate between the blood and lymph, and larger cells that originate in the lymph nodes and migrate to the thymus, where they develop into T cells. Lymphocytes and other immune system components travel to the body's cells via the bloodstream and return from the body's cells via the lymph vessels (see Chapter 8 for more information).

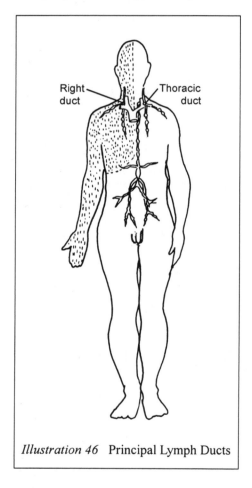

Illustration 46   Principal Lymph Ducts

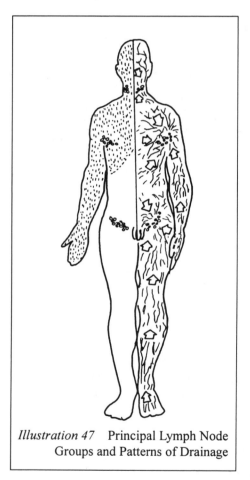

Illustration 47   Principal Lymph Node Groups and Patterns of Drainage

ASSESSMENT: OBSERVATION AND PALPATION

There are six main areas to consider in assessing the circulatory system. These are:

- skin color and temperature,
- nailbed color and shape,

  • presence of unusual veins,
  • edema,
  • swollen lymph nodes with or without tenderness, and
  • presence of anti-coagulant medication in the person.

In addition, if you feel it fits into your practice, checking the pulse(s) and blood pressure before and after the bodywork can provide useful information in some cases.

There are three main ways of getting this assessment information:

  • asking for this information in the health history,
  • observing the client's body during the bodywork, and
  • palpating the body.

As previously described in Chapter 4, the skin can take on four distinct abnormal colorations: pallor, cyanosis, erythema, and jaundice. *Pallor* (paleness) can be indicative of moderate lack of oxygen and is most often caused by *vasoconstriction* due to stress, disease, or cold temperature or to a lack of oxygen in the blood. *Cyanosis* (blueness) is due to the presence of deoxygenated blood and excess carbon dioxide, is a progression of pallor, and is indicative of severe lack of oxygen. The two areas where pallor and cyanosis are first evident are usually around the mouth and in the nail beds. Pallor and cyanosis are also usually accompanied by a the client feeling cold, and the extremities may be cold to the touch.

Erythema (redness) is caused by *vasodilation* as a result of inflammation or infection, a nervous mechanism in the body, or an external influence such as friction, pressure, heat, cold, or radiation. Bodywork itself can cause erythema. However, working on erythema that is present before you have worked in that area should be avoided. *Jaundice* (yellowness) can be present in the sclera (whites) of the eyes as well as in the skin and urine and is due to excess bilirubin in the blood, usually caused by an obstruction of the bile pathways, excess destruction of red blood cells, or liver dysfunction.

Other discolorations that relate to the circulatory system are:

  • *bruises* (bluish spots changing to greenish-brown or yellow as they begin to fade)
  • *brawny induration* (brown or bronze areas of thickened tissue) usually from chronic inflammation
  • *petechiae* (small reddish or purplish spots on the skin or mucous membrane) from capillary hemorrhages
  • *mottling* (pink, purple, or white splotches) from poor oxygenation and circulation; occurs most often on the feet, legs, and hands.

Healthy nails are pink and grow at a slightly upward angle from the cuticle. Nailbed color changes first to pale and then to cyanotic with lack of oxygen. Over time, when a person has been chronically oxygen deprived, the finger and toe tips enlarge, and the nails' angle straightens (see *Illustration 48* next page). This condition is called "*clubbing*" because it makes the finger and toe tips look like clubs. Inequality of temperature between the two arms or two legs can indicate circulation problems.

The presence of pain in the chest often indicates either a lack of blood supply to the heart or a lung problem (see specific illnesses). Pain in the calf muscles can indicate a lack of either arterial blood supply or venous return (see specific illnesses). Enlarged, swollen, or twisted veins (*varicose*) can occur in almost any part of the body but are most often

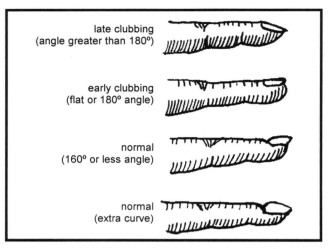

late clubbing
(angle greater than 180°)

early clubbing
(flat or 180° angle)

normal
(160° or less angle)

normal
(extra curve)

Illustration 48   Clubbing

observed in the feet and legs. Varicose veins occur because of severe pressure against the normal venous flow (see Varicose veins and Spider veins).

Edema means swelling and can be localized or systemic. Tissues swell because they contain excess fluid. The most common locations of edema are the feet, ankles, and lower legs, however, any area can swell if venous circulation is restricted or if inflammation is present. Aside from inflammations, the most common causes of edema are venous obstruction, congestive heart failure, renal failure, and protein deficiency. The most severe type of edema is called "*pitting*" edema. This term describes edema that forms pits, or indentations, when the skin is pressed gently with the fingertips. Bodywork is locally contraindicated in areas of pitting edema because even light pressure can damage the swollen, fluid-filled cells. If the edema is non-pitting, gentle bodywork, such as light effleurage, can be beneficial (see *Illustration* page 59).

The presence of swollen lymph nodes with tenderness can indicate an infection in a nearby part of the body. Swollen lymph nodes without tenderness can indicate lymphoma. In both cases, bodywork is locally contraindicated. Refer the client to a physician for assessment and diagnosis.

MEDICATIONS RELATED TO THE CARDIOVASCULAR SYSTEM

The main cardiovascular medications to consider before giving bodywork are *anti-coagulants*, also called *blood thinners*. Physicians prescribe anticoagulants when a person has a harmful blood clot or has the potential for one, because the anticoagulants interfere with the blood's clotting mechanisms. As a drug treatment, anticoagulants are often able to dissolve small blood clots before damage is done. As a prevention, smaller doses may prevent dangerous clots from forming. However, while a person is taking an anticoagulant drug, s/he may bleed or bruise easier than usual. Unless you know for certain that the person's clotting time is normal, methods such as compression, friction, skin rolling, and deep sustained pressure point work should be avoided. Common anticoagulant names are: warfarin, Coumadin, heparin, and Persantine. Aspirin also has significant anti-coagulant effects and can be taken by itself or as an ingredient in Alka-Seltzer, Bufferin, Ecotrin, etc. If you choose to ask about medications on your health history form, you might want to list anticoagulants specifically.

GENERAL CIRCULATORY SYSTEM CONDITIONS

The following are definitions and descriptions of general circulatory findings. Information on more specific circulatory disorders follows in the next section. As a general rule, refer clients with the following findings to a physician for assessment and diagnosis:

- pulse over 90 or under 60 beats per minute
- blood pressure over 140 systolic (top number) or over 90 diastolic (bottom number)
- pallor, cyanosis, erythema, or jaundice
- unexplained bruising, browning or mottling of the skin
- unexplained chest or calf pain
- swollen lymph nodes, with or without tenderness
- pitting edema
- bulging neck veins
- positive Homan's sign (see thrombophlebitis)
- if legs are visibly unequal in circumference
- if limbs are palpably unequal in temperature

SPECIFIC CIRCULATORY SYSTEM CONDITIONS

Anemia: This is a symptom of various diseases, rather than being a specific disease, and is a deficiency in the number of circulating red blood cells and/or hemoglobin in the blood that can occur as a result of blood loss from any of a variety of causes. If the onset of anemia is very slow, the body may adjust so that there are no signs or symptoms. Otherwise, the symptoms are pallor, weakness, fatigue, dizziness, headache, difficulty breathing (dyspnea), heart palpitations or racing, and digestive disturbances. Clients with these symptoms are advised to consult with a physician for assessment and diagnosis of the cause. The following are the most common types of anemia:

- blood cell destruction (*hemolytic anemia*). This can be caused by genetics or from exposure to poisons. Bodywork is systemically contraindicated without a physician's verification that the client can tolerate the work.
- decrease in red blood cell production (*pernicious anemia*). This can be fatal if not treated with vitamin B12, iron, and diet. Bodywork is generally beneficial to persons being treated, but clients are advised to monitor their progress with a physician.
- dietary deficiency of iron (*iron deficiency anemia*). This is the most common form of anemia and affects approximately 20% of people living in the U.S. and 50% of people in living in developing countries. Bodywork is beneficial.

• inhibition or failure of bone marrow to produce red blood cells (*aplastic anemia*). Bodywork is systemically contraindicated without a physician's verification that the client can tolerate the work.

• chronic or acute loss of blood that exceeds the body's ability to replace it (*hemorrhagic anemia*). Bodywork is beneficial after the cause has been identified and treated.

Aneurysm: This is a localized abnormal dilation of a blood vessel, usually an artery, due to a congenital defect or weakness of the vessel wall that can be caused by arteriosclerosis in the presence of hypertension, bacterial infection, or injury. The most common location is in the *abdominal aorta*, where symptoms are shortness of breath (dyspnea), cough, difficulty swallowing, and inequality of left and right radial pulses. Clients with these symptoms are immediately referred to a physician for assessment and diagnosis. Surgical removal and repair is the usual treatment. If an aneurysm is not treated, it will eventually rupture, causing sudden hemorrhage and death. Another type is the *cerebral aneurysm*. When this ruptures, it causes a stroke (CVA). An abrupt severe headache can be a warning symptom of a cerebral aneurysm. Bodywork is systemically contraindicated for persons with a known aneurysm, unless a physician verifies in writing that the person can tolerate the increase in circulation and pressure. However, bodywork is locally contraindicated for any abdominal aneurysm.

Angina pectoris: This is chest discomfort caused by a temporary insufficiency of blood supply to the heart muscle. It is often triggered by exertion and relieved by rest. Symptoms are mild to severe pain and/or mild to moderate pressure in the chest, often radiating to the left shoulder and down the left arm, jaw or back, and rarely radiating to the abdomen or right arm. The pain is often accompanied by anxiety and pallor. The episode can be brief or last for several minutes. It is important to stay with the client since angina is sometimes a precursor to heart attack (see heart attack). If the person has nitroglycerin tablets with him/her, one should be placed under the tongue as soon as possible. If the pain is not gone in five minutes, the client should take another nitro tablet. If pain persists another five minutes, give another nitro and call 911. Also, if the person at any time turns gray (ashen), becomes nauseous, or begins perspiring, call 911 immediately, even if only one nitro has been taken. Bodywork is systemically contraindicated during an episode of angina but can resume if the symptoms were relieved without complication.

Arrhythmia, dysrhythmia or fibrillation: These terms mean general irregularity or loss of rhythm of the heartbeat. In some cases, it is also used to indicate a heartbeat that is abnormally fast or slow. Arrhythmia is a symptom, not a disease, and can be caused by the heart spasming or quivering, instead of beating forcefully. This can provoke symptoms ranging from mild tiredness or dizziness, in the case of atrial arrhythmia, to loss of consciousness and death in ventricle arrhythmia. Bodywork is beneficial for persons with atrial arrhythmia, and clients are advised to consult a physician for assessment and diagnosis of the underlying problem if they have not yet done that.

Arteriosclerosis: This is a thickening, hardening, and loss of elasticity in walls of the arteries, and results in reduced blood flow to whatever body part the artery serves. The etiology is unknown, but risk factors are: age (men over 35 and women after menopause), stress, genetics, hypertension, smoking, high blood lipids (e.g., cholesterol over 200 mg.), obesity, diabetes, physical inactivity, and being male. Symptoms are intermittent chest pain (angina), intermittent claudication, changes in skin temperature, headache, and dizziness. Bodywork is beneficial to facilitate relaxation, general circulation, and body awareness, but clients with these symptoms who have not consulted a physician are urged to do so.

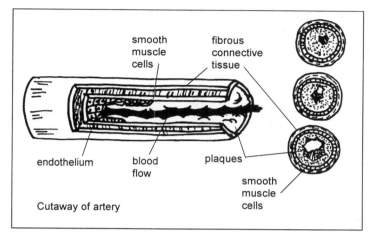

Illustration 49   Atherosclerosis

Atherosclerosis: This is a form of arteriosclerosis (see above), characterized by fibrous tissue, lipids and calcium deposits, which cause the walls of the arteries to fill with plaques (see illustration). The etiology is unknown, and the risk factors and symptoms are the same as for arteriosclerosis. Bodywork is beneficial to facilitate relaxation, general circulation, and body awareness, but clients are urged to consult a physician for assessment and diagnosis.

Cardiomyopathy: This is a disease of the heart muscle (myocardium), and can be caused by a variety of factors, including: alcoholism, congestive heart failure, parasites (worms) in the heart, and inflammation of the sack around the heart (pericarditis). Bodywork is beneficial with a physician's verification that the client can tolerate it.

Congestive heart failure (CHF): This is a condition where the heart does not maintain an adequate circulation of the blood (pump failure), and may result from either right or left-sided failure, each of which has its own distinct set of problems. Causes can include: hypertension, infection, insufficiency of heart valves, congenital malformations, arteriosclerosis, atherosclerosis, and hyperthyroidism. Symptoms can include: difficulty breathing (dyspnea), cardiac asthma, slowing of systemic or liver circulation, edema, cyanosis, and enlargement of the heart (see *Illustration*). Bodywork is beneficial except for local contraindications for pitting edema. Some persons

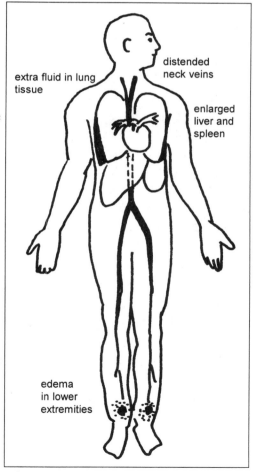

Illustration 50
Right-sided Congestive Heart Failure

with CHF have difficulty breathing when they lie flat. If so, body support would be needed.

Coronary bypass surgery: This surgery opens the entire chest, cutting through the sternum or ribs, and creates a new artery to go around, or bypass, an artery in the heart muscle that has become blocked by atherosclerosis. The new artery is made from a piece of vein that has been taken from elsewhere in the body, most often from the saphenous vein or the internal mammary artery. During recovery, bodywork is locally contraindicated for the vessel removal and chest incision sites until the tissues can tolerate the work. It is best for client, physician, and bodyworker to collaborate closely on this. Clients can expect to feel weak and easily fatigued for between six weeks and one year after their bypass surgery.

CVA Embolus (see Stroke): This is a mass of undissolved material traveling through a blood or lymph vessel. It can be solid, liquid, or gas, and may consist of a bit of tissue, a small glob of fat, an air bubble, a clump of bacteria, or a blood clot. If the embolus gets stuck in a blood vessel, the body will not get circulation through the blockage. An embolus, or embolism, is one of the causes of stroke (CVA) and heart attack (myocardial infarction, or MI) and can cause paralysis or death. Bodywork is systemically contraindicated (see *Thrombus*).

Heart attack (Myocardial infarction, MI): This is caused by blockage of one or more of the coronary arteries (the arteries that supply the heart muscle with nutrition and oxygen). The main symptom is sudden and intense pressure or squeezing pain in the center of the chest, behind the sternum. The pain may spread to the left shoulder, neck, arm and hand, the back, teeth, or jaw. Women often experience gastrointestinal distress, fatigue, and a vague heavy feeling in the arms, without severe chest pain. Typically, the person will be pale and perspiring, and s/he may have trouble breathing or be nauseated. A common reaction is denial that anything is wrong. However, if you observe these symptoms in anyone, it is imperative that you call 911 immediately. Do not try to transport the person to the hospital yourself. About half of the people with heart attack will experience cardiac arrest (complete heart stoppage) before reaching the hospital. If that occurs, CPR (cardio-pulmonary resuscitation) is needed immediately. After the acute and initial recovery phases are over, clients may benefit from bodywork but should consult with their physician to verify that they can tolerate it.

Heart murmur: This is a general term referring to any abnormal heart sounds. Murmurs are produced by the blood passing over a roughened valve (*rheumatic heart disease*); by flowing through a constricted opening (*mitral stenosis*); flowing through defect in the wall between the ventricles, or flowing backwards through a valve that does not close correctly (*mitral regurgitation*). Bodywork is beneficial for general relaxation and body awareness.

Hemophilia: This is a hereditary blood disorder characterized by prolonged bleeding time, but it may also cause joint swelling. Hemophilia occurs almost exclusively in males. There is no cure, however medication can be given to control bleeding episodes. Bodywork is systemically contraindicated unless a physician verifies that a client can tolerate the work.

Hypercholesterolemia (high cholesterol in the blood): This is a general term that usually refers to an abnormal increase in the low-density lipoproteins (LDL) while the high-density lipoproteins (HDL) are normal. There are many possible causes, and medical assessment and diagnosis of each individual case is important. In many cases, dietary changes that reduce or eliminate saturated fats will help lower LDL. Bodywork is beneficial for general relaxation, body awareness, and an increase in circulation.

Hypertension (high blood pressure): Also known as "the silent killer," this is defined as an increase in either the systolic (top number) or diastolic (bottom number) blood pressure above normal (140-100/90-60). The main factor in this disorder is an increase in peripheral resistance resulting from vasoconstriction of peripheral blood vessels, which causes a pressure increase in the whole circulatory system. However, the exact cause can usually be identified in only a small number of people. In those cases there are definite treatments that can cure the underlying problem. In most cases, hypertension is medically controllable, even if it is not curable. If left uncontrolled, hypertension can lead to arteriosclerosis, stroke, and death. Risk factors for hypertension include obesity, stress, lack of exercise, and genetics. Bodywork is beneficial for general relaxation and body awareness up to a blood pressure of 160/90. If either number in a client's B/P is higher than that, bodywork may be given with a contraindication against deep abdominal work, and advice to the client to consult a physician for assessment and treatment. If the B/P is over 190/100, bodywork is systemically contraindicated, and the client is referred to a physician.

Hypotension (low blood pressure): This is defined as either a decrease in the systolic (top number) or diastolic (bottom number) blood pressure below normal (140 to 100/90 to 60). It occurs in shock, hemorrhage, infection, fever, cancer, anemia, and various other diseases. People can have a consistently low blood pressure and adjust to it well. They can also have a type that occurs only when they suddenly stand from a lying position (ortho-static hypotension), causing them to feel light-headed. Bodywork is beneficial for general relaxation, body awareness, and an increase in circulation.

Intermittent claudication: This is a general term describing severe pain in the calf muscles that occurs during walking or exercise but subsides during rest. It results from inadequate blood supply to the legs and can be due to arterial spasm, atherosclerosis, arteriosclerosis, or blockage from a clot (thrombus).

Leukemia: There are many varieties of leukemia, but all involve excessive growth of leukocytes (white blood cells). Leukemia can be either chronic or acute, with a prognosis of 3 to 10 years in most cases, depending on the type and severity of disease. The etiology is unknown. General symptoms include fatigue, weight loss, anemia, and pallor. Bodywork is systemically contraindicated unless a physician verifies that the person can tolerate the work.

Lymphoma: This is a general term for malignant growth of new tissue in the lymphatic system. It is important to refer anyone with painless enlarged lymph nodes to a physician for assessment and diagnosis. There are many types of lymphoma. The two main types are:

- *Hodgkin's disease*: this is the most common form of lymphoma. The etiology is unknown. It involves painless enlargement of lymph nodes, beginning in the cervical region and progressing to the axillary, inguinal, mediastinal, and mesenteric regions. Also, signs of pressure and enlargement occur in the spleen and liver (see illustration). Other symptoms include skin rashes, itchiness, fever, chills, night sweats, loss of appetite, and weight loss. Bodywork is systemically contraindicated unless a physician verifies that the person can tolerate the work.

- *Non-Hodgkin's disease*: this is also called lymphocytic leukemia. This also involves painless enlargement of lymph nodes and many of the same symptoms as Hodgkin's. Non-Hodgkin's is more malignant and faster growing, often with a prognosis of only 4 to 6 months. Bodywork would be indicated only in terms of terminal caring.

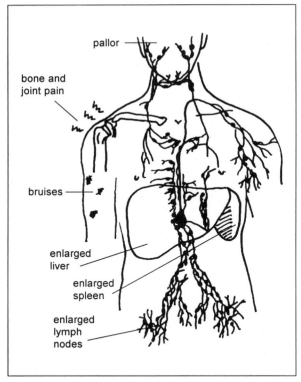

Illustration 51   Signs Associated with Lymphoma

Mononucleosis: this is an infectious disease that mainly affects the lymph nodes, liver, and spleen, often making them enlarged and tender. Additional symptoms include fever, fatigue, sore throat, and foul breath. It is associated with the Epstein-Barr virus. Incubation period may be as long as 4 to 7 weeks, in some cases. Treatment is rest and support of the immune system. Bodywork is beneficial except for local contraindications for the abdomen and all areas of enlarged lymph nodes.

Peripheral vascular disease: this is a general term referring to diseases of the arteries and veins of the extremities, especially those conditions that interfere with adequate blood flow to or from the extremities, such as atherosclerosis, diabetes, etc. There are two main types:

- *arterial insufficiency:* symptoms are sharp pain that increases with exercise (intermittent claudication), cool, pale skin with absent or diminished pulses in that area, and painless sores on the feet or toes.
- *venous insufficiency* symptoms are aching, cramping type of pain, edema, mottled or brown pigmented skin, and in some severe cases, an open, oozing ulcer near the ankle.

Venous insufficiency can be prevented or reduced by wearing support stockings, walking daily, changing leg position frequently, weight control, and elevating the legs at least 12 inches above the heart when lying down. Bodywork is beneficial to clients with either arterial or venous insufficiency except for local contraindications for pitting edema, open sores, ulcers, and persistent pain.

Phlebitis: This term means inflammation of a vein. Symptoms are pain and tenderness along a vein, erythema, swelling and acute edema distal to the vein, rapid pulse, mild temperature elevation, and pain in nearby joints. The etiology is unknown, but it often occurs during infections or following childbirth or surgery. Bodywork is locally and distally contraindicated.

Raynaud's disease or phenomenon: This is a peripheral vascular disorder that occurs most often in women ages 18 to 30. It is caused by abnormal vasoconstriction of the extremities when the person is under stress or is exposed to cold temperatures. A history of symptoms for at least two years is required for diagnosis. Pallor or cyanosis is intermittent, bilateral, and symmetrical, pulses are normal, and there is no evidence of circulatory obstruction. There may be burning, tingling, or numbness during the episode. Tissue turns erythematous before returning to normal. Clients with these symptoms are advised to consult with a physician for assessment and diagnosis of the underlying cause. Bodywork is beneficial for general relaxation and body awareness prior to local bodywork. In some cases, local massage is contraindicated. It is best to discuss your style and techniques with the client and physician prior to giving the session.

Rheumatic heart disease: This is a general term referring to symptoms of chest discomfort and heart murmur that is caused by a past episode of *rheumatic fever*, which is an episode of fever and joint pain with other various symptoms, that follows a strep infection (such as a strep throat, etc.). The etiology is unknown, but it occurs most often in children making the person susceptible to subsequent episodes. Prevention is to promptly treat strep infections. Bed rest is required for persons experiencing signs of active rheumatic fever, in order to prevent heart valve damage. During the acute phase, bodywork is systemically contraindicated unless a physician verifies that the client can tolerate the work. After recovery, bodywork is indicated without restriction.

Spider veins: These are areas of dilated superficial venules or capillaries that are small, thin, and dark red or purple. They are usually located on the leg and radiate out from a central point. They are not varicose veins, and gentle, attentive bodywork is indicated unless the area is complicated with pain or bulging varicosities.

"Stroke" (CVA; cerebrovascular accident): This is a sudden loss of consciousness followed by paralysis or death, and is caused by a hemorrhage, an embolus, or a thrombus in the brain (see illustration). In each case, some portion of the brain is suddenly without its necessary blood supply. In the case of hemorrhage, there is an additional problem of pressure on the brain from the bleeding. Symptoms include: unusual breathing, pupil inequality,

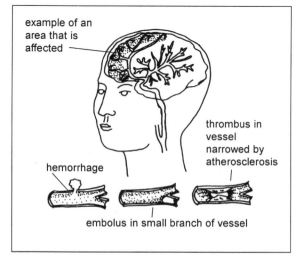

example of an area that is affected

thrombus in vessel narrowed by atherosclerosis

hemorrhage

embolus in small branch of vessel

Illustration 52 Three principal causes of CVA ("stroke")

one-sided paralysis involving the face, arm and/or leg, a clammy sweat, and slurred speech. If you witness these symptoms, keep the client warm and either in a prone or side-lying position and call 911 immediately, followed by calling a friend or family member, if possible. After the acute phase is over, the person usually has some measure of deficit in speech, vision, and/ or motor function, and will benefit from physical therapy and bodywork that focuses on strengthening and re-patterning the neuromuscular pathways. Often the person will feel a lot of grief and will need consistent emotional support. Deficits that are still present six months after the stroke are likely to remain permanently (see also *TIA*, or mini-stroke).

Thrombocytopenia: This is an abnormal decrease in the number of blood platelets, which are the cells that clot the blood. Symptoms are bruising easily, small reddish or purplish spots on the skin or mucous membranes (*petechiae*), and abnormally long bleeding time when cut. This acute condition requires careful monitoring. Bodywork is systemically contraindicated unless a physician verifies that the client can tolerate the work.

Thrombophlebitis: This is the inflammation of a vein (phlebitis) with the added presence of a *thrombus*, which is a blood clot. A blood clot is a normal and functional thing when it prevents a person from bleeding, but it is abnormal and can be life-threatening when it occurs in a blood vessel, because it will slow or even stop the circulation to the nearby body part. If the thrombus breaks loose, it becomes an embolus and can travel through the vessel until it becomes lodged in a smaller diameter vessel, blocking the circulation there. The main causes of either thrombus or thrombophlebitis are: injuries, surgery, childbirth, cardiovascular disorders, obesity, heredity, age, and systemic infection (sepsis), however, they can occur anytime a person has been very sedentary and/or had an injury, especially in the legs. Symptoms include: inequality in the color, temperature, or circumference of two matching limbs (see illustration), pain in the limb, and a positive Homan's sign. To assess Homan's sign, ask the client to extend the leg and dorsiflex the foot (point the toes back toward the face). If the client has calf pain on dorsiflexion, the sign is positive. Bodywork is locally contraindicated to the entire affected limb if any of these symptoms are present. Urge the client to seek immediate assessment from a physician.

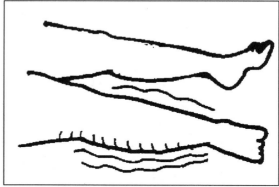

Illustration 53   Signs of Thrombophlebitis: Inequality in Color, Temperature and Circumference Between the Two Legs

TIA ("mini-stroke"): TIA is an acronym for transient ischemic attacks, which are temporary interferences to the brain's blood supply. The symptoms are sudden and brief weakness or numbness in an arm, leg, or face on one side of the body. Symptoms can be slight, usually lasting only five to 30 minutes, and leaving no permanent effects. After the episode, no brain damage is evident. One or more TIAs can signal an impending "stroke" (CVA). Bodywork is contraindicated only during the acute episode.

Varicose veins: This is enlarged, swollen, or twisted (varicose) veins that can occur in almost any part of the body, but are most often observed in the feet and legs (see illustration). Two other common locations are internal: the esophagus and the rectum (hemorrhoids). Varicose veins result from severe back pressure against the normal venous flow, such as occurs in

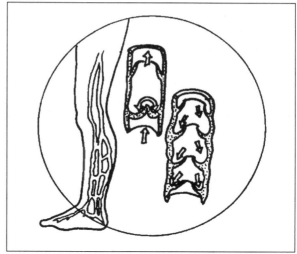

- an obese or pregnant abdomen that restricts blood flow up the Vena Cava;
- occupations that require extended periods of standing;
- straining at passing hard stool (in the rectum), or
- by increased portal vein pressure (near the liver) that affects the veins in the esophagus.

Illustration 54 Varicose Veins Caused by Increased Back Pressure Against Valves Inside the Veins

Elastic hose, elevating the feet, and surgery are treatments. Bodywork is locally contraindicated for all varicosities.

COMMON EFFECTS OF AGING ON THE CIRCULATORY SYSTEM

Cardiac (heart) output generally decreases by 50% from age 25 to age 75, causing decreased blood flow to the vital organs (brain, heart, kidneys, liver, etc.). Arteries lose their elasticity, which increases peripheral vessel resistance, causing the extremities to get less blood supply and the blood pressure to increase. Heart valves thicken and become more rigid, causing murmurs and less efficient movement of blood through the heart. The heart muscle (myocardium) loses elasticity, causing it to adapt more slowly to stress and change. Resting and average heart rate remains the same as during younger years, but reaches a lower maximum rate during exercise. Endurance decreases.

CASE PRESENTATIONS

1/31/96: Surgery-childhood; tired-overworked; heart problems; Dec. '95 heart racing (atrial fibrillation); no continued problem since then; said is released from MD.

2/3/96: Phone call to check client's response to massage. Client has bruising on left arm. Said she bruises easily, and I used too much pressure on last visit. Said massage got rid of a headache that was starting that day. Says she takes prescription meds for her heart. I check health history, no note of headache, meds, or bruising easily.

2/16/96: Client requests another massage. Says thinks she's pregnant. I inform her I need consent from her MD, and I will not work on her again without it. She doesn't want to do that and doesn't want to see another massage therapist. I reaffirm my position.

1/13/96: 38 yo woman, bookkeeper. Goal: help control B/P

History: hypertension since '81, from "stress & diet"; not under MD care now; he recommended using exercise & diet to control B/P, which she does; checks & records B/P every other month. Most recent reading 2/95: 126/88. Also says R arm & hand go numb occasionally.

Referral: Dr. S. Zore D.C. for R limb numbness

Treatment: Swedish & breathing techniques for relaxation & movement of fluids. Suggested she add relaxation techniques to home care routine.

Outcome Summary: Over six months of seeing this client monthly, there's a marked difference in her ability to relax. At first she was rigid and resisted everything. Now she breathes deeply and lets her limbs be heavy and limp. B/P is now 121/78.

STUDY QUESTIONS

What questions would you have asked that were not asked?

What bodywork techniques would you have done?

What referral(s)?

What other ways could the therapeutic outcome have been evaluated?

How might you have changed the format or way the cases were written?

What were the indications for massage/bodywork?

What were the contraindications?

REFERENCES

Fritz, S. (1995). Mosby's fundamentals of therapeutic massage. St. Louis: Mosby Lifeline.

Jarvis, C. (1992). Physical examination and health assessment. Philadelphia: W. B. Saunders Co.

Juhan, D. (1987). Job's body: A handbook for bodywork. Barrytown, NY: Station Hill Press.

Kapit, W. & Elson, L.M. (1977). The anatomy coloring book. NY: Harper & Row.

Kapit, W., Macey, R.I., & Meisami, E. (1987). The physiology coloring book. NY: Harper & Row.

Lowe, Whitney W. (1995). Functional assessment in massage therapy. Corvallis, OR: Pacific Orthopedic Massage.

Malasanos, L., Barkauskas, V., & Stoltenberg-Allen, K. (1990). Health assessment. St. Louis, MO: C.V. Mosby Co.

Mulvihill, M.L. (1995). Human diseases: A systemic approach (4th ed.) Norwalk, CT: Appleton & Lange.

Newton, D. (1995). Pathology for massage therapists. Portland, OR: Simran Publications.

Romero, R. R. (1995). Massage and damage to the lymphatics. Nurse's Touch, 1(1), 11.

Sameulson, P. (1994). Pathophysiology for massage: The travel guide. Overland Park, KS: Mid-America Handbooks, Inc.

Thomas, C.L. (1989). Taber's cyclopedic medical dictionary (16th ed.). Philadelphia: F.A. Davis Co.

Zerinsky, S. S. (1987). Introduction to Pathology for the Massage Practitioner. (S. Weinstein & J. E. Thompson, eds.) The Swedish Institute.

CHAPTER REVIEW

1. The circulatory system consists of the _____

2. The heart muscle is called the_____

3. The four chambers in the heart are the left and right _____ and the left
   and right _____.

4. The main force of the heartbeat comes from the contraction of the _____

5. A healthy adult heart rate averages between _____ and _____ beats/minute.

6. Blood in the arteries is bright red because it_____
   Blood in the veins is purplish or blue because it _____

7. With one exception, _____ carry oxygenated blood away from the heart.

8. With one exception, _____ carry deoxygenated blood to the heart.

9. The exchange of nutrients and wastes that pass between the body and the blood occurs in
   the _____.

10. _____ differ from arteries in that they are larger in diameter, greater in number,
    have thinner walls, lower pressure, and periodically have valves inside to prevent back-
    flow of blood.

11. A healthy adult blood pressure averages between _____ and _____ on the top
    number and between _____ and _____ on the bottom.

12. Lymph from the majority of the body empties into the thoracic duct, which then empties
    into the _____

13. The main lymph node groups are located in the _____

14. The lymph nodes, _____, _____ and are all made prima-
    rily of lymphatic tissue.

15. Lymphocytes travel to the body's cells via the _____ and return from the body's
    cells via the _____.

16. The five main areas to consider in assessing the circulatory system are: _____
    _____
    _____

17. Pallor is most often caused by _____ , or a _____

18. Cyanosis is due to the presence of deoxygenated blood and excess carbon dioxide, and is a progression of _____

19. The most severe type of edema is called _____ edema.

20. As a general rule, refer clients with the following findings to a physician for assessment and diagnosis: _____

_____

21. _____ is a deficiency in the number of circulating red blood cells and/or hemoglobin in the blood.

22. _____ is a localized abnormal dilation of a blood vessel, usually an artery, due to a congenital defect or weakness of the vessel wall.

23. _____ is caused by a temporary insufficiency of blood supply to the heart muscle.

24. _____ means general irregularity or loss of rhythm of the heartbeat.

25. _____ is a thickening, hardening, and loss of elasticity in walls of the arteries, and results in reduced blood flow to whatever body part the artery serves.

26. _____ is a form of arteriosclerosis with fibrous tissue, lipids, and calcium deposits, which cause the walls of the arteries to fill with plaques.

27. _____ is a condition where the heart does not maintain an adequate circulation of the blood.

28. _____ is a mass of undissolved material traveling through a blood or lymph vessel.

29. The symptoms of _____ are sudden and intense pressure or squeezing pain in the center of the chest, behind the sternum, often radiating to the left shoulder, neck, arm and hand, the back, teeth or jaw.

30. Risk factors for hypertension include: _____

_____

31. Symptoms of _____ are: sharp pain that increases with exercise, cool, pale skin with absent or diminished pulses in that area, and painless sores on the feet or toes.

32. Symptoms of _____ are: aching, cramping pain, edema, mottled or brown pigmented skin, and in some severe cases, an open, oozing ulcer near the ankle.

33. _____ is caused by a hemorrhage, an embolus, or a thrombus in the brain that blocks and artery.

34. Symptoms of either a _____ or _____ include: inequality in the color, temperature, or circumference of two matching limbs (arms or legs), pain in the limbs, and a positive Homan's sign.

35. _____ result from severe back pressure against the normal venous flow.

ANSWERS TO CHAPTER REVIEW

1. heart, blood, blood vessels, lymph, lymph nodes & vessels

2. myocardium

3. atriums; ventricles

4. ventricles

5. 60 to 80

6. contains a lot of oxygen; has little oxygen and a lot of carbon dioxide

7. arteries

8. veins

9. capillaries

10. veins

11. 140 and 100; 90 and 60

12. left subclavian vein

13. neck, armpit, and groin

14. spleen, tonsils, and thymus

15. blood vessels (arteries or capillaries); lymph vessels

16. 1) skin color and temperature, 2) nailbed color and shape, 3) presence of pain or unusual veins, 4) edema, and 5) swollen lymph nodes, with or without tenderness

17. vasoconstriction; lack of oxygen in the blood

18. pallor

19. pitting

20. pulse over 90 or under 60 beats per minute
    blood pressure over 140 systolic (top number) or over 90 diastolic (bottom number)
    pallor, cyanosis, erythema, or jaundice
    unexplained bruising, browning, or mottling of the skin
    unexplained chest or calf pain
    swollen lymph nodes, with or without tenderness
    pitting edema
    bulging neck veins
    positive Homan's sign (see thrombophlebitis)
    if legs are visibly unequal in circumference
    if limbs are palpably unequal in temperature

21. anemia

22. aneurysm

23. angina

24. arrhythmia

25. arteriosclerosis

26. atherosclerosis

27. CHF/congestive heart failure

28. embolus

29. myocardial infarction, MI, or heart attack

30. obesity, stress, lack of exercise, and genetics

31. arterial insufficiency

32. venous insufficiency

33. CVA or cerebrovascular accident

34. thrombus or thrombophlebitis

35. varicose veins

CHAPTER 7

IMMUNE SYSTEM: IMMUNITY, ALLERGIES AND COMMUNICABLE DISEASES

ANATOMY AND PHYSIOLOGY REVIEW

The immune system does much more than help us recover from a cold or flu. It is an awesome network involving neuro-transmitter and neuro-endocrine chemicals, white blood cells (WBCs, leukocytes), lymph nodes, thymus, liver, spleen, intestinal tissue, and bone marrow, and it locates and tries to eliminate anything that is not identified as being "You." In health care, the term *immune* means having or producing antibodies. *Antibodies* are specific immune system proteins that are capable of responding to, and mediating, specific antigens. *Antigens* are protein or polysaccharide substances that stimulate the body to produce antibodies. This antigen-antibody reaction forms the basis for immunity.

Neuro-transmitter chemicals are substances that are released when the axon terminal of a neuron is excited. The substance then travels across the synapse to act on the target cell to either inhibit or excite it. Neuro-transmitters are part of the autonomic nervous system, but they interact with the immune system by stimulating the bone marrow, thymus, lymph nodes, skin, and spleen. Neuro-transmitters include: acetylcholine, norepinephrine, enkephalins, dopamine, and substance P.

Neuro-endocrine chemicals include ACTH, vasopressin, oxytocin, and adrenal cortical hormones. These substances are part of the endocrine system, but they interact with the immune system by stimulating the receptors of the immune cells (see chapter 9).

Leukocytes are white blood cells (WBCs). Although there are several types of leukocytes, they all help defend the body against microbial infections. Anatomically, leukocytes are divided into two types: 1) granulocytes (which have specific granules in their cytoplasm, i.e., neutrophils, basophils and eosinophils) and 2) agranulocytes (which do not have granules, i.e., macrophages, lymphocytes, and monocytes). Granulocytes are formed in the bone marrow; and lymphocytes are formed in both the bone marrow and the lymph nodes; monocytes are formed in the cells lining the capillaries of the spleen.

Granulocytes are more numerous than agranulocytes. Functionally, the granulocytes, monocytes, and macrophages have the power of phagocytosis, that is, they can ingest bacteria, protozoans, cell debris, dust particles, and colloids. The lymphocytes are not phagocytic (see the immune response, below). In general, a greatly increased number of leukocytes in the blood is indicative of bacterial infection somewhere in the body.

IMMUNITY AND THE IMMUNE RESPONSE

The term *immunity* means being *immune* (or protected) to a disease such as occurs after a person is exposed to a *pathogen,* or is immunized, or is vaccinated. Pathogens are organisms capable of causing communicable disease. There are four types of pathogens: bacteria, viruses, fungi, and parasites (see page 146). There are two main types of immunity:

- *active immunity* results from the body's development of antibodies in response to a pathogen that the person either was exposed to naturally (e.g., chicken pox or mumps) or was injected with as a vaccine (e.g., smallpox, polio, DPT). Active immunity takes time to develop because it takes time for the body to make the antibodies to the pathogen.
- *passive immunity* results from antibodies that have been transferred directly into a person, either by being passed from a mother to a fetus through the placenta, or by being injected into a person as an immunization (e.g., hepatitis, rabies, tetanus). In either case, passive immunity is effective immediately.

The *immune response* is defined as the body's reaction to substances that are foreign or are interpreted as being foreign. There are three principal categories of immune response: 1) natural immunity, 2) acquired immunity, and 3) auto-immunity.

1) Natural (or non-specific) immunity involves the inflammation response and phagocytosis, but not antibody production. In general, the process is: a pathogen invades the body, and the local cells release histamine that promotes vasodilation and vascular permeability. Plasma proteins and fluids flow in, causing local edema. Fibrin formation clots this fluid, trapping the bacteria, protozoa, or whatever foreign particles are present. The stationary macrophages in the local tissues begin to phagocytize the pathogen. (This step is called the first line of defense.) Next, neutrophils migrate to the injured area, squeeze through the spaces between the capillary cell walls, and begin massive phagocytosis (the second line of defense). If these two steps do not adequately neutralize the infection, the monocytes migrate to the site, transform themselves into macrophages, and help the neutrophils eliminate the bacteria (this is the third line of defense). If bacteria are present, a pus sac containing dead cells and debris develops and is either extruded or gradually cleared away during tissue repair by the macrophages. Generally, this whole process takes between 24 and 72 hours. If the natural (non-specific) immunity responses are not sufficient to eliminate the infection, toxins invade the blood system and activate more defense responses, such as fever and activation of the lymphocytes and antibodies, which is the second category of immune response, *acquired immunity.*

2) Acquired immunity is a slower and more complicated process than natural immunity. It takes two different forms: antibody-mediated (or humoral-mediated) immunity, and cell-mediated immunity.

- The <u>antibody-mediated (humoral) immune response</u> begins when special receptor sites on the surface of the B lymphocytes (also called B cells) sense the presence of a pathogen, most commonly bacteria. *B Cells* are made in the bone marrow and normally circulate in the blood, lymph, and connective tissues (see illustration). Antigens are protein or polysaccharide substances on the surface of pathogens. Each type of B cell contains only one specific kind of receptor and can respond only to that specific type of antigen. When stimulated (or sensitized), the B cells transform into plasma cells, which divide and make clones identical to the original cell. The clones produce antibodies that circulate in the lymph and blood, attaching to the antigens and deactivating them. In some cases, the antibodies promote additional inflammatory responses, which brings in more granulocytes, causing more phagocytosis. Also during sensitization, some plasma cells transform to memory cells, which lie dormant in the lymph nodes until the person has a second exposure to the antigen. At that time, the memory cells produce antibodies intensively, rapidly deactivating the antigens. The memory cell response is the basis of immunization and vaccination practices. The antibody-mediated response can produce immunity or hypersensitivity (also called allergy).

• In cell-mediated immune response, the T lymphocytes (T cells) directly attack and destroy foreign cells. *T cells* are lymphocytes, made in the bone marrow, that migrate to the thymus, where they develop into lymphoid cells and begin to mature. The *thymus* is a small organ located in the mediastinal cavity anterior to and above the heart. From the thymus the T cells go to the peripheral lymphoid tissues, and from there they circulate between blood and lymph. T cells sometimes live for up to 5 years in the body. They defend against cancer cells, viral and fungal pathogens, some slow-acting bacteria (such as tuberculosis), and tissue or organ transplants. In general, their process is: The antigens on the surface of the pathogens sensitize the T cells, which multiply and form three sub-populations of T cells:

> • cytotoxic or killer T cells, which contain antibody-like molecules, enabling them to attach to antigens, swell, and inject the pathogen with a toxin that causes it to die and/or causes transplant rejection;
> • helper T cells enhance antibody production by the B cells and may also produce lymphokines, which are strong antibody-like substances, and
> • suppressor T cells, which suppress the actions of the helper cells to homeostatically regulate the immune responses.

3) In the case of *auto-immunity*, the body produces antibodies against its own tissues, as if they were foreign substances, to such an extent that tissue injury is caused. Auto-immune diseases may affect whole organs or parts of them. At this time, it is not clear why the body mistakes part of itself for a foreign substance. Some researchers believe that exposure to viruses, bacteria, parasites, x-rays and/or certain drugs sometimes causes a profusion of antigens that sometimes are very similar, or even identical, to antigens on the surface of some cells of the body. When this happens, the body's antibodies attack those cells. Auto-immune diseases are one of the great challenges facing mainstream and alternative medical research. Examples of auto-immune diseases include: rheumatoid arthritis (Chapter 4), lupus erythematosus (Chapter 3), multiple sclerosis (Chapter 4), myasthenia gravis (Chapter 4), and scleroderma (Chapter 3).

ALLERGIES

The term *"allergy"* means a hypersensitivity to a substance that normally does not cause any reaction. An allergy is essentially a disorder of the immune system that results in an antibody-antigen reaction, but in some cases the antibody can not be found. Most hypersensitivity (allergic) reactions are immediate, with the response occurring in a few seconds or minutes.

The etiology of allergies is not completely understood. Some people may have a genetic predisposition to certain allergies. Another factor is that repeated exposures to an allergen can eventually cause the body to produce enough antibodies to cause an allergic response. Symptoms most often involve the respiratory tract, digestive tract or the skin. Some common allergic conditions include: allergic rhinitis, hay fever and bronchial asthma (Chapter 8), eczema and hives (Chapter 3), and food allergies (see next page).

The substance that causes an allergic reaction is called an *allergen*. Allergens are a type of antigen. Pollen, dust, hair, fur, feathers, wool, chemicals, drugs, insect bites and stings, eggs, chocolate, milk, wheat, and citrus fruits are common allergens. Common allergy symptoms are: rash, swelling, sneezing, wheezing, itching, abdominal cramps, vomiting, headache, ringing in the ears, a rapid pulse, and fainting. Coughing, congestion, and other respiratory problems are commonly associated with exposure to airborne allergens. In addition, when the respiratory system is being challenged by airborne allergens, the body/mind is more vulnerable to respiratory infections, such as strep throat, bronchitis, or pneumonia, and to spasm and mucosal edema, which can lead to asthma or respiratory distress.

In general, a substance is an allergen if you feel better by avoiding it, it makes you ill when you re-expose yourself to it, and no other cause can be shown. Specific allergens, and the degree to which you react to them, can be identified by allergy specialists.

When some body tissue comes into contact with an allergen (also called an antigen), the cells respond by producing antibodies (also called abnormal immunoglobulins, or abnormal IgE) against the allergen. These antibodies attach themselves to the mast cells, stimulating the mast cells to release *histamine* and other chemicals (see *Illustration* 56). When histamine is released locally, the capillaries dilate and release plasma, causing an immediate red

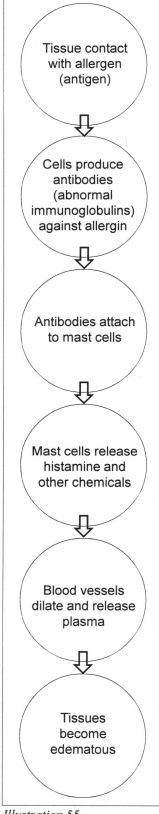

Illustration 55
Allergic Chain of Events

flush in the area, followed by localized edema. When histamine is released systemically, blood pressure drops temporarily, skin is flushed, smooth bronchial muscles constrict, and gastric (stomach) secretions increase. Some of the other chemicals that are released can cause the local mucous membranes to produce excessive mucus.

Foods may cause adverse reactions through a variety of mechanisms, including "classic" allergic reactions, non-allergic mediated reactions, and a wide range of mind/body responses not yet well understood. Immunological reactions to foods are commonly divided into two groups: allergic mediated and non-allergic mediated. With the allergic mediated reactions, symptoms usually appear within a few minutes to a few hours after eating the food, and may manifest as hives, swelling or fluid retention, rash, asthma, lowered blood pressure, diarrhea, vomiting, abdominal pain, "irritable bowel" or other anaphylactic symptoms. Clinical studies have shown the most common food allergens to be: cow's milk, wheat, corn, nuts, eggs, chocolate, strawberries, soy products, and yeasts. Less prevalent, but still common are shellfish, fungi, tropical fruits, tomatoes and food colorings.

Non-allergic mediated reactions, often called food intolerance, are reactions that are mediated by other immunological mechanisms and can occur from several hours to a few days after the food has been eaten. This delay makes it much more difficult to establish a clear association between the symptoms and the food eaten. It also lends support to the theory that the body may be reacting to a by-product produced by faulty digestion, rather than to the food, itself. Symptoms are primarily gastrointestinal irritation or inflammation and its associated malabsorption syndromes, which cause micronutrient deficiency and can lead to a host of other tissue and organ system dysfunctions.

When an allergic reaction is extremely severe, it is called *anaphylaxis*, or *anaphylactic shock*. Anaphylaxis can cause any of these signs: dyspnea, hoarseness, dizziness, rash, and large amounts of mucus, loss of consciousness, and, if severe enough, death. If a client suddenly develops one or more of these signs, call 911.

COMMUNICABLE DISEASE

A *communicable disease* is a contagious disease. This means that it is caused by *pathogens* that are easily spread from person to person. Pathogens are organisms capable of causing communicable diseases. Maintaining a healthy immune system and clean, intact skin are the primary ways to prevent pathogens from entering the body. There are four types of pathogens: bacteria, viruses, fungi, and parasites.

- *Bacteria* are primitive cells without nuclei that 1) secrete toxins that damage body tissues, 2) become parasites inside cells, or 3) form colonies that disrupt normal body function. Bacteria thrive in warm, dark, moist places and in areas where the skin or mucous membrane is *open*, including rashes, cuts, scrapes, hangnails, etc. Bacteria can usually be killed by antibiotics, disinfectants, sunlight, and dryness.

- *Viruses* are protein capsules made of DNA or RNA. They invade healthy cells and replicate there. Viruses can lie dormant for years until conditions support their activation. Viruses are unaffected by antibiotics. They enter the body through the respiratory system, through open skin, and through breaks in the mucous membranes. *Mucous membranes* are the thin, fragile tissues that line most of the body's openings and passages. Mucous membranes protect the body by secreting mucus, which keeps the tissues moist and elastic and contains antibacterial, antiviral, antifungal chemicals.
- *Fungi* are plant-like organisms without chlorophyll. Most live on the skin or mucous membranes. Like bacteria, fungi thrive in warm, dark, moist areas.
- *Parasites* include one-celled or multi-celled organisms that feed off another animal's tissue. Most are worms, tiny insects, or amoebas.
- *Contamination* is the process by which an object or an area becomes inhabited by pathogens. In order to affect a person's health, the pathogens must have some physical contact with the person. There are three main ways, or routes, through which this can happen:

  - *oral route*: ingesting contaminated foods or fluids
  - *airborne route*: breathing pathogens into the lungs
  - *direct contact route*: touching or being touched by contaminated fluids or objects

In most cases, *blood and body fluids* are the most likely vehicles for transmission of serious communicable diseases. The term "blood and body fluids" is generally defined as including blood, semen, vaginal fluid, urine, feces, vomit, nasal and lung mucous, saliva, breast milk, and wound drainage. (Tears and perspiration are usually not considered carriers of significant pathogens, but if they contact another person's circulatory system, e.g., through an open skin area, it is possible that they can transmit disease.)

When pathogens are present and replicating in or on the body, we call the condition an *infection*. The presence of any local inflammation increases the chances of a person developing a local infection in that same area. Infections usually have the same symptoms as inflammations, plus, when bacteria is involved, may have white, yellow, or green pus. A local infection can spread and become systemic if it overwhelms the body's defenses. The most common symptoms of systemic infection are fever, chills, fatigue, and pain, although people whose immune systems are deficient may not show these symptoms until their infection is severe.

For your convenience, the names, symptoms, and routes of transmission for many common communicable diseases are listed in the table on page 152. It is important to note that pathogens travel both ways so both the client or the bodyworker can transmit pathogens to each other unless appropriate precautions are maintained.

In order to prevent the spread of communicable diseases, the U.S. Center for Disease Control (CDC) has issued a set of standards, called *Universal Precautions*, that outlines requirements that all health care personnel must follow. The following is a summary of those standards with applications for bodyworkers:

- Avoid all contact with clients' blood, body fluids, or any area of local infection. Wear gloves if contact is needed.
- Wash hands before and after client contact (See *Hand Washing*).
- Do not eat, drink, smoke, handle contact lenses, or apply makeup without washing hands first.
- Clean and disinfect all client contact surfaces on a regular basis (See *Disinfection*).
- Immediately clean and disinfect equipment that has been in contact with blood or body fluids. Clean blood off of equipment with a solution of 1 part bleach to 9 parts water. Mix the bleach/water solution and use the same day, as it loses its effectiveness if stored. To clean blood off linens, add 1/4 cup bleach to wash cycle, wash on hot (minimum 160 degrees) for 25 minutes, and dry on high. Any other body fluids can be cleaned off equipment with germicidal sprays or alcohol; linens can be simply washed with detergent on hot and dried on high.
- Linens and towels must be changed between each client, must be stored in a separate, closed container until washed.
- Disposable articles contaminated by blood or body fluids must be placed in leak-proof containers, labeled as a bio-hazard.
- If you have any open skin area on your hands, it must be completely covered before you give bodywork. Gloves or finger cots can be used.
- If using lotion or oil bottles without pumps, the bottle should be washed after each session.

The single most effective way to prevent infection is *hand washing*. Bodyworkers are required to wash their hands with hot water, friction, and anti-bacterial soap before and after eating, before and after each massage, and after nose-blowing, coughing, and using the toilet. Thorough hand washing includes vigorous scrubbing for 10-30 seconds, including the areas between the fingers, the thumbs, under the nails, the wrists, and the forearms if exposed. Use a fingernail brush or orange stick to clean under the nails. Dry with a clean towel. Disposable towels are preferred because then pathogens are not passed to the next person who dries his/her hands. Use the towel to turn off the faucet and open the doorknob, before throwing it away (see *Illustration 56*).

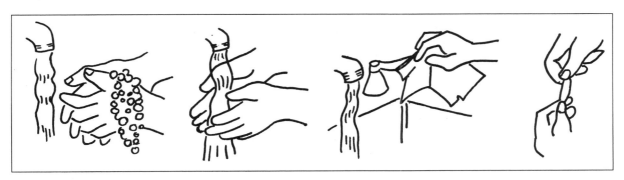

1. Lather with germicidal soap, hot water, and friction.

2. Rinse

3. Turn off faucet using towel to contact knob.

4. Clean under nails.

| *Illustration 56* | Hand Washing Procedure |

Always wear *gloves* when contact with blood or body fluids is likely. The use of gloves is an additional infection precaution, but never replaces the need for thorough hand washing. Either vinyl or latex gloves can be used, however, the latex is made more permeable when exposed to oil based products. Use only water-based products when using latex gloves. Sterile gloves can be worn when there is concern for protecting the client from infection. Some people with severe illnesses can feel very vulnerable. Wear gloves whenever so requested by your client. You might also feel vulnerable to infection when working with some clients. In those instances, explain to the client that you are most comfortable working with them while wearing gloves, and get agreement with them that it is all right before proceeding.

Always cover your mouth when you cough and wash your hands after each coughing episode. Ask your clients to cover their mouths and offer them tissues to cough into. Avoid touching the client's used tissues by presenting a receptacle for them. If you are working with a person who is under evaluation for TB, wear a mask until the MD verifies that the infective period is over (usually about two weeks after treatment has begun).

Disinfection is the chemical destruction and/or removal of pathogens. Most disinfectants are used on equipment or surfaces rather than in or on the body. Bodyworkers are required to disinfect all equipment, including linens, tables, etc., that come in contact with clients. Some of the most common disinfectants are alcohol, iodine, and chlorine (bleach). Disinfection does not usually destroy 100% of the pathogens present, but it does reduce their number so significantly as to render the object or area safe to use.

The only process that destroys 100% of the pathogens present is *sterilization*, which can only be accomplished through subjecting an object to high temperature dry or steam heat, or to toxic gas. Bodyworkers are not required to sterilize equipment unless it will be used to pierce or invade the body, such as the needles used in acupuncture.

ASSESSMENT: OBSERVATION AND PALPATION

As you might be gathering by now, there are a large number and variety of signs and symptoms associated with allergies and other immune system disorders. As always, listen closely to the client's description of their health experience and read the intake form with your knowledge of the immune system in mind. Be sure to ask questions to clarify or add to the information the client gives.

Observe for skin color and condition, hives and rashes, fever, fatigue, irritability, mood swings, insomnia, headaches, variable joint and muscle aches or pains, fluid retention, bladder irritation and recurrent infections, chronic sinusitis, cough, and asthma. Palpate gently if assessing for swollen lymph nodes.

GENERAL CONDITIONS RELATED TO THE IMMUNE SYSTEM

The following are definitions and descriptions of general immune system findings. Information on more specific immune disorders follows in the next section. As a general rule, refer clients with the following findings to a physician for assessment and diagnosis:

- history of chronic fatigue
- history of recurrent skin, digestive or respiratory ailments
- history of food intolerance
- failure to gain weight
- unexplained weight loss
- rashes, hives, or itching of unknown origin
- enlarged lymph nodes, with or without tenderness
- excessive or persistent skin dryness or scaliness

SPECIFIC COMMUNICABLE DISEASES

BODYWORK IS LOCALLY CONTRAINDICATED TO ANY AREAS OF LOCAL RASH, SKIN INFLAMMATION, LESION, OR OPEN AREA. Systemically, promoting a deep clearing (physically or energetically) in a person whose body/mind is challenged by infection can temporarily overload the body with toxins, which can increase or intensify symptoms such as high fever, vomiting, diarrhea, dizziness, confusion, or uncontrollable emotional release. An increase in symptoms can be scary, can further deplete the client's energy, or can require medication to reduce the symptoms. Gentle approaches best serve to support and nurture the person's health during infection. Therefore, BODYWORK IS SYSTEMICALLY CONTRAINDICATED FOR PEOPLE WITH FEVER, CHILLS, PERSISTENT FATIGUE OR DIAGNOSED SYSTEMIC INFECTIOUS DISEASE unless there is a physician's verification that the stimulation will not negatively affect the client. In that case, bodywork is still systemically limited to the most gentle and non-stimulating forms (see table on the next page for a summary of common communicable diseases).

For the protection of their clients and themselves, many bodyworkers choose to not work on any clients who have infectious illnesses. Unless your state or city has legal guidelines that require otherwise, it is up to each bodyworker to determine who he/she works on and when. In all cases, bodyworkers must follow universal precautions, be knowledgeable about the routes of transmission of common communicable diseases, and protect themselves from contact. The following are summaries of information about the types of communicable disease most common in adult bodywork clients. If you plan to work with children, consult a pediatric reference.

AIDS (see *HIV Infection*)

CMV, or cytomegalovirus: This is a type of herpes virus that commonly inhabits the salivary glands and can lie dormant for years in a healthy immune system, then be activated by preg-

Common Communicable Diseases

Name	Signs and Symptoms	Mode of Transmission
COLDS	Runny nose, watery eyes, fever & fatigue	Viral: airborne and oral routes Bacterial: airborne
STREP THROAT	Pain, fever, white plaques	Bacterial: oral routes
FLU (influenza)	Chills, fever, sore throat, runny nose, muscle aches, diarrhea, vomiting	Viral: airborne and oral routes
HEPATITIS A	Fever, fatigue, diarrhea, vomiting, liver tenderness, jaundice	Viral: oral route
HEPATITIS B	Same as hepatitis A plus liver failure	Viral: contact with blood/body fluids through a break in the skin or intact membranes
HIV	Stage 1: flu-like symptoms, rash Stage 2: no symptoms Stage 3: swollen lymph glands, weight loss, diarrhea, dyspnea, night sweats, neuropathy, fevers, weakness, fatigue, yeast infections Stage 4: (AIDS) all of stage 3 symptoms become more severe plus pneumocystis, Kaposi's and other opportunistic infections	Viral: contact with blood/body fluids through a break in the skin or intact mucous membranes
STAPH (staphylococcus) acne, boils, abscesses	Local inflammation with pus: carbuncle, fever, chills	Bacterial: contact through a break in the skin or intact mucous membranes
FUNGI yeast, thrush, Candida, ringworm, thick nails, athlete's foot, jock itch	Inflammation with plaque and/or blisters in mouth, genitals, groin, under breasts, axillae, between toes, under nails	Fungal: contact
HERPES simplex (cold sores & fever blisters) zoster (shingles, chicken pox)	Inflammation with oozing or crusts on lip and/or face Inflammation with painful blisters that follow nerve	Viral: contact through a break in the skin or intact mucous membranes
SCABIES	Intense itching, small bites	Parasite: contact w/contaminated items
LICE (pediculosis)	Nits in hair, itching, inflamed bites	Parasite: contact w/contaminated persons or articles
TB (tuberculosis)	Weight loss, fever, fatigue, cough with sputum, night sweats	Bacterial: airborne through droplets
PNEUMONIA	Chest pain, cough, fever, chills, fatigue, dyspnea	Bacterial, viral or fungal: airborne

nancy, multiple blood transfusions, or immune suppression. Can cause mental or motor retardation in infants and can cause dementia, bowel problems, and blindness in people with AIDS. Bodywork is contraindicated unless a physician verifies that the stimulation will not negatively influence the client. Universal precautions should be followed and pregnant women are advised to avoid direct contact with persons with CMV.

Common Cold, or *Coryza*: This is a general term for acute inflammation of any or all parts of the respiratory tract, including the nasal mucosa, sinuses, throat, larynx, trachea, and bronchi. It is caused by any of a number of viruses and is highly contagious by the oral and airborne routes for over a week after onset of symptoms. The incubation period is 12 to 72 hours. Symptoms include nasal congestion, clear or white watery nasal discharge, sneezing, tearing, chilliness, and just feeling bad (malaise). Fever is rare, so, if it is present, then influenza (flu) or other infection may be involved. Symptoms usually resolve, regardless of treatment, in two to ten days, depending on the strength of the person's immune system.

Flu or *Influenza*: This is a highly contagious acute respiratory infection, caused by any of a number of viruses, and transmitted by the oral and airborne routes. It is characterized by sudden onset, fever, chills, headache, muscle aches, and fatigue. Cough, sore throat, and clear or white nasal discharge are also common. Less frequently, digestive system symptoms occur, including loss of appetite (anorexia), nausea, vomiting, and diarrhea. The incubation period is 1 to 3 days. Probably as many or more infected people are asymptomatic as are symptomatic. Symptoms usually resolve, regardless of treatment, in 2 to 7 days, depending on the strength of the person's immune system. The influenza virus is the only organism that still causes acute nationwide epidemics. Flu can be fatal for weakened, very old, and very young people. Vaccines are available each fall for the virus strains that are expected to be most prevalent that winter.

Fungi: See Chapter 3 and table on page 152.

Hepatitis: This is inflammation of the liver. It can be caused by a variety of agents, including viral infections, bacterial infection, and physical or chemical agents (e.g., alcohol and drugs). The symptoms usually include fever, weakness, diarrhea, jaundice, and an enlarged liver. Recent advances in detection, vaccination, and treatment are decreasing the numbers of new infections, however, 10-20% of cases are still caused by viruses that have not yet been identified. Bodywork is locally contraindicated to the abdomen, due to liver fragility and enlargement. There are three main types, as follows:

- *Hepatitis A*, also called *infectious hepatitis*: This usually occurs in children and young adults. Is carried in the feces and taken into the body through eating or drinking contaminated food or water. Is common in places where sanitation systems are deficient, but outbreaks also occur occasionally through restaurants. Symptoms may appear two to six weeks after contact, and usually subside in less than two months. Can be prevented by a vaccine available through physicians and public health departments.
- *Hepatitis B*, also called *serum hepatitis*: Route of transmission is through the

blood and body fluids, so it usually occurs in IV drug abusers, health care workers, and sexual partners of people in these groups. It is also passed from mother to child at birth. Approximately 90% of cases are acute and resolve in three to four months. The other 10% become chronic, and then have increased risk for cirrhosis (see chapter 11), liver failure, and liver cancer. Can be prevented by a vaccine, which is routinely given to infants and health care workers, and is available to others through physicians and public health departments.

- *Hepatitis C*: Route of transmission is thought to be through the blood and body fluids. Approximately 15-25% of cases are acute, but 75-85% are chronic, and many cases develop into cirrhosis.

Herpes: This is a general term that refers to vesicular eruptions on the skin and/or mucous membranes, caused by the group of viruses that includes herpes simplex, herpes zoster, CMV, and Epstein-Barr (mononucleosis). In lay language, it most commonly refers to herpes simplex I, otherwise known as cold sores or fever blisters (see below).

- *Herpes simplex I, cold sores* or *fever blisters*: This is a highly contagious infection that causes inflammation and vesicles that may ooze or crust. It usually affects the border between the skin and the mucous membrane at the mouth but also may occur inside the mouth, throat, gingiva (gums), or conjunctiva (lining of the eyelids). It is transmitted by direct contact with either the lesion or its drainage. It can be present and dormant until the person has sun exposure and/or is under excessive stress. Caffeine intake may also increase susceptibility to vesicle eruption.
- *Herpes simplex II*: This is a highly contagious infection of the genital and anorectal skin and mucosa, that is transmitted by direct contact with either the lesion or its drainage. It is classified as a sexually transmitted disease, but can also be transmitted to an infant during delivery and can be fatal to the infant. Adult symptoms include itching and soreness immediately before a small patch of erythema appears, which develops into a painful vesicle that opens and heals in about 10 days.
- *Herpes zoster*, or *Shingles*: This is a highly contagious infection and inflammation of the posterior spinal or cranial root ganglia and appears mainly in adults. (Children exposed to herpes zoster usually get chicken pox.) It is characterized by painful vesicles that erupt along the course of the affected nerve and is almost always unilateral. The incubation period is 7 to 21 days. The total duration from onset of vesicles to their disappearance varies from 10 days to 5 weeks, but pain may last much longer. This infection is spread by direct contact with the lesions or their drainage.

HIV Infection, or *Human Immunodeficiency Virus*: As its name suggests, this virus weakens the immune system, causing an immune deficiency that destroys T cells and makes the person susceptible to serious opportunistic infections, malignancies (cancers), and neurologic diseases. Many people with HIV infection experience a roller-coaster disease progression, with dramatic remissions and exacerbations, rather than an orderly or sequential progression. Once thought to be 100% fatal, some people with HIV infection are now living without symptoms for 10 or more years, and hope to continue doing so. The disease progresses to *AIDS (acquired immune deficiency syndrome)* when the T cell count is below 200 per cubic mm of blood, that is about 1/5 of the level in a healthy adult. AIDS is characterized by severe and disabling symptoms that end in death.

Before beginning any bodywork for persons with HIV infection, take a full assessment of the client's health and medications. Encourage open communication and feedback, and reassess during and after each session. Modify your work to match the person, and expect that each session might be different, because having HIV infection often means having ongoing body/mind changes. Also, avoid touching any open skin areas [sores, cuts, abrasions, and puncture wounds (e.g., recent IV or blood test areas)] even with gloved hands, because these are vulnerable areas for an immunodeficient client, and because the areas will be tender. Other painful areas may be acknowledged by gently placing a hand there without pressure or stroking.

The following is a brief summary of recommended guidelines for bodywork with persons with HIV infection. For more detailed information, consult the FURTHER RESOURCES listed at the end of this chapter.

- Stage 1 (*Flu-like symptoms*): Some people experience flu-like symptoms and/or a rash immediately after becoming infected, however, most people do not, and so the person will probably not know s/he is infected. Tests for the HIV antibody usually do not show positive for up to six weeks after exposure. Bodywork would be systemically contraindicated if fever, chills, or persistent fatigue is present, and locally contraindicated in the area of rash.
- Stage 2 (*Asymptomatic/no symptoms*): These clients are leading healthy, productive lives, but an HIV antibody test would be positive. They may or may not know they are infected. All forms of bodywork are appropriate, unless the client is involved with an *experimental drug treatment*. In that case, advise him/her to consult with the physician before receiving bodywork. Some drug treatments are highly toxic, and may not be easily filtered from the body. Promoting a deep clearing (physically or energetically) in a person whose body/mind is weakened by illness can temporarily overload the body with toxins, which can increase or intensify symptoms such as high fever, vomiting, diarrhea, dizziness, confusion, or uncontrollable emotional release. An increase in symptoms can be scary and/or can further deplete the client's energy, or require more medication to reduce the symptoms. Gentler approaches would better serve to support and nurture the person's health.
- Stage 3 (*Mild symptoms*): Mild symptoms are defined as aggravating but not often physically restricting, and can include swollen lymph glands, weight loss, diarrhea, difficulty breathing (dyspnea), night sweats, neuropathy, fevers, weakness, fatigue, and yeast infections. All forms of bodywork are appropriate, with the following exceptions:
    a) If the client is fatigued, gentle nurturing bodywork is needed, rather than stimulating forms, so as to conserve and help replenish the client's energy.
    b) If the client is experiencing neuropathy (numbness, tingling, or sharp pain in

the extremities), s/he may not want to be touched in the affected areas. If touch is wanted there, be very gentle, because pressure or vigorous work can increase pain or damage nerves. If the client has numbness, touch very gently to avoid causing damage that is not felt by the client.

c) As always, avoid rashes and bruises (see Chapters 4 and 6).

d) If the client is taking an experimental drug, follow the recommendations given earlier under Stage 2.

e) Often people with HIV infection will bruise or bleed easily, even severely, as a result of minor injuries. Advise clients who are experiencing unusual bleeding or bruising to be seen by a physician to assess their clotting time, and treat if necessary, before getting bodywork.

• Stage 4 *(Serious symptoms/AIDS)*: During this stage, the virus has severely depleted the person's ability to produce T cells, and so s/he is extremely vulnerable to infections of all types. The client may experience several mild symptoms occurring simultaneously or any one symptom's chronic occurrence, plus may also experience dementia (see Chapter 2), prolonged bleeding time, bruising easily, and/or *opportunistic infections* such as pneumocystis (see Chapter 8), Kaposi's (see Chapter 12), cytomegalovirus (CMV), tuberculosis (TB) (see Chapter 8), shingles (see Chapter 3), and others. Opportunistic infections are caused by pathogens (usually fungi and bacteria), that occur almost everywhere in our environment but would not cause infection in healthy people. Opportunistic infections are usually not contagious unless a person's immune system is suppressed by a long illness, by taking certain antibiotics or steroids for a long time, or by HIV. For clients in stage 4, follow the recommendations given earlier under "experimental drugs," even if this client is not taking any, because his/her system will be fragile and easily overloaded. At this stage, only gentle, nurturing bodywork is indicated, and it is better to under-do than over-do. If the client is not expected to live long, follow the additional recommendations for working with terminally ill persons, given in Chapter 12.

Lice or *Pediculosis*: See Chapter 3 and table on page 152.

Pneumonia: See Chapter 8 and table on page 152.

Scabies: See Chapter 3 and table on page 152.

Staph, staphylococcus, abscesses, boils, or acne: These are discussed in Chapter 3, under carbuncles and furuncles. See also table on page 152.

Toxemia: This is a general term meaning the distribution throughout the body of the poisonous products of bacteria that are growing in a local site. It results in systemic symptoms including fever, diarrhea, vomiting, increased pulse and respirations, and, in severe cases, shock.

TB or *Tuberculosis*: See Chapter 8 and table on page 152.

CARE OF THE IMMUNE SYSTEM

As a bodyworker, it is likely that clients will frequently ask you questions about how they can care for, or strengthen, their immune systems. The following is general information for health maintenance. As always, if symptoms are progressively worsening or persisting, advise clients to consult with a physician.

Excessive antibiotics, unwholesome food and drink, poor hygiene, environmental toxicity, and constant mental/emotional stressors weaken the immune system. Supportive friendship, rest, relaxation, laughter, play, touch, the arts, self expression, and a diet of fresh, whole foods strengthen the immune system.

In addition, it is wise to apply some of the basic tenets of traditional, or indigenous, philosophies of health, which have been developed through centuries of human observation and care. One of these tenets is that exposure to cold moving air has a diminishing effect on the immune system. Another is that warm clothes, warm foods, and self-reflective activities are naturally in tune with health during the colder months, when the immune system is more easily overwhelmed.

High-quality rest, supportive relationship, and nutrition are the primary approaches to boosting immunity naturally. From an American, bio-chemical perspective, vitamins A, E, and C; minerals such as zinc, iron, and selenium, and coenzyme Q_{10} have been found to strengthen immunity. Whole or unrefined herbs can also add important nutritional components, as can refined or concentrated herbs, although, as these become more concentrated, they will act more as drugs than as foods. Echinacea, garlic, goldenseal, shiitake mushrooms, essential oils, and homeopathy are some common food/herb concentrations used to boost immunity during bacterial, viral, fungal, and parasitic infections.

Hands-on healing in the form of caring touch stimulates the body's healing and immune defense mechanisms. Therapeutic massage/bodywork and chiropractic approaches can influence neurologic function, release of neuro-peptides, lymphatic drainage, blood flow, and muscle tension. Acupuncture, Therapeutic Touch, Shiatsu, Reiki, and other energetic approaches can stimulate the immune system by opening or balancing the flow of chi, or vital energy. Prayer has been demonstrated in controlled, double-blind studies to positively benefit health.

COMMON EFFECTS OF AGING ON THE IMMUNE SYSTEM

In general, the immune system often begins to weaken after the age of 70. This may be due to decreased nutrition, exercise, and social support as much as to aging, but has not, at this point, been studied thoroughly. Common changes can include fewer signs and symptoms of inflammation or infection (fever, redness, pain, swelling), due to a decreased ability to mobilize immune defenses, until the infection is severe. Recovery from infection can also be slower, and older people may be more susceptible to infections than younger people with the same exposure.

CASE PRESENTATIONS

11/13/96: 48 yo woman; normal height & weight. Says she has a sore throat, feels tired & has a cough. Normal temperature.

Goal: Get relief from her cold symptoms.

History: Salivary glands removed 10 yrs ago. Chronically tight upper back and neck muscles. Gets massage regularly every 2 wks. Taking no medications.

Assessment: No visible deformities. Gait & ROM normal. Face is slightly pale; wrist pulse strong and regular at 88/min.

Indications: Clear heat from sore throat. Stimulate descending and dispersing of lung energy to stop coughing. Tonify general energy levels.

Contraindications: Protect client from losing heat.

Application: Kept room warm & provided blankets. Massaged upper back & chest with Vic's Vapo Rub & put heating pad on upper back while massaging legs. Effleurage, petrissage, and friction to back & neck to produce erythema, which releases interior heat. Used deep sustained acupressure on Bladder 12. Pressed on Bladder 13. Held & pressed on Governor Vessel 16 & 14, Gallbladder 20 & 21, Large intestine 4 & 11, Lung 11.

Outcome: Said she could breathe better, her throat was less sore, and she felt warm & relaxed. Pulse 80/min.

Referral: Suggested she consult her physician if cold symptoms get worse.

STUDY QUESTIONS

> Would you have worked on this client?
> What questions would you have asked that were not asked?
> What bodywork techniques would you have done?
> What other ways could the therapeutic outcome have been evaluated?
> How might you have changed the format?

FURTHER RESOURCES

AIDS Massage Project
> c/o Stuart Holland
> 3601 14th Avenue South
> Minneapolis, MN 55407

AIDS: The Ultimate Challenge
> plus other books, tapes & seminars
> Elisabeth Kubler Ross Center
> South Route 616

Headwaters, VA 24442
(703)396-3442

Audio and Video Tapes available through:
Innerlight Productions
PO Box 21478
Oakland, CA 94620
(800)537-6767

Massage for People with AIDS: The Well, the Unwell, and the Dying.
Stuart Holland
National AMTA Office
820 Davis Street, Suite 100
Evanston, IL 60201-4444
(708)864-0123

Workshops and Guidelines for Massaging HIV Infected Persons available through:
Service Through Touch
Irene Smith
41 Carl Street #C
San Francisco, CA 94117
(415) 564-1750

REFERENCES

Fritz, S. (1995). Mosby's fundamentals of therapeutic massage. St. Louis: Mosby Lifeline.
Kapit, W. & Elson, L.M. (1977). The anatomy coloring book. NY: Harper & Row.
Kapit, W., Macey, R.I., & Meisami, E. (1987). The physiology coloring book. NY: Harper & Row.
Mulvihill, M.L. (1995). Human diseases: A systemic approach (4th ed.) Norwalk, CT: Appleton & Lange.
Newton, D. (1995). Pathology for massage therapists. Portland, OR: Simran Publications.
Sameulson, P. (1994). Pathophysiology for massage: The travel guide. Overland Park, KS: Mid-America Handbooks, Inc.
Smith, I. & Bridgeman, K. (1992). Guidelines for massaging people with AIDS. (Out of print until revised).
Thomas, C.L. (1989). Taber's cyclopedic medical dictionary (16th ed.). Philadelphia: F.A. Davis Co.

CHAPTER REVIEW

1. Communicable diseases can be spread by: (3 routes) _____
_____

2. The immune system can be supported and strengthened by: _____
_____

3. Antibiotics are used to neutralize which pathogen(s)? _____
_____

4. Define phagocytosis: _____

5. What is the progression of tissue changes in allergy? _____
_____

6. _____ is the single most effective way to prevent spread of communicable diseases.

7. List the conditions when you would refer a client to a physician, based on this chapter: __
_____
_____

8. List 4 airborne communicable diseases: _____
_____

9. List 4 contact communicable diseases: _____
_____

10. Define contaminated: _____

11. What are the four pathogens? _____

12. Natural (or non-specific) immunity involves _____
_____ and _____, but not _____

13. Acquired immunity involves the activity of _____ cells and _____ cells, which are two types of lymphocytes.

14. In auto-immunity, the body _____

15. List the symptoms of systemic infection: _____
_____

16. Common allergy symptoms are: _____
_____

17. Hepatitis is inflammation of the _____

18. Define opportunistic infections: _____

ANSWERS TO CHAPTER REVIEW

1. oral, direct contact, airborne

2. Supportive friendship, rest, relaxation, laughter, play, touch, exposure to the arts, self expression, and a diet of fresh, whole foods

3. bacteria

4. when WBCs (or leukocytes) ingest & digest pathogens

5. histamine is released, capillaries dilate, erythema & edema

6. hand washing

7. history of chronic fatigue
    history of recurrent skin, digestive or respiratory ailments
    history of food intolerance
    failure to gain weight
    unexplained weight loss
    rashes, hives or itching of unknown origin
    enlarged lymph nodes, with or without tenderness
    excessive or persistent skin dryness or scaliness

8. colds, flu, TB, pneumonia

9. hepatitis B, HIV, staph, fungi, herpes, scabies, lice

10. the process by which an object or an area becomes inhabited by pathogens

11. bacteria, viruses, parasites & fungi

12. phagocytosis, inflammation; antibodies

13. B; T

14. makes antibodies against its own tissue

15. fever, chills, fatigue & pain

16. rash, swelling, sneezing, wheezing, severe abdominal cramps,   vomiting, rapid pulse, fainting

17. liver

18. caused by pathogens that occur almost everywhere in our environment, that would not cause infection in healthy people

Chapter 8

RESPIRATORY SYSTEM

ANATOMY AND PHYSIOLOGY REVIEW

The respiratory system provides oxygen to the circulatory system to distribute. The two systems work so closely together that sometimes they are referred to as one cardio-pulmonary system. For our purposes, they are discussed separately.

The respiratory system consists of a tubular air passageway, made of smooth muscle tissue, that is coated with cilia and mucous membrane (see *Illustration 58*). *Cilia* are hair-like projections in the epithelial cells that propel mucus, pus, and dust particles in the direction of the nose and mouth, to help the body expel foreign particles. The *mucous membrane* is the lining of all passages and body cavities that contact the outside world. It consists of an epithelial layer, a basement membrane, and an underlying layer called the lamina propria. Mucus-secreting cells or glands usually are present. The mucous membrane is normally moist with *mucus*, a clear viscous fluid that lubricates and provides a protective immune barrier to pathogens.

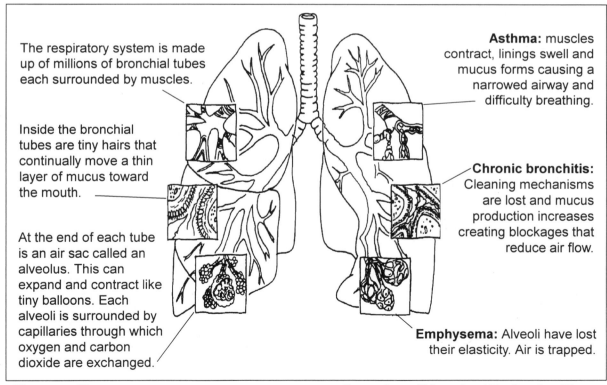

The respiratory system is made up of millions of bronchial tubes each surrounded by muscles.

Inside the bronchial tubes are tiny hairs that continually move a thin layer of mucus toward the mouth.

At the end of each tube is an air sac called an alveolus. This can expand and contract like tiny balloons. Each alveoli is surrounded by capillaries through which oxygen and carbon dioxide are exchanged.

Asthma: muscles contract, linings swell and mucus forms causing a narrowed airway and difficulty breathing.

Chronic bronchitis: Cleaning mechanisms are lost and mucus production increases creating blockages that reduce air flow.

Emphysema: Alveoli have lost their elasticity. Air is trapped.

Illustration 57   Comparison of Normal and Dysfunctional Lung

The tubular air passageway consists of the *nose, sinuses,* and *pharynx* (throat), with the *epiglottis* forming a gateway that prevents food and fluids from entering the *trachea* (windpipe). The nose, sinuses, pharynx, and epiglottis form a bridge between the external environment and the internal environment of the *tracheo-bronchial tree* and *lungs*. Inert particles, bacteria, fungi, and viruses enter with each inhalation, stimulating the immune response when needed. Illnesses from the nose to the epiglottis are called *upper respiratory diseases*. Since upper respiratory pathogens are airborne, most are highly contagious.

Directly after the epiglottis is the *larynx* (voice box), followed by the *trachea*, which branches out into two *bronchi*, one going to each lung. The bronchi branch out into smaller and smaller tubes called *bronchioles*, until they eventually end in small air sacs called the *alveoli*. The alveoli are very thin-walled sacs that are surrounded by capillaries. When air is inhaled, oxygen diffuses from the alveoli to the capillaries, and, at the same time, waste gases diffuse from the capillaries to the alveoli. *Carbon dioxide*, which is a waste product of cellular metabolism, is the primary waste gas. The waste gases are expelled from the alveoli during exhalation. Illnesses of the larynx, trachea, bronchi, bronchioles, alveoli, and remaining lung tissues comprise the *lower respiratory diseases*.

Respiration is controlled by the medulla in the brain. The signals that the medulla sends to the body to make it breathe are stimulated by the level of *carbon dioxide* in the blood. The more carbon dioxide, the greater the need to breathe. Breathing causes oxygen to come into the lungs and wastes, such as carbon dioxide, to be expelled from the lungs. The *diaphragm* is the large muscle directly under the lungs that contracts to expand the lungs (*inhalation*) and relaxes to compress the lungs (*exhalation*). Small muscles between the ribs (the external intercostals) assist the breathing process. When people are very ill and the diaphragm and external intercostals are not strong enough to perform adequate breathing, the abdominal and internal intercostal muscles assist. These muscles can also be trained to assist in healthy breathing, such as occurs in many Eastern body/mind exercises, such as yoga, Qi Gong, Tai Chi, and others.

The lungs are enveloped by a double membrane, consisting of two layers of *pleura*. The inner layer covers the lungs and the outer layer lines the chest (or thoracic) cavity. The space between these two membranes is called the pleural space, and has a small amount of lubricating fluid in it.

ASSESSMENT: OBSERVATION AND PALPATION

As always, listen closely to the client's description of their health experience and read the intake form with your knowledge of the respiratory and circulatory systems in mind. Ask questions to clarify or add to the information the client gives. Observe the skin color and temperature, rate and pattern of respiration, chest movements, upper body lymph nodes, and chest pain. Count the respiration rate by counting each inhalation/exhalation pair as one. The *normal adult respiration rate* is 16 breaths per minute, at rest. If you count for 15 seconds, there should be approximately 4 respirations. Tiredness, anxiety, irritability, confusion, pallor, and/or cyanosis around the lips or in the nail beds are signs of too little oxygen.

Wheezing is a whistling or sighing sound that is caused by narrowed airways. It is often heard with a stethoscope, but can sometimes also be heard without one. Wheezing often occurs in asthma, coryza, hay fever, and some more serious cardio-pulmonary illnesses, such as bronchial spasm, pulmonary tumor, obstruction, edema, or tuberculosis.

Crackles (also called rales or rattles) are abnormal breathing sounds that sound like dry crackling, popping, or moist gurgling. They are usually heard with a stethoscope, but sometimes also heard without one, and are usually caused by the air being breathed through mucous or other secretions inside the airways.

GENERAL CONDITIONS RELATED TO THE RESPIRATORY SYSTEM

The following are definitions and descriptions of general respiratory findings. Information on more specific respiratory disorders follows in the next section. As a general rule, refer clients with the following findings to a physician for assessment and diagnosis:

- dyspnea (difficult or labored breathing)
- tachypnea (rapid breathing; 24 or more per minute at rest)
- flaring of nostrils on inspiration
- pursed lips on exhalation
- pallor or cyanosis around lips or in nail beds
- enlarged, tender lymph nodes
- chest pain
- cough productive of thick greenish sputum
- wheezing

SPECIFIC RESPIRATORY CONDITIONS

COMMUNICABLE RESPIRATORY ILLNESSES

These illnesses are caused by: 1) airborne pathogens, 2) orally transmitted pathogens, and 3) contact with secretions from the upper airways, thus they are easily spread to the therapist and to other clients who will use the room that day. Bodywork is systemically contraindicated for clients with a fever. If the client has respiratory symptoms and does not have a fever, and if the work is very gentle, bodywork is not contraindicated. To protect yourself, however, it is best to stay 12" to 18" away from the mouth and nose of the client and not to handle their paper tissues. Thorough disinfection of all equipment that comes in contact with the client's exhalations, such as the face rest, is recommended before another client uses the equipment.

Common Cold (Coryza): This is an acute inflammation of the mucous membrane lining the upper respiratory areas and/or the trachea and bronchi. It can be caused by any of thousands of different viruses, so having one cold usually does not give immunity to the next one you are exposed to. It is highly contagious by the oral and airborne routes for over a week after onset of symptoms. The incubation period is 12 to 72 hours. Symptoms include nasal congestion, clear or white watery nasal discharge, sneezing, tearing, chilliness, and just feeling bad (malaise). Fever is rare, so, if it is present, then influenza (flu) or other infection may be involved. Symptoms usually resolve, regardless of treatment, in 2 to 10 days, depending on the strength of the person's immune system. When a person has a viral infection, their general immune responses are often overwhelmed for up to four weeks afterward, thus making the person more susceptible to other infections during that time. When bacterial infection accompanies the viral infection, it causes the nasal discharge to be thick and yellow or greenish.

Flu or *Influenza*: This is a highly contagious acute respiratory infection, caused by any of a number of viruses and transmitted by the oral and airborne routes. It is characterized by sudden onset, fever, chills, headache, muscle aches, and fatigue. Cough, sore throat and clear or white nasal discharge are also common. Less frequently, digestive system symptoms occur, including loss of appetite (anorexia), nausea, vomiting, and diarrhea. The incubation period is 1 to 3 days. Probably as many or more infected people are asymptomatic as are symptomatic. Symptoms usually resolve, regardless of treatment, in 2 to 7 days, depending on the strength of the person's immune system. The influenza virus is the only organism that still causes acute nationwide epidemics. Flu can be fatal for weakened, very old, and very young people. Vaccines are available each fall for the virus strains that are expected to be most prevalent that winter.

Fungal Infections of the lung: These are generally not infectious unless the person's immune system is in a weakened condition. Symptoms may have sudden or gradual onset and include dyspnea, fever, fatigue, and weakness. Common types include candidiasis, histoplasmosis, and coccidioidomycosis, which are each named for their causative fungus. Bodywork is contraindicated if fever is present. Transmission of infection is through mouth, nose, and chest secretions, so take appropriate precautions to avoid contact with these.

Laryngitis: This is an inflammation of the larynx (voice box). *Acute laryngitis* develops quickly (hours to days) and symptoms include hoarseness, decreased ability to make sounds, and, occasionally, pain on talking and/or swallowing. The etiology is improper use of overuse of the voice; exposure to cold and wet conditions; extension form nasal and/or pharyngeal infections; inhalation of irritating vapors or dust, or association with systemic diseases such as measles or bronchitis. Bodywork is contraindicated if a fever is present. *Chronic laryngitis* can be due to chronic irritation or can follow an acute episode. Symptoms include tickling in the throat, voice huskiness, and difficulty in speaking. It is often secondary to sinus or nasal pathology, such as polyps, improper use of the voice, smoking, drinking or neoplasms. Bodywork is indicated for relaxation and body awareness.

Pharyngitis: This is a general term meaning inflammation of the pharynx (throat). In *acute pharyngitis*, symptoms develop quickly (hours to days) and include fever, difficulty swallowing, throat pain, postnasal secretions, and malaise. If white or yellow plaques are present, testing should be done to determine if strep bacteria are present. If so, medical treatment is indicated. Bodywork is contraindicated if fever is present. In chronic pharyngitis, symptoms develop slowly (days to weeks) and include dryness and irritation of throat. *Chronic pharyngitis* is caused by smoking, mouth breathing, and chronic tonsillitis. Bodywork is indicated for relaxation and body awareness.

Pneumonia: This is a general term for the acute inflammation of the alveoli and bronchioles, and there are over 50 different causes. The most common causes are bacteria, viruses, and certain chemical irritants, although radiation, fungi, and protozoa (a type of parasite) also can cause pneumonia. It decreases the lung's ability to exchange oxygen and carbon dioxide and causes severe chest pain, fever, chills, pallor and/or cyanosis, coughing, and a thick, purulent sputum. The term "double pneumonia" refers to both lungs being affected. Risk factors include smoking, alcoholism, and weakened health from other illness, old age, or stress. Pneumonia is often severe and/or fatal in very young, very old, and very weakened persons. Immunization is available for elderly and weakened people, is effective for life, and includes antibodies for the most common forms of pneumonia.

- *Bacterial Pneumonia*: This causes a sudden (acute) onset of symptoms, including chills, fever, chest pain, cough, and yellow or greenish sputum that sometimes is also bloody. Antibiotics are an important treatment for bacterial pneumonia, which can be fatal in severe cases. Bodywork is contraindicated if fever is present. Transmission of infection is through mouth, nose and chest secretions, so take appropriate precautions to avoid contact with these.
- *Pneumocystis Carinii Pneumonia (PCP):* This is a rare form of bacterial pneumonia that is rarely encountered in otherwise healthy people, but its presence is a major defining characteristic for AIDS diagnosis, accounting for over half of all AIDS deaths. Symptoms are a persistent cough and severe chest pain, weakness and dyspnea. It is often accompanied by chills, fever, increased pulse and respirations.
- *Viral Pneumonia*: This has a sudden (acute) onset, characterized by symptoms that range from ones resembling the common cold to severe and progressive dyspnea and respiratory insufficiency. The etiology can be influenza or any of a number of systemic viral infections. Bodywork is contraindicated if fever is present and may need to be modified if the client has dyspnea or is in a weakened condition.

Sinusitis: This is a general term meaning inflammation of the paranasal sinuses. The etiology can be viral, bacterial, or allergic, and the condition can be acute or chronic. The most common symptoms are nasal congestion and painful pressure in the sinuses, but malaise, sore throat, headache, and/or fever can also be present. Bodywork is contraindicated only if fever is present.

Tonsillitis: This is an inflammation of the tonsil, a mass of lymphatic tissue located in a ring that encircles the pharynx, which acts as a filter to protect the body from invasion of bacteria and which aids in the production of white blood cells. Etiology may be bacterial or viral. Tonsillitis is usually acute, but may be recurrent. The onset is sudden, usually accompanied by chills, fever, malaise, headache, muscle aches, and pain in the throat, especially on swallowing. Tonsils may appear enlarged and red with white or yellow plaques. If plaques are present, testing should be done to determine if strep bacteria are present. If so, medical treatment is indicated. Bodywork is contraindicated only if fever is present, but care should be taken to avoid contact with oral secretions.

Tuberculosis or *TB*: This is a highly infectious disease worldwide and was once considered of minimal threat in the U.S. However, TB is significantly on the rise in the U.S. It is caused by a specific bacteria, and characterized by inflammatory responses in the lung tissue, formation of pockets in the lung that become encased and then die, forming abscesses and calcified holes in the lung tissue. TB also can affect the digestive and genitourinary tracts, the bones, joints, nervous system, lymph nodes, and skin. Infection usually occurs as a result of contact with an infected person's sputum or from inhaling air droplets produced by an infected person who is speaking or coughing close by or in a shared, closed environment. It can also be contacted by drinking contaminated, unpasteurized milk. Symptoms include night sweats, fatigue, weakness, weight loss, and a deep cough that is productive of thick, sometimes blood-tinged sputum. TB is effectively treated medically, but cure requires taking daily medication for a year. People being treated are not infectious after about two weeks of treatment. Bodywork is contraindicated unless the physician verifies that the infection is not contagious and the person can tolerate the stimulation without adverse effects.

CHRONIC OBSTRUCTIVE PULMONARY DISEASES

This group of diseases involves restriction of air flow in the bronchial tubes. They are all caused by irritants, such as industrial fumes, auto exhaust, cigarette smoke, and pathogens, and include *bronchitis, emphysema, bronchial asthma*, and *bronchiectasis* (see illustration on page 163). The symptoms generally involve dyspnea (difficulty breathing), wheezing, thick mucus in the lungs, and increased susceptibility to lung infection. COPD begins gradually and gets progressively worse over the years. After many years, the person develops a "barrel chest" appearance from his/her prolonged efforts to get air in and out. As the carbon dioxide level builds up in the blood, the fingers, toes, and lips often turn cyanotic (bluish).

Asthma, bronchial: This is an intermittent, reversible form of COPD, involving sudden onset of dyspnea and wheezing caused by muscle spasms that contract the bronchial tubes, swelling of the bronchial mucous membrane, and an increased production of mucus that clogs the airways. An "attack" may last a few minutes or up to several hours. Asthma affects about 7% of the U.S. population and occurs most often in children or young adults. When the etiology is external (also called atopic), it is caused by allergens that are inhaled in the air and/or ingested in food or drugs. Atopic asthma usually, but not always, begins in childhood. When the etiology is internal (also called nonatopic), it typically begins after age 35, and the cause is not known, but it is believed to be an over-reaction of the immune system. With both types of asthma, recurrence and severity of attacks are greatly influenced by the presence of infection, mental or physical fatigue, exposure to cold air or fumes, endocrine changes at various periods in life, and emotional stress. Bodywork is only contraindicated during acute episodes and/or if fever is present. If a client has asthma symptoms, stop the bodywork and assist him/

her to sit up, to use his/her inhaler, to breathe through pursed lips, to close the eyes, and to use any relaxation techniques s/he is familiar with. If symptoms continue to get worse, call for emergency medical help. A severe, prolonged asthma attack can develop into status asthmaticus, which can lead to death.

Bronchiectasis: This is a form of COPD, involving chronic dilation of the bronchi or bronchus, with a secondary infection that usually involves the lower portion of the lung. Dilation may be in an isolated segment or spread throughout the bronchi. Etiology can be congenital, but is usually secondary to obstruction or infection, such as pneumonia, chronic bronchitis, or tuberculosis. Symptoms include cough, dyspnea, and production of foul sputum (especially in the morning or when changing position). Bodywork is contraindicated unless the physician verifies that the stimulation will not adversely affect the client. Be sure to avoid touching lung secretions, which are contaminated with pathogens.

Bronchitis: This is inflammation of the mucous membrane lining of the bronchial tubes. The etiology can be viral, bacterial, allergic, or from chronic physical irritation from dusts or fumes. Predisposing factors are exposure to cold, wet weather, fatigue, and malnutrition. *Acute bronchitis* develops suddenly (hours to days) and is characterized by chills, malaise, pain and constriction behind the sternum, coughing and fever. *Chronic bronchitis* is a form of COPD and is a risk factor for emphysema and lung cancer. A productive cough is usually present for at least three months a year for two consecutive years, and there is hypertrophy and hyperplasia of the mucus-secreting glands in the tracheo-bronchial tree. Bodywork is contraindicated only if fever is present. Positioning may need to be modified if the client has difficulty breathing in a supine or prone position.

Emphysema: This word comes from the Greek word for "to inflate." It is a form of COPD, characterized by an abnormal increase in the size of the alveoli, with destructive changes to their walls, causing them to break down and lose their elasticity. This causes dead air to accumulate in the enlarged alveoli blocking the delivery of oxygen to the bloodstream. The etiology is usually smoking or long-term inhalation of airborne irritants. Symptoms include dyspnea and cough. People with emphysema have a high risk for respiratory infection, chronic bronchitis, and eventual lung collapse. Bodywork is indicated unless a secondary infection is present. Positioning may need to be modified if the client has difficulty breathing in a supine or prone position.

Pneumoconiosis: This is a condition of the respiratory tract due to inhalation of dust particles, and is commonly an occupational disorder from mining, farming, carpentry, etc. Two examples are described below.

  • *Asbestosis*: This is a form of pneumonoconiosis resulting from inhalation of asbestos particles. Exposure to asbestos has been associated with the later development of cancer of the lung with a latency period of 20 or more years. Bodywork is indicated for relaxation and body awareness, unless a secondary infection is present.
  • *Silicosis*: This is a form of pneumonoconiosis resulting from inhalation of silica (quartz) dust, characterized by formation of small discrete nodules in the lung. In

advanced cases, a dense fibrosis and emphysema with impairment of respiratory function may develop. Bodywork is indicated for relaxation and body awareness, unless a secondary infection is present.

MISCELLANEOUS RESPIRATORY ILLNESSES

Hay fever (seasonal allergic rhinitis): This is a hypersensitivity (allergy) to airborne pollens from plants, especially grasses, trees, and other plants in bloom. When the pollens contact the mucous membranes in the upper respiratory areas, the immune system releases antibodies, and then histamine is released, which stimulates inflammation. This is not an infection, but the presence of inflammation makes the area more susceptible to the growth of pathogens so a secondary infection is more likely. Symptoms of hay fever are watery, itching eyes and nose, sneezing, and nasal congestion. Secondary bacterial infection can cause the nasal secretions to become thick, yellow or greenish. Bodywork is indicated if no other contraindicated condition is present.

Lung Cancer (Bronchogenic Carcinoma): This is the main cause of cancer death in American adults, with men affected twice as often as women. The main cause is tobacco smoking. It develops slowly over decades of time but often metastasizes to other organs when this cancer is advanced, it interferes with the delivery of oxygen into the circulation, and symptoms of breathlessness develop. The person may require oxygen administration via a nasal canula or a mask. Also, the person may be most comfortable in a seated or supine position, depending on his/her breathing (see Chapter 12).

Pleurisy: This is an inflammation of the pleural lining around the lungs. It can be unilateral or bilateral, primary or secondary; acute or chronic. Symptoms generally include: intense chest pain (sometimes referred into the abdomen), anxiety, and difficulty breathing. If a bacterial infection is present, fever, chills, and pallor are common. Bodywork is contraindicated unless a physician verifies that the stimulation will not adversely affect the person.

Sleep Apnea: This term means that breathing stops (apnea) off and on during sleep. It is not an illness, per se, but is a symptom of certain sleep disorders. To be medically diagnosed, the apnea must last at least 10 seconds and occur 30 or more times during a seven hour sleep period. Etiology can include: obstruction of the upper airway; absence of respiratory muscle activity, or a mixture of both. It mainly affects middle-aged, obese men with a history of loud snoring and daytime sleepiness. Bodywork is indicated, and the client is likely to sleep during the session.

GENERAL EFFECTS OF AGING ON THE RESPIRATORY SYSTEM

Between the ages of 25 and 75, there is usually a 30% loss of overall pulmonary functioning, resulting in shallower breathing, less ability to cough and breathe deeply, more air remaining in the lungs after exhalation, and more carbon dioxide retention, which all contribute to more limited mobility and more overall anxiety. Some of the decrease in pulmonary functioning is due to atrophy and increasing rigidity of chest muscles (diaphragm and intercostals). Other related factors are: the alveoli and capillary tissues become thicker and less elastic, which causes less efficiency in oxygen and waste gas diffusion; the mucous membranes get drier, the cilia decrease in number and motility, and the immune system has slower responses, which all contribute to making the lungs more susceptible to pathogens. The overall rate of respirations decreases, there is increased mouth breathing, and snoring becomes more common. Also, lifetime exposures to cigarette smoking and other air pollutants has usually taken some toll on delicate lung tissues by the elder years.

CASE PRESENTATIONS

11/25/96: 50 yo male. Goals: stress relief, relaxation, & reduce upper body stiffness & soreness.
History: Has bronchial asthma & uses inhalers and frequent antibiotics. Otherwise in good
    health. Exercises 3-4 times/wk.
Subjective: Feels stiff & sore around chest and shoulders.
Objective: Normal posture & gait. No major deformities.
Indications: Swedish massage for relaxation & to improve flexibility & circulation in chest &
    shoulder tissues.
Contraindications: Prolonged prone or supine positions could cause difficulty breathing.
Application: Effleurage, tapotement & petrissage to back, neck, chest, and arms, with the
    main focus on upper back, chest, neck and shoulders. Worked 30 minutes. Positioning
    was in a chair, with client leaning forward on pillows, as needed.
Outcome: Client said he felt great(!) & will return monthly.

STUDY QUESTIONS

    Which parts of the above case presentations are subjective?
    Which parts are objective?
    What questions would you have asked that were not asked?
    What bodywork techniques would you have done?
    What referral(s)?
    What other ways could the therapeutic outcome have been evaluated?
    How might you have changed the format or way the cases were written?

REFERENCES

Fritz, S. (1995). Mosby's fundamentals of therapeutic massage. St. Louis: Mosby Lifeline.
Jarvis, C. (1992). Physical examination and health assessment. Philadelphia: W. B. Saunders Co.
Kapit, W. & Elson, L.M. (1977). The anatomy coloring book. NY: Harper & Row.
Kapit, W., Macey, R.I., & Meisami, E. (1987). The physiology coloring book. NY: Harper & Row.
Malasanos, L., Barkauskas, V., & Stoltenberg-Allen, K. (1990). Health assessment. St. Louis,
    MO: C.V. Mosby Co.

Mulvihill, M.L. (1995). Human diseases: A systemic approach (4th ed.) Norwalk, CT: Appleton & Lange.

Newton, D. (1995). Pathology for massage therapists. Portland, OR: Simran Publications.

Sameulson, P. (1994). Pathophysiology for massage: The travel guide. Overland Park, KS: Mid-America Handbooks, Inc.

Thomas, C.L. (1989). Taber's cyclopedic medical dictionary (16th ed.). Philadelphia: F.A. Davis Co.

CHAPTER REVIEW

1. Illnesses from the _____ to the _____ are called upper respiratory diseases.

2. The _____ are thin-walled sacs that are surrounded by capillaries.

3. The _____ are where the diffusion of oxygen and wastes gases takes place.

4. The _____ and _____ muscles can be trained to assist in healthy breathing.

5. The normal adult respiration rate at rest is _____/minute.

6. Tiredness, anxiety, irritability, confusion, pallor, and/or cyanosis around lips or in the nail beds are signs of (too little/too much) oxygen. (circle one)

7. _____ is a whistling or sighing sound in the lungs.

8. _____ sound like dry crackling, popping, or moist gurgling sounds in the lungs.

9. In general, refer the following findings to a physician:

_____

_____

_____

10. Communicable respiratory illnesses are transmitted through _____

_____

11. Bodywork is systemically (indicated/contraindicated) for people with fever. (circle one)

12. List at least 5 common communicable respiratory illnesses: _____

_____

13. If a client has asthma symptoms that are not relieved within a few minutes, _____ should be sought.

14. Define dyspnea: _____

ANSWERS TO CHAPTER REVIEW

1. nose, epiglottis

2. alveoli

3. alveoli

4. abdominal and internal intercostals

5. 16

6. too little

7. wheezing

8. crackles

9. dyspnea (difficult or labored breathing)
   tachypnea (rapid breathing; 24 or more per minute at rest)
   flaring of nostrils on inspiration
   pursed lips on exhalation
   pallor or cyanosis around lips or in nail beds
   enlarged, tender lymph nodes
   chest pain
   cough productive of thick greenish sputum
   wheezing

10. airborne and orally transmitted pathogens

11. contraindicated

12. common cold, flu, fungal infections, laryngitis, pharyngitis, pneumonia, sinusitis, tonsillitis, tuberculosis

13. emergency medical help

14. difficulty breathing

CHAPTER 9

ENDOCRINE SYSTEM

ANATOMY AND PHYSIOLOGY REVIEW

The *endocrine system* is comprised entirely of ductless glands that secrete *hormones* into the blood or lymph systems. These hormones produce effects on tissues in all parts of the body. Hormones may be steroids, proteins, or modified amino acids.

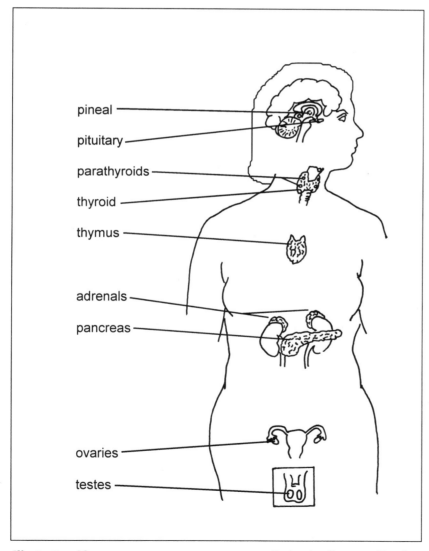

pineal

pituitary

parathyroids

thyroid

thymus

adrenals

pancreas

ovaries

testes

Illustration 58   Endocrine System: Glands

The *endocrine glands* include the pituitary gland, the thyroid gland, parathyroid glands, adrenal glands, the islands of Langerhans in the pancreas, and the gonads (ovaries and testes) (see *Illustration*). The *hypothalamus* produces special hormones that exert an effect on the production and release of hormones in the other endocrine glands. The *pineal* and *thymus* glands have not been definitively proven to produce any hormones, but this is controversial. Other structures, such as the gastrointestinal mucosa and the placenta also have endocrine functions, but these go beyond the scope of this text.

Some endocrine hormones have a specific local effect on an organ or tissue and some have a systemic effect on the entire body.

Among the physiological processes affected by hormones are:

- rate of metabolism and metabolism of specific substances;
- growth and development;
- the secretory activity of other endocrine glands;
- the development and functioning of the reproductive organs;
- sexual characteristics and libido;
- the development of personality and higher nervous system functions;
- resistance to disease, and the ability of the body/mind to meet conditions of stress. In addition to their endocrine function, some endocrine glands also produce an exocrine, or external secretion.

Most glandular activity in the endocrine system is controlled by the *pituitary*, which is sometimes called the master gland. The pituitary gland is a small, gray, rounded body attached to the base of the brain by a stalk, which is a downward extension of the brain's third ventricle. The pituitary gland has two distinct parts, the anterior and the posterior, and each secrete different hormones.

The *anterior pituitary* secretes seven different hormones, affecting six different parts of the body. The hormones secreted by the anterior pituitary are:

- growth hormone (*GH*, or somatotropin) which promotes growth and development of muscles, bones and organs;
- thyroid stimulating hormone (*TSH*, or thyrotropin) which stimulates the thyroid gland to produce thyroxine, which regulates body metabolism;
- adreno-corticotropic hormone (*ACTH*) which controls the functions of the adrenal cortex;
- follicle stimulating hormone (*FSH*) which stimulate egg and sperm development of the ovaries and testes;
- luteinizing hormone (*LH*) which, in conjunction with FSH, stimulates secretion of estrogen, ovulation and development inside the ovaries;
- *prolactin* which stimulates the breast to produce milk and induces secretion of progesterone, and
- melanocyte stimulating hormone (*MSH*) which stimulates production of melanin in the skin.

Both the anterior and posterior pituitary are controlled by the *hypothalamus*, which is a small chamber in the brain's third ventricle. This gland directs which hormones are secreted by the anterior pituitary at any particular time, by sending hormone stimulating and releasing chemicals through blood vessels that connect the two glands.

The *posterior pituitary* works differently. The hormones it receives from the hypothalamus travel over nerve fibers that connect the two glands. Then it stores them for later release. The posterior pituitary secretes two hormones:

- oxytocin, which increases the tone and contractions of the smooth uterine muscles during and immediately after labor, and
- vasopressin (also called anti-diuretic hormone, or *ADH*), which stimulates contraction of the smooth muscles of the blood vessels and prevents excessive water loss through the kidneys as urine.

The *thyroid gland* is located in the neck, directly inferior to the larynx, with one lobe on each side of the trachea, and a connecting strip anterior to the trachea between the two lobes. Thyroid functions affect the whole body. Although the thyroid secretes more than one hormone, for clarity the thyroid hormones will be referred to here as *thyroxine* (also called T4), because that hormone is secreted in the largest quantity. Thyroxine stimulates gastrointestinal movement and digestive juice secretion; increases body temperature; increases cellular metabolism (the rate at which energy/calories are burned); increases respiration rate; and stimulates heart rate and output.

The *adrenal glands* are stimulated in response to stress (sympathetic nervous system) and are located at the top of each kidney, each resembling a cap. Each gland has two distinct parts: the cortex (outer layer) and the medulla (inner layer). The adrenal glands are stimulated by ACTH, which is secreted by the anterior pituitary gland. The *adrenal cortex* secretes many steroid hormones, and all are synthesized from cholesterol. They can be classified into three groups:

- mineralocorticoids (the main hormone in this group is *aldosterone*)
- glucocorticoids (the main hormone in this group is *cortisol*, or *hydrocortisone*)
- sex hormones, which include *androgens*, *estrogens* and *progestins*.

Aldosterone acts on the kidney, where it regulates the sodium and potassium balance in the blood. The sex hormones will be discussed in Chapter 11.

Cortisol, or *hydrocortisone*, regulates carbohydrate, lipid, and protein metabolism. It also has an anti-inflammatory action. During prolonged stress, an excess of cortisol can contribute to the spread of infection because the body's normal inflammatory response that barricades the infected area is suppressed. Also, nonpathogenic organisms that normally live in the respiratory tract, the intestines, or on the skin become dangerous when the body's defenses against them are reduced.

Medically, a closely related chemical called *cortisone* is often used to treat non-bacterial inflammatory diseases, such as rheumatoid arthritis, bursitis, and asthma. It can greatly relieve pain, but it only relieves the symptoms, not the cause of the inflammation. Long-term use can cause many side effects, including a puffiness in the face, referred to as a "moon face" appearance, high blood pressure, peptic ulcers, and an electrolyte imbalance that affects the heart. When either cortisone or natural cortisol are present in the body, the overall inflammatory response is suppressed, so symptoms of bacterial or viral infection can go unnoticed until the infection is widespread.

Anabolic steroids, which are closely related to the male sex hormone, *testosterone*, were used at one time by athletes to build muscle tissue. Their use is now illegal because their side effects include serious and sometimes fatal kidney damage, increased risk of heart disease, and development of liver cancer. Other, less serious side effects include increased irritability and aggressive behavior, deepening of voice, growth of facial hair, and diminished sperm production.

The *adrenal medulla* is particularly related to body/mind responses to stress, and secretes three chemicals called catecholamines: 1) norepinephrine, 2) epinephrine, and 3) dopamine.

- *Norepinephrine* is released when the person anticipates stressful events. It constricts the arterioles and venules, which causes an increase in blood pressure and a slowing of the heart.
- *Epinephrine* (also called adrenaline) is released during intense fight or flight situations when additional energy and strength are needed. Epinephrine raises blood pressure, stimulates heart activity, dilates blood vessels in skeletal muscles, dilates the bronchi, diminishes gastrointestinal activity, and causes an increase in blood sugar (glucose) by stimulating the release of glycogen from the liver.
- *Dopamine* is actually a precursor of norepinephrine. It dilates the systemic arteries, increases the heart's output, increases blood flow to the kidneys, and increases urinary output. These three catecholamines are also produced in other parts of the body.

The *parathyroids* are four tiny glands located on the posterior side of the thyroid gland. They secrete *parathormone*, which regulates the level of circulating calcium and phosphate in the blood. Ninety-nine percent of the body's calcium is in its bones, but the remaining one percent must be kept within a narrow, constant range in order for normal blood-clotting, heart muscle contraction/relaxation, and skeletal muscle contraction/ relaxation to be maintained. Whenever the blood calcium level falls, even by a small fraction, parathormone is released and raises the blood calcium level again, mostly by stimulating a release of calcium from the bones. Parathormone can also prevent calcium loss from the kidneys, increase the amount of calcium that is absorbed from the food in the digestive tract, and often is associated with the formation of kidney stones.

The *pancreas* controls the blood sugar (glucose) level by secreting two hormones: insulin and glucagon. These hormones are secreted by different cells within the pancreas, and they work antagonistically (opposite) to each other, like a seesaw. *Insulin* lowers the blood sugar level and *glucagon* raises it. When a meal is eaten, the process of *digestion* changes sugars, starches, and other foods into glucose, which is carried through the blood to the cells of the body, particularly the skeletal muscle and fat cells because they absorb the most energy. Insulin is secreted when the blood sugar level is going up and helps change the glucose in the cells into quick energy for immediate use. Normal blood sugar level is about 90 milligrams (mg) per milliliter (ml) of blood. This is sometimes expressed as 90 mg percent, or, a blood sugar of 90. When exercise or inadequate food intake cause the blood sugar level to fall below normal, the pancreas releases glucagon, which circulates to the liver, where it releases glucose from storage, raising the blood sugar level back to normal.

Abnormally excessive secretion of sex hormones in childhood (before puberty) causes early sexual development. In males, this causes rapid growth of the long bones, but because the bones are not ready, normal height is never attained. In females, this occurrence is rare, because of a built-in feedback mechanism that prevents severe hypersecretion of the sex hormones. Abnormally deficient secretion of sex hormones causes late or no sexual development.

Principle Endocrine Glands

Name	Position	Function	Endocrine Disorders
Thyroid	Two lobes in anterior portion of neck	Influences basal metabolic rate; indirectly influences growth and nutrition	Hypofunction—cretinism in young; myxedema in adult; goiter Hyperfunction— goiter; thyrotoxicosis
Parathy-roid	Four or more small glands near the thyroid	Calcium and phosphorus metabolism; indirectly affects muscular irritability	Hypofunction—tetany Hyperfunction—resorption of bone; renal calculi
Adrenal Cortex	One above each kidney	Steroid hormones regulating carbohydrate metabolism and salt and water balance; some effects on sexual characteristics	Hypofunction—Addison's disease Hyperfunction—adrenogenital syndrome; Cushing's syndrome
Adrenal Medulla	The inner portion of the adrenal gland. It is surrounded by the adrenal cortex	Effects on sympathetic nervous system and carbohydrate metabolism	Hypofunction—almost unknown Hyperfunction—pheochromocytoma
Anterior Pituitary	Small gland at the base of the brain	Influences grown, sexual development, skin pigmentation, thyroid function, adrenocortical function through effects on other endocrine glands (except for growth factor, which acts directly on cells)	Hypofunction—dwarfism in child; decrease in all other endocrine gland functions except parathyroids Hyperfunction—acromegaly in adult; diabetes, gigantism in child
Posterior Pituitary	Attached to the anterior pituitary	Oxytocic factor influencing some aspects of uterine contraction Antidiuretic factor influences absorption of water by kidney tubule	Unknown Hypofunction—diabetes insipidus
Testes and Ovaries	Testes: in the scrotum Ovaries: in the pelvic cavity	Development of secondary sex characteristics; some effect on metabolism	Hypofunction—lack of sex development or regression in adult Hyperfunction—abnormal sex development
Pancreas (endocrine portion)	Abdominal cavity. Head adjacent to duodenum; tail close to spleen and kidney	Secretes insulin and glucagon, which regulate carbohydrate metabolism	Hypofunction—diabetes mellitus Hyperfunction—if a tumor produces excess insulin, hypoglycemia; if excess glucagon, diabetes mellitus

Table 6

ASSESSMENT: OBSERVATION AND PALPATION

Listen closely to the client's description of his/her health experience and read the intake form with your knowledge of the endocrine system in mind. Ask questions to clarify or add to the information the client gives. Observe for fluid retention, menstrual dysfunction, sexual dysfunction, nervousness, fatigue, depression, agitation, hypervigilance, and changes in mood, energy level, sleep pattern, skin, hair, or personal appearance as possible indicators of endocrine problems.

GENERAL CONDITIONS RELATED TO THE ENDOCRINE SYSTEM

The following are definitions and descriptions of general endocrine system findings. Information on more specific endocrine disorders follows in the next section. As a general rule, refer clients with the following findings to a physician for assessment and diagnosis:

- cold, clammy skin
- numbness in fingers, toes, or mouth
- rapid heartbeat
- faintness; dizziness; light-headedness
- open, but painless foot sores
- tremors
- dyspnea
- thyroid nodule
- unusually warm hands and feet
- excessive perspiration
- lethargy; weakness
- unexplained weight loss
- excessive thirst
- excessive urination
- pigment changes in skin or mucous membranes
- recurrent skin, gum, or bladder infections

SPECIFIC ENDOCRINE CONDITIONS

Endocrine dysfunction may result from *hyposecretion*, in which an inadequate amount of the hormone is secreted, or *hypersecretion*, in which excessive amounts of hormones are secreted. As described earlier, endocrine gland secretion may be controlled by the nervous system, by chemical substances in the blood, or, in some cases, by other hormones. Many pathological conditions are the result of, or associated with, the malfunctioning of the endocrine glands. In general, tumors of the endocrine glands produce hypersecretion of hormones (see *Table* on previous page).

Diabetic Crises (see next page for a *Quick Reference Guide*). There are two different kinds of diabetic crises that can occur: 1) when the blood sugar gets critically *high (hyperglycemia)*, and 2) when the blood sugar gets critically *low (hypoglycemia).*

- *Hypoglycemia* (also called *insulin reaction* or *insulin shock*) occurs suddenly if too little food is eaten, if too much insulin is injected, or if too much exercise is done. Hypoglycemia must be treated quickly with a simple sugar, such as juice, sugared soft drink, candy, etc. If untreated, hypoglycemia can lead to unconsciousness. Symptoms of hypoglycemia are feeling cold, clammy, nervous, shaky, weak, and/ or very hungry. Some people also get pale, irritable, or act strangely. If the person becomes unconscious, do not try to get them to swallow food or fluid. Instead, glucagon must be injected. Call 911.

- *Hyperglycemia* (also called *diabetic coma*, in severe cases) occurs more slowly if too much food is eaten or if not enough insulin is taken. Illness, especially infection, and emotional stress can also cause hyperglycemia. In severe hyperglycemia, ketones accumulate in the blood over several hours or days, eventually causing a type of poisoning. Signs and symptoms of severe hyperglycemia include dry mouth, great thirst, loss of appetite, excessive urination, dry and flushed skin, labored breathing, fruity-smelling breath, abdominal pain, vomiting, and eventually unconsciousness. If any of these last six signs are present, immediately get the client to a physician or call 911.

Diabetes Insipidus: This is caused by hypoactivity of the posterior pituitary gland. In the absence or deficiency of anti-diuretic hormone (ADH), water is lost from the kidney, through the urine. Excessive urination (polyuria) results. This excessive water loss can quickly lead to dehydration, however, the body often compensates through producing insatiable thirst. Medical treatment is possible through administration of ADH. Bodywork is indicated and clients are encouraged to maintain contact with a physician to monitor and support health maintenance.

Diabetes Mellitus: This is caused by an absence and/or an ineffectiveness of insulin (a hormone produced by the pancreas), making the blood sugar (glucose) unavailable to the cells for energy. Instead of being used by the cells, the glucose collects in the blood, leading to the high sugar levels (*hyperglycemia*) that are characteristic of untreated diabetes. Untreated and poorly controlled diabetes results in blood vessel and nerve changes throughout the body, which can progress to serious tissue damage and/or death. It is estimated that 14 million Americans have diabetes (approximately 10%). Unfortunately, another estimated six million have diabetes and do not know it.

Approximately 13 million Americans are diagnosed with the most common type of diabetes (*Type II* or *non-insulin dependent*). In this type, the pancreas produces some insulin but either it is not enough or it is not used effectively (or both). People who are over 40, overweight, and have a family history of diabetes are most at risk for this type. In another type of diabetes (*Type I* or *insulin dependent*), the pancreas stops making insulin or makes only a tiny amount. Since insulin is necessary to life, it must be injected into the subcutaneous tissue one or more times every day. This type occurs most often in children and young adults, but it can occur at any age. Regular exercise and a well-balanced diet, low in simple and concentrated sugars, are essential to treatment of all types of diabetes.

There are other types of diabetes, but these are less common: 1) *gestational diabetes* occurs during pregnancy. It usually disappears after the birth although nearly 50% of these women develop diabetes within 5 to 10 years, and 2) *secondary diabetes* is caused by damage to the pancreas from chemicals, certain medicines, or diseases of the pancreas (such as cancer) or other glands. *Impaired glucose tolerance* is when a person's blood sugar falls between "normal" and "diabetic" levels. This condition used to be called *borderline diabetes*, but it is no longer considered a form of diabetes. People with impaired glucose tolerance have an increased risk of developing diabetes.

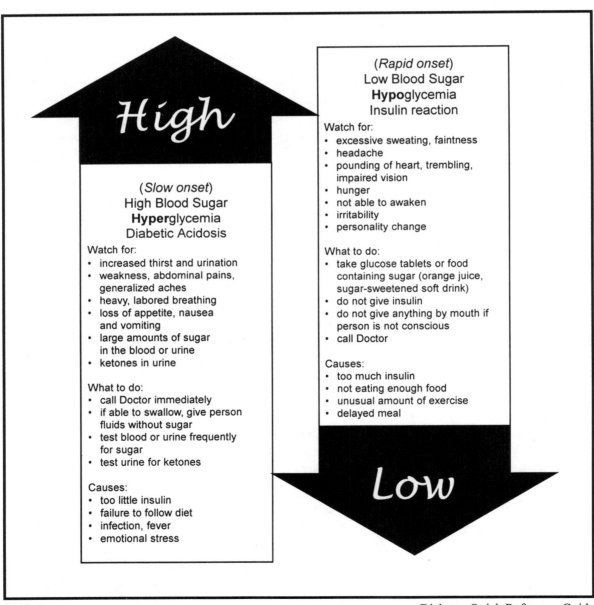

High

(*Slow onset*)
High Blood Sugar
Hyperglycemia
Diabetic Acidosis

Watch for:
- increased thirst and urination
- weakness, abdominal pains, generalized aches
- heavy, labored breathing
- loss of appetite, nausea and vomiting
- large amounts of sugar in the blood or urine
- ketones in urine

What to do:
- call Doctor immediately
- if able to swallow, give person fluids without sugar
- test blood or urine frequently for sugar
- test urine for ketones

Causes:
- too little insulin
- failure to follow diet
- infection, fever
- emotional stress

(*Rapid onset*)
Low Blood Sugar
Hypoglycemia
Insulin reaction

Watch for:
- excessive sweating, faintness
- headache
- pounding of heart, trembling, impaired vision
- hunger
- not able to awaken
- irritability
- personality change

What to do:
- take glucose tablets or food containing sugar (orange juice, sugar-sweetened soft drink)
- do not give insulin
- do not give anything by mouth if person is not conscious
- call Doctor

Causes:
- too much insulin
- not eating enough food
- unusual amount of exercise
- delayed meal

Low

Table 7

The following signs and symptoms are typical in diabetes, although some people with non-insulin dependent diabetes have symptoms so mild that they go unnoticed:

- unusually large amounts of urine (polyuria)
- excessive thirst (polydipsia)
- chronic hunger (polyphagia)
- increased sugar (glucose) in the blood and urine
- dramatic weight loss
- irritability
- weakness and fatigue
- recurring or hard to heal infections in the skin, gums, or bladder
- drowsiness
- blurred vision
- numbness or tingling in hands or feet

The signs and symptoms of diabetes are caused because the body's cells can not get enough glucose to feed their activity, and so the body's fat is burned instead. This often causes weight loss and increases blood lipid (fat) levels, which in turn can lead to atherosclerosis and increased risk of ischemia, thrombus, and embolism formation. These conditions can lead to heart attack, stroke, kidney failure, blindness, poor wound healing, pain, numbness and weakness in the hands and feet (neuropathy), and serious foot sores that develop into gangrene.

Bodywork is indicated if the client's condition has been stable, and you follow these four guidelines:
- avoid working on or near any areas of recent insulin injection
- refer clients with any diabetic symptoms to a physician for assessment
- pay close attention to the client's feet and refer if any open sores are present
- be familiar with the signs of *diabetic crises* and be prepared to stop work and help the person with the appropriate action, if necessary (see *Diabetic Crises*).

Goiter: This is a general term meaning enlargement of the thyroid gland. It can be due to many causes, including: lack of iodine in the diet, thyroid infection, thyroid inflammation (thyroiditis), tumor, hypofunction or hyperfunction of the thyroid. In some cases, the gland can enlarge up to 30 times its normal size. The most common type of goiter occurs in geographic inland areas isolated from salt water, where iodine is not naturally plentiful in the food or water. Since iodine is needed by the thyroid to produce thyroxine, people whose diets are iodine deficient, including the unborn fetuses, often have goiter. Iodized salt can be used to prevent the condition. Bodywork is indicated for people with goiter, but locally contraindicated to the neck area.

Hyperadrenalism or *Cushing's syndrome*: This is results from a hypersecretion of glucocorticoids from the adrenal cortex. The most common cause is overproduction of ACTH by a pituitary tumor, but adrenal tumor and prolonged treatment with cortisone or other adrenocortical hormones will also cause this syndrome. Symptoms include protein loss, increased fatty tissue, fatigue, weakness, osteoporosis, loss of menstrual flow, impotence, edema, excess hair growth, fragile capillaries, and skin discoloration. Also, a rounded "moon face" and hypertension are common. Bodywork is systemically contraindicated unless a physician verifies that the client can tolerate the stimulation.

Hypoadrenalism or *Addison's disease*: This is a hyposecretion of all the adrenocortical hormones and can be caused by infectious disease, hemorrhage, cancer, or under-secretion of ACTH by the anterior pituitary gland. Symptoms include increased pigmentation of skin and mucous membranes, irregular patches of vitiligo, black freckles over the head and neck, weakness, fatigue, nausea, hypotension, vomiting, anorexia, weight loss, and sometimes hypoglycemia. Bodywork is systemically contraindicated unless a physician verifies that the client can tolerate the stimulation.

Hypoglycemia: This is a general term meaning an abnormally low blood sugar (glucose) level and results from either not enough food taken into the body in relation to energy being burned or from too much insulin secretion or administration. Tumor in the pancreas, liver diseases, and hypoadrenalism can also cause hypoglycemia. Mild symptoms include: hunger, fatigue, malaise, nervousness, irritability, sweating, trembling, headache, and tachycardia. There may also be central nervous system problems such as blurred vision, confusion, and weakness. Serious cases can lead to convulsions, and coma (see *Diabetic Crises* page 181). Bodywork is indicated for people with a history of hypoglycemia unless symptoms are currently present, and, in that case, the client is advised and/or assisted to consume food. Gentle bodywork can be resumed if symptoms are mild and easily relieved.

Hyperparathyroidism: This is an excess of the parathyroid hormone (parathormone), most often a result of a benign tumor. This excess causes hypercalcemia (too much calcium in the blood, primarily because it is being pulled from the bones). Kidney stones often result from the excess calcium being filtered in the kidneys, and osteoporosis is also common. Symptoms include muscle weakness, reduced muscle tone, and general hypo-excitability in the nervous system. Bodywork is systemically contraindicated unless a physician verifies that the client can tolerate the stimulation.

Hypoparathyroidism: This is a deficiency of parathyroid hormone (parathormone), most often a result of excessive radiation or accidental surgical removal during thyroid treatment. This deficiency causes hypocalcemia (not enough calcium in the blood). Symptoms include hyperexcitability of the nervous system, hypertonic, and in severe cases, sustained contraction in the skeletal muscles (tetany), which can lead to death by asphyxiation. Bodywork is systemically contraindicated unless a physician verifies that the client can tolerate the stimulation.

Hyperpituitarism: This relates to excessive secretion of any of the hormones of the anterior pituitary gland. The most common cause is a benign tumor. Signs and symptoms are created by whichever hormone is being hypersecreted, plus the tumor may produce headaches and/or visual disturbances. The hormone most frequently involved is growth hormone (GH). If present before puberty, it causes the person to grow very tall, resulting in *gigantism*. If it occurs during adulthood, it causes enlargement of soft tissues, facial, hand and feet bone, and is called *acromegaly*. Bodywork is indicated unless pain is present, and then the client is advised to consult with the physician about his/her present condition, first.

Hypopituitarism: This most commonly involves hyposecretion of the growth hormone, which impedes growth and development in children, causing *dwarfism* and low or no functioning in thyroid, adrenals, and sex glands. Bodywork is indicated unless there is another contraindicating condition present.

Hyperthyroidism: This is an excess of thyroxine, which causes rapid heartbeat, rapid respirations, increased body temperature, intolerance to hot environments, nervousness, excessive perspiration, increased appetite, increased metabolic rate and weight loss. Severe hyperthyroidism is also called *Graves' disease*. Graves' disease is an autoimmune condition in which antibodies to a thyroid antigen stimulate hypersecretion of thyroxine. Graves' disease is sometimes treated with radioactive iodine, which destroys some of the gland, or by surgical removal of the gland. If the gland is removed, thyroxine must be taken daily, as a medicine, for the rest of the person's life. In some cases of untreated Graves' disease, edema occurs in the tissue behind the eyeballs, giving the person a fixed, staring expression and protruding eyeballs. This is called exophthalmos. Bodywork is locally contraindicated for the anterior neck area, but otherwise is indicated for relaxation and body awareness. Refer the client who is having symptoms to a physician for assessment.

Hypothyroidism: This is a deficiency of thyroxine, which causes slow heart rate, slow respirations, decreased body temperature, intolerance to cold environments, decreased appetite, decreased metabolic rate, slow digestion, dry skin and hair, fatigue, and weight gain. If severe hypothyroidism occurs during childhood, cretinism occurs, which produces mental and physical retardation. If it occurs in adulthood, myxedema occurs, which produces swollen, thickened skin, lethargy, slowed mental processes, thick tongue, puffy eyes, and bloated face. Myxedema can be caused by surgical or radiation treatments to correct hyperthyroidism, or it can result from an autoimmune disorder. Bodywork is locally contraindicated to the anterior neck area but otherwise is indicated for relaxation and body awareness. Refer the client who is having symptoms to a physician for assessment.

COMMON EFFECTS OF AGING ON THE ENDOCRINE SYSTEM

Advancing age generally decreases endocrine function. Dysfunctions that are commonly associated with aging include: hypoglycemia, hypothyroidism, hypopituitarism, and hypothermia. Signs and symptoms of these dysfunctions are often overlooked or excused as part of "being old."

CASE PRESENTATIONS

9/28/96: 30 yo female, enlarged thyroid gland
Goal: relaxation & relief of lower back pain (3 on 0-5 scale)
History: Graves' disease; fractured lumbar vertebra 5 yrs ago; recently severe weight loss,

rapid pulse, diarrhea, insatiable thirst; insomnia with long periods of bed rest; taking heart medication; has MD order for massage.

Assessment: enlargement at base of neck, perspiring, hand tremors, nervous & excitable, rapid respirations, no exophthalmos, hypertonic lumbar erectors

Treatment: relaxation massage avoiding pressure around anterior throat; acupressure points held at C5, 3 times for 10 seconds each; reflexology to feet for neck area; effleurage & pressure point work to erector insertions

Outcome: low back pain relieved (0 on 0-5), says feels relaxed

Follow up 2 days later: client slept well night after massage

STUDY QUESTIONS

Which parts of the above case presentations are subjective?

Which parts are objective?

What questions would you have asked that were not asked?

What bodywork techniques would you have done?

What referral(s)?

What other ways could the therapeutic outcome have been evaluated?

How might you have changed the format or way the cases were written?

What were the indications for massage/bodywork?

What were the contraindications?

FURTHER RESOURCES

American Diabetes Association
Diabetes Information Service Center
1660 Duke Street
Alexandria, VA 22314
(800) 232-3472

REFERENCES

Fritz, S. (1995). Mosby's fundamentals of therapeutic massage. St. Louis: Mosby Lifeline.

Jarvis, C. (1992). Physical examination and health assessment. Philadelphia: W. B. Saunders Co.

Kapit, W. & Elson, L.M. (1977). The anatomy coloring book.. NY: Harper & Row.

Kapit, W., Macey, R.I., & Meisami, E. (1987). The physiology coloring book. NY: Harper & Row.

Malasanos, L., Barkauskas, V., & Stoltenberg-Allen, K. (1990). Health assessment. St. Louis, MO: C.V. Mosby Co.

Miller, C. A. (1990). Nursing care of older adults: Theory and practice. Glenview, IL: Little, Brown Higher Education.

Mulvihill, M.L. (1995). Human diseases: A systemic approach (4th ed.) Norwalk, CT: Appleton & Lange.

Newton, D. (1995). Pathology for massage therapists. Portland, OR: Simran Publications.

Sameulson, P. (1994). Pathophysiology for massage: The travel guide. Overland Park, KS: Mid-America Handbooks, Inc.

Thomas, C.L. (1989). Taber's cyclopedic medical dictionary (16th ed.). Philadelphia: F.A. Davis Co.

CHAPTER REVIEW

1. The endocrine glands include the: _____
   _____ (6 glands)

2. The _____ is called the master gland.

3. The hormones secreted by the anterior pituitary are the: _____
   _____
   _____(7 hormones)

4. The anterior pituitary is controlled by the _____

5. The posterior pituitary secretes two hormones: _____
   _____

6. Thyroxine stimulates: _____
   _____

7. During prolonged stress, an excess of _____
   can suppress the body's normal inflammatory response.

8. Anabolic steroids are closely related to the hormone: _____

9. The use of anabolic steroids is illegal because their side effects include: _____
   _____

10. The adrenal glands are controlled by the _____

11. the actions of adrenaline (epinephrine) are: _____
    _____
    _____ (6 actions).

12. The parathyroid glands regulate: _____
    _____

13. Ninety-nine percent of the body's calcium is in its bones, but the remaining one percent is essential to _____
    _____

14. The _____ secretes insulin and glucagon.

15. _____ lowers the blood sugar level and raises it.

16. Normal blood sugar level is about _____

17. In general, refer the following findings to a physician: _____

_____

_____

_____

18. Tumors of the endocrine glands produce _____

ANSWERS TO CHAPTER REVIEW

1. pituitary, thyroid, parathyroid, adrenals, pancreas, & gonads (ovaries and testes)

2. pituitary

3. growth hormone (GH), thyroid stimulating hormone (TSH), adreno-corticotropic hormone (ACTH), follicle stimulating hormone (FSH), luteinizing hormone (LH), prolactin, and melanocyte stimulating hormone (MSH)

4. hypothalamus

5. oxytocin; vasopressin or antidiuretic hormone (ADH)

6. gastrointestinal movement; digestive juice secretion; increases body temperature, cellular metabolism, respiration rate, heart rate and output.

7. cortisol or cortisone

8. testosterone

9. kidney damage, heart disease, liver cancer, aggression, etc.

10. sympathetic nervous system

11. raises blood pressure, stimulates heart activity, dilates blood vessels in skeletal muscles, dilates the bronchi, diminishes gastrointestinal activity, & causes an increase in blood sugar (glucose)

12. the level of circulating calcium and phosphate in the blood

13. blood-clotting, heart muscle contraction/relaxation, and skeletal muscle contraction/relaxation

14. pancreas

15. insulin; glucagon

16. 90

17. cold, clammy skin
    numbness in fingers, toes or mouth
    rapid heartbeat
    faintness; dizziness; light-headedness
    open, but painless foot sores
    tremors
    dyspnea
    thyroid nodule
    unusually warm hands and feet
    excessive perspiration
    lethargy; weakness
    unexplained weight loss
    excessive thirst
    excessive urination
    pigment changes in skin or mucous membranes
    recurrent skin, gum, or bladder infections

18. hypersecretion of hormones

CHAPTER 10

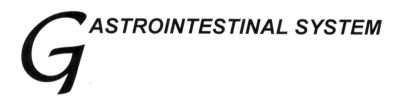

GASTROINTESTINAL SYSTEM

ANATOMY AND PHYSIOLOGY REVIEW

The gastrointestinal system serves two main purposes: 1) it takes in and breaks down the foods we eat into units we can use for energy and regeneration (*digestion*) and 2) it eliminates whatever materials can not be used (*elimination*). These functions take place within a flexible hollow tube that begins at the lips and runs continuously through the center of the body, ending at the anus. This entire tube is made of smooth muscle and lined with mucous membrane, but along the way are highly specialized cells that perform the functions needed at each point in the process. This chapter focuses on all the various parts of the gastrointestinal system, including "the tube" and the organs near it which support its functions.

Digestion is the process by which food is broken down mechanically and chemically and converted into absorbable forms. Salt, the simplest sugars (e.g., glucose), and water can be directly absorbed, but starches, fats, and proteins generally are not absorbable until they are split into smaller molecules. Even table sugar (sucrose) must first be split into glucose and fructose in order to be absorbed.

The path of digestion begins at the *mouth* with chewing (see *Illustration 59*). Chewing is a very important and often overlooked part of the digestive process as it chops the food and moistens it with *saliva* and an *enzyme* (amylase) that immediately begins breaking down *carbohydrates* (starches and sugars). The chopped and moistened food is then swallowed and passes through the *pharynx*. When the food enters the *esophagus*, it begins being moved by the rhythmical, wavelike contractions of the smooth muscle tube, called peristalsis. *Peristalsis* is an involuntary wavelike reflexive movement stimulated by distention of the walls of the tube. The wave consists of contraction of the circular smooth muscle above the distention, with relaxation and opening of the area immediately below the distention. This simultaneous contraction and relaxation causes the contents of the tube to be moved forward. This process goes on day and night when food is present, and a minor amount continues even without the presence of food, moving small amounts of mucus and digestive fluids along the tube. Usually, peristalsis is only interrupted during severe sympathetic stimulation or deep central nervous system anesthesia. Peristalsis occurs in the reverse direction immediately before a person vomits.

As the food leaves the esophagus, it passes through the entry sphincter muscle (called the *cardiac sphincter*) that prevents reflux. *Reflux* is any backward flow of food into the esophagus, after it has entered the *stomach*. The stomach is a saclike pouch in the tube that lies

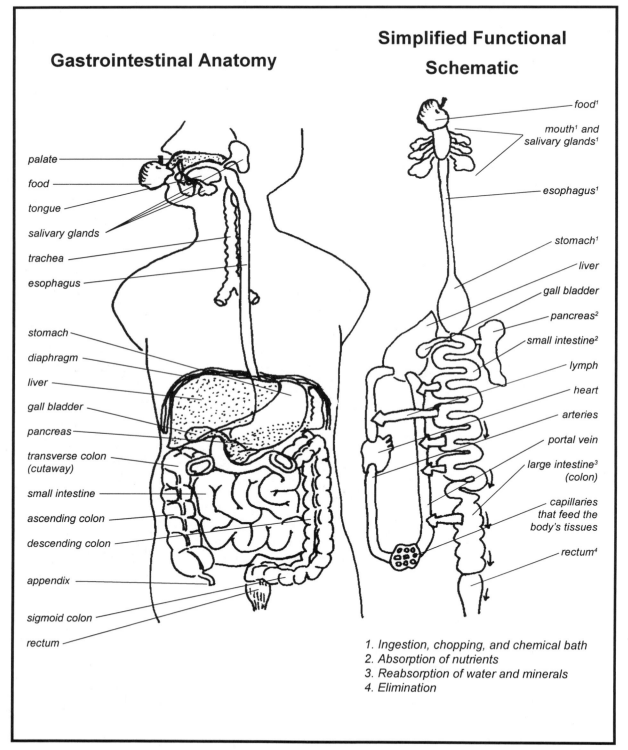

Gastrointestinal Anatomy

palate
food
tongue
salivary glands
trachea
esophagus
stomach
diaphragm
liver
gall bladder
pancreas
transverse colon (cutaway)
small intestine
ascending colon
descending colon
appendix
sigmoid colon
rectum

Simplified Functional Schematic

food[1]
mouth[1] and salivary glands[1]
esophagus[1]
stomach[1]
liver
gall bladder
pancreas[2]
small intestine[2]
lymph
heart
arteries
portal vein
large intestine[3] (colon)
capillaries that feed the body's tissues
rectum[4]

1. Ingestion, chopping, and chemical bath
2. Absorption of nutrients
3. Reabsorption of water and minerals
4. Elimination

Illustration 59

Path of Digestion

inferior to the diaphragm and has walls with several layers of smooth muscle, each running in a different direction, plus a thick mucous membrane layer on the inside. A great deal more moistening and mixing occurs in the stomach. The stomach secretes gastric juice (made of an enzyme [pepsin] and hydrochloric acid) which destroys or neutralizes a large amount of the microbes (bacteria, viruses and parasites) if they are present in the food; provides an intrinsic factor that acts on the vitamin B12 in the food, and provides a highly catalytic and acidic chemical environment that begins the digestion of *proteins*. This chemical mix would be very damaging to the stomach tissues, except that it is lined with a particularly thick mucus covering.

When the food is ready to be moved out of the stomach, nerve and hormonal signals cause relaxation of the exit sphincter of the stomach (called the *pyloric sphincter*) and the food moves into the small intestine. The food/chemical mixture is now in liquid form, and we call it *chyme*. The chyme continues being moved along by peristalsis. The greatest amount of *digestion* occurs in about the first 10 inches of the small intestine (called the duodenum). In the *duodenum*, the chyme mixes with pancreatic juice, intestinal juices, and bile from the liver and gallbladder.

Bile is a thick, bitter-tasting fluid that is produced in the liver and passes into the duodenum as needed. Extra bile is stored in the gallbladder and secreted into the duodenum when fatty foods enter there. Bile contains salts, cholesterol, lecithin, and other substances. It stimulates peristalsis, is an antiseptic (prohibits the growth of microorganisms), is a purgative (laxative), and is an emulsifier of *fats*, meaning it breaks the fats into smaller units, allowing them to be mixed with water. The bile from the liver is straw colored, while that from the gallbladder varies from yellow to brown and dark green.

Bile's action on the fats enables a pancreatic enzyme (lipase) to dissolve them further into small, absorbable nutrients. Other pancreas enzymes (trypsin and amylase) further digest the protein and carbohydrates in the chyme. The intestinal juices complete the chemical changes so that the food nutrients are ready to be absorbed. Bile, pancreatic juice, and intestinal juices neutralize the acidity of the chyme with their alkalinity.

By the time this process is complete, the nutrients have moved past the duodenum and are moving into the *jejunum*, which is another section of the small intestine and is about 9 feet long. The jejunum, in turn, joins the *ileum*, which is about 13-14 feet long, making the total length of the small intestine about 23 feet. As the chyme moves along inside the small intestine, the nutrients and water are gradually absorbed into the capillaries and lymph vessels through the inner surface of the walls. The walls are specially constructed to provide the greatest amount of surface area possible to maximize the absorption of nutrients. This surface presents millions of tiny fingerlike projections (called *villi*) each containing capillaries and lymph vessels through which nutrients and water can be absorbed. The total surface area of the inside of an average adult's small intestine is estimated to be close to 1000 square yards.

The ileum ends in the lower right quadrant of the abdomen, where it joins with the large intestine (also called the *colon*). At this point of junction there is a valve called the *ileocecal valve*, which allows the passage of the chyme into the colon while preventing it from back-flowing into the ileum again. Once inside the colon, the material is called *feces*, or *stool*.

The purpose of the colon is to absorb water and minerals out of the feces so they become progressively firmer as they approach their exit at the anus. The inner surface of the colon is covered with a mucous membrane similar to that found in the rest of the gastrointestinal tube, but without the villi to absorb nutrients. The colon's total length is about 5 feet.

Starting at the ileocecal valve, the first part of the large intestine is called the *cecum*. This is a small pouch-shaped area, and it catches the feces and diverts them upward, into the *ascending colon*. At the inferior part of the cecum is a smaller, fingerlike tube that is about 3-4 inches long. This is the *appendix*, and it catches and stores seeds and other bits of indigestible materials.

The first portion of *ascending colon* extends from the cecum to the undersurface of the liver where it turns to the left and becomes the *transverse colon*. The transverse colon passes horizontally to the left to the region of the spleen where it turns downward and becomes the *descending colon*. The descending colon continues downward on the left side of the abdomen until it reaches the pelvic brim and curves like the letter S, becoming the *sigmoid colon*. The *rectum*, which is immediately anterior to the sacrum, is about 4-5 inches long and passes downward to end in the final part, the *anus*, which is a tight muscular sphincter that opens externally.

Elimination is the process of excreting gastrointestinal waste products (*stool* or *feces*) via the colon. The terms "*defecation*" and "*evacuation of the bowels*" are synonymous with the term elimination. The amount and character of the feces depends on the amount and composition of food ingested. However, even when a person does not eat, s/he will have bowel movements because a large quantity of cellular material is sloughed from the lining of the gastrointestinal tract each day and passes out of the body through the colon. When food is eaten, the food residues cause an urge to defecate when they reach the rectum. Usually, when a person eats a well-balanced diet, drinks approximately one to two liters of fluids, performs a moderate amount of exercise, and heeds his/her natural urge to defecate, s/he can expect to have one or more soft, easy bowel movements every day or two.

Other organs that assist in the process of digestion include the liver, gallbladder, and pancreas. The *liver* is the largest glandular organ of the body, and is located on the right side of the abdomen, inferior to the diaphragm, level with the lower tip of the sternum. The undersurface of the liver is concave and it lies against the stomach, duodenum, colon, and right kidney. It is completely covered with a tough fibrous sheath and has four lobes.

The liver performs many vital jobs including immunologic, metabolic, coagulatory, and digestive functions. The liver's immunologic functions include the filtering and detoxifying the blood by removing and neutralizing bacteria, cellular debris, and foreign particles by means of the phagocytic cells attached to the liver sinus walls. The liver derives its blood supply from the hepatic artery and the portal vein. The portal vein carries the nutrient-rich blood from the absorbing villi of the small intestines directly to the liver. The liver removes the glucose, turns it into glycogen, and then stores it for future energy needs. The liver also uses some glucose to form amino acids, and incorporates amino acids into protein synthesis, including fibrinogen and prothrombin, which are blood components essential for clotting. The liver is the body's source for heparin (an anti-coagulant), albumin, and plasma proteins. It stores vitamins B12, A, D, E and K; is important in fat (lipid) metabolism; plays a vital role in the regulation of blood volume; and is one of the main sources of body heat.

The liver's digestive functions include the secretion of 800 to 1000 ml of bile every 24 hours. The bile leaves the liver through many intrahepatic (intra-liver) passages that converge and empty into the hepatic duct, which converges into the common bile duct that empties into the duodenum. However, the sphincter at the end of the common bile duct ordinarily is closed, forcing the bile to enter the gallbladder, where it is concentrated and stored until needed.

The *gallbladder* is a pear-shaped sac on the undersurface of the right lobe of the liver. The gallbladder stores and concentrates bile by removing water from it. When bile is needed in the small intestine, the gallbladder contracts, and a sphincter in the common bile duct relaxes, permitting the bile to pass into the duodenum.

The *pancreas* is a gland located posterior to the stomach, and anterior to the 1st and 2nd lumbar vertebrae, in a horizontal position, with its head attached to the duodenum and its tail touching the spleen. The area between the head and tail is called the body of the pancreas. The pancreas is made of lobules that form lobes connected by strands of tissue with ducts that lead from the lobules into the main pancreatic duct, which then connects with the duodenum. The pancreas produces both an external and an internal secretion. The external secretion, called pancreatic juice, passes through the pancreatic duct into the duodenum, where it assists digestion (see duodenum, above). The internal secretion is produced by differentiated masses of cells scattered throughout the gland, called "the islets of Langerhans." These internal secretions include the hormones insulin and glucagon (see *Chapter 9*).

EFFECTS OF DIET ON HEALTH

The term *nutrition* includes all the processes involved in taking in and using food, so that the growth, repair, and maintenance of the body can occur. This process includes ingestion, digestion, absorption, and metabolism. *Malnutrition* literally means "bad nutrition," and includes both undernutrition and overnutrition. Again, in diet there is presently no theory that holds true for all people at all times. The USDA food pyramid is one model of a healthful diet (see *Illustration*), but many other valuable models, or theories, are available, as well. Despite much controversy, many nutritionists agree that most Americans consume too much

Food Pyramid: A Guide to Healthy Eating
Source: U.S. Department of Agriculture and
the U.S. Department of Health and Human Services

red meat, fat, refined sugars, sodium, preservatives, and additives, and too few fresh vegetables, fruits, whole grains, pure water, and fiber.

Depending on the expert consulted, somewhere between 50 and 100 nutrients are needed to maintain human health. The major groups of nutrients are *protein, carbohydrates* (which include starches and sugars), *fats* (also called lipids), *vitamins, minerals, water,* and *fiber.* Some nutrients are capable of being stored in the body and drawn upon when food intake is insufficient, but most nutrients are needed every day or two. Deficiencies in nutrients can occur from poor diet, poor digestion, poor absorption of the nutrients through the intestinal walls and into the blood, loss of nutrients from diarrhea, and increased demands on the body during illness, trauma, stress, smoking, chronic exposure to pollution, pregnancy, and growth.

PROTEINS

Proteins occur naturally in animal tissues and in many plants. Proteins are a source of heat and energy for the body. When digested, proteins yield *amino acids*, which are essential for the growth, maintenance, and repair of human tissues. Amino acids form an essential part of the protoplasm of every cell in the body. Different numbers and kinds of amino acids are present in different foods. The average adult woman needs about 40-45 grams of protein per day, and the average adult man needs about 50-60 grams.

Protein is considered "complete" when all ten essential amino acids are present. In general, animal proteins, as found in eggs, meat, poultry, fish, cheese, and milk are complete, and plant proteins are incomplete (do not have all ten amino acids). However, when a variety of vegetable protein sources is eaten, the body gets all the essential amino acids during the course of the day. When a variety of vegetable proteins are eaten in the same meal, there is a significant increase in the amount of usable protein. To accomplish this, the most common vegetable protein combinations are:

- grains (rice, corn, wheat, barley, etc.) + legumes (peas, beans, lentils)
- grains + dairy products (milk, cheese, yogurt, etc.)
- seeds (sesame or sunflower) + legumes

Children and people who are pregnant, breast-feeding, healing wounds, or under excessive stress need more protein than usual. In general, protein needs decrease as people get older, and elderly people need less than the "average" adult. Excess protein intake can result in decreased calcium absorption and increased nitrogen excretion in the urine.

CARBOHYDRATES

Carbohydrates are a group of nutrients that include sugars, starches, and fibers. Common sources of carbohydrates are whole grains and grain products (pasta, bread, crackers, crusts, etc.), vegetables, fruits, legumes, honey, and sugar. Alcohol, sugar, pop, and candy are called "empty" sources, because there are no vitamins, minerals, or essential amino acids in these foods.

Carbohydrates are present in digestible and indigestible forms. The forms that are not digestible (called *insoluble* fiber), are beneficial in adding bulk to the chyme and feces. This helps stimulate peristalsis and bowel movement and helps reduce the risk of colon cancer. Common sources of insoluble fiber are the whole-grain foods, wheat bran, fruits, and vegetables.

Soluble fibers, which do digest, are found in legumes, oat bran, whole grains, fruits, and vegetables. Soluble fibers help the body keep the cholesterol balanced, keep blood sugar at a more even level, and add some bulk to the chyme and feces. Freezing foods causes some breakdown of fiber. Grinding and cooking cause more. Drying fruits (such as raisins, prunes, figs, etc.) does not affect the fiber content.

The World Health Organization recommends a daily intake of 30 to 35 grams of fiber. The average American diet provides only about half of that. The American Dietetic Association recommends that at least 5-9 grams per day be the soluble type. The main symptom of fiber deficiency is constipation, and chronic fiber deficiency can be a risk factor for colon cancer. Excess intake of fiber can produce loose stools.

If given adequate chewing time, the body is able to digest and absorb certain sugars and starches in the mouth, by the action of the saliva. The other sugars and starches, and the soluble fibers, are digested and absorbed in the small intestine, where they are broken down into their most simple form, *glucose*. Glucose is used by the body for heat and energy. Glucose is made of only carbon, hydrogen, and oxygen molecules, and is the most abundant organic chemical compound on earth.

FATS

Fats occur naturally in many foods, and are essential nutrients for human health. Fat provides insulation, padding, and a stored supply of energy for emergency use. However, fats are higher in Calories than proteins and carbohydrates, and saturated fats contribute to too much cholesterol in the blood.

Cholesterol is made in the liver and ingested through animal products, such as meat and dairy. Cholesterol is what makes up most of the atherosclerotic plaques that block arteries. However, cholesterol is not a fat. It is an alcohol (sterol) material. The large size of the cholesterol molecule gives it a solid, waxy characteristic. In addition to being a major component of bile, it is also a precursor for the adrenal corticoid and sex hormones.

An elevated blood cholesterol level is a risk factor for coronary artery disease. Total blood cholesterol is primarily made up of low-density lipoproteins (LDLs), which carry large fatty particles, and high-density lipoproteins (HDLs), which are smaller and which help carry fat and cholesterol to the liver for reprocessing, thus reducing the amount of circulating fat. After the age of 30, the desirable total cholesterol level is 200 mg/dl or less. However, having a high LDL ratio can still increase risk of coronary artery disease and atherosclerosis. A desirable ratio between total cholesterol level and HDL is 4.5, which is figured by dividing the total cholesterol level by the HDL. For example, if the total cholesterol level is 200 mg/dl, and the HDL is 45 mg/dl, divide 200 by 45. This turns out to be 4.4; within desirable range.

A *calorie* is a unit of heat that can be equated to work or energy. Nutritional calories are measured in kilocalories, identified with a capital C. Protein and carbohydrates supply 4 Calories per gram and fats supply 9 Calories per gram. Normal caloric intake for an average adult male between 23 and 50 years old is approximately 2700 Calories per day, with 8.3% (56 grams) of that coming from protein sources, 62% coming from carbohydrates, and no more than 30% coming from fats. Normal caloric intake for an average adult female between 23 and 50 years old is 2000 Calories per day, with 8.8% (44 grams) of that coming from protein sources, 61% coming from carbohydrates and no more than 30% coming from fats.

Caloric needs increase with pregnancy, lactation, trauma, stress, exercise, and certain illnesses, and decrease with a sedentary lifestyle, age, and certain illnesses. The most health-producing diet is to eat a variety of fresh foods that you enjoy, in about the same amounts each day, avoiding highly sweet, fat, or salty foods. Yo-yo dieting (losing then gaining weight again) is harmful and should be avoided.

VITAMINS

There are four *fat-soluble vitamins: A, D, K and E*. The fat-soluble vitamins are stored in the body's fat tissues, so supplies are built slowly and depleted slowly. With the exception of Vitamin E, these vitamins can build up to toxic levels. Vitamins A, D, E, and C (C is not fat soluble) are considered anti-oxidants. *Anti-oxidants* have electrons that bind to the free-radical molecules in your body. Free radicals are atoms or groups of atoms that can cause damage to the body's cells and possibly lead to immune system impairment and degenerative diseases. A diet rich in anti-oxidants helps certain enzymes in the body act as free radical scavengers, keeping oxidation in check.

Vitamin A deficiency can cause decreased vision at night and, if severe, causes complete blindness. This is the leading cause of blindness in the world. Vitamin A is plentiful in dark green leafy vegetables (e.g., chard, kale, spinach, etc.) and dark orange vegetables (e.g., carrots, winter squashes, etc.). In foods, Vitamin A is derived from beta-carotene. In vitamin supplements, Vitamin A can be toxic and/or cause birth defects if taken at doses of 15,000 IU or more per day. Symptoms of Vitamin A toxicity include headache, gastrointestinal upset, pain, and liver and blood abnormalities. Beta-carotene has not been found to be toxic at any dose because the body only converts it to Vitamin A as it is needed. Excess beta-carotene sometimes causes a yellowing of the skin that is different from jaundice, in that it does not affect the sclera (whites) of the eyes or the mucous membranes.

Vitamin D deficiency causes malabsorption of calcium, which leads to calcium deficiency, which leads to weak bones, osteoporosis, clotting problems, and poor muscle and nerve function. Vitamin D is available as an additive to most milks purchased in the grocery stores, and in many vitamin supplements. Symptoms of Vitamin D toxicity include digestive upset, excessive thirst and urination, weakness, nervousness, and high blood calcium levels, with development of calcium deposits in the soft tissues. The human body manufactures adequate Vitamin D if the person gets at least 20 minutes of sunlight per day, at least five days per week.

Vitamin K deficiency causes prolonged bleeding time and contributes to easy bruising. In the U.S., deficiency is usually caused by liver disease, alcoholism, chronic use of anti-coagulant drugs, or persistent diarrhea. Vitamin K is available in foods from dark green leafy vegetables and in many vitamin supplements.

Vitamin E is available in foods from whole grains, wheat germ and fish oils, dark green leafy vegetables, nuts, seeds, eggs, sweet potatoes, legumes, and in many vitamin supplements. Vitamin E is a potent anti-oxidant and is needed for tissue maintenance, tissue repair, blood clotting, and many other normal functions. At this time, no deficiency and no toxicity levels are known.

There are seven *water-soluble vitamins: C, B1, B2, B3, B6, B12*, and *folic acid*. These vitamins are balanced by the body continuously, and excess intakes are excreted daily through the urine and feces. Therefore, toxicity is rare. However, heat and dehydration greatly decrease the water-soluble vitamin content of foods, and cooking with water causes the vitamins to transfer from the food to the water. *Vitamin C* deficiency causes poor wound healing, fragile capillaries (which leads to easy bruising and bleeding), susceptibility to infection, and poor collagen formation. Vitamin C is also required for iron absorption, so a Vitamin C deficiency can contribute to anemia. Smokers require up to 10 times more Vitamin C intake to maintain normal levels. Vitamin C is available in foods in fresh fruits and vegetables, especially the highly acidic ones (see chart).

Most of the B vitamins are required for carbohydrate metabolism, healthy nerve function, and muscle tone. Deficiencies, therefore, are noticed in symptoms of fatigue, lack of energy, and feeling stressed. The B vitamins are available in fresh, whole grains; liver; eggs; and processed grain foods that have been enriched with the B vitamins (read the labels). They are also available in many vitamin supplements and will cause the urine to be bright yellow when taken as a supplement.

Vitamin B1 (thiamine) deficiency contributes to muscle weakness, nervous system problems, and decreased acuity in the four senses. *Vitamin B2 (riboflavin)* deficiency contributes to pain and cracks at the corner of the mouth, inflamed tongue and gums, and skin and cornea lesions. Severe deficiency can contribute to bone marrow malfunction and anemia. *Vitamin B3 (niacin)* deficiency contributes to skin hypersensitivities (dermatitis), diarrhea, and mental confusion. When taken as an immediate release vitamin supplement, niacin causes rapid vasodilation, resulting in a temporary drop in blood pressure and a hot, flushed experience. *Vitamin B6 (pyridoxine)* is essential to protein and fat metabolism. Deficiency contributes to dermatitis, sore tongue and mouth, diarrhea, anemia, muscle weakness, and decreased acuity of the senses. *Vitamin B12* is essential for nervous system and bone marrow functions. It is abundant in meat, eggs, dairy products, and tempeh. Deficiency contributes to muscle weakness, anemia, sore tongue, diarrhea, fatigue, and sensory and motor problems. Severe deficiency causes *pernicious anemia*, which is common among people who do not eat any meat and those whose stomachs lack "intrinsic factor," a chemical required for Vitamin B12 absorption. *Folic acid* is essential for red blood cell production and normal fetal development. Deficiency causes problems similar to those listed for Vitamin B12.

Water is an essential and often overlooked nutrient. Our bodies are approximately 2/3 water, and we need approximately one and one-half liters of fresh, pure water each day; more if we have a fever, are vomiting, having diarrhea, are in a hot or windy environment, or are taking certain drugs. Symptoms of deficiency include dry mouth, eyes, and skin, small urine output, and constipation. Symptoms of over-hydration (water intoxication) include drunken-like behavior, electrolyte imbalance, and, in some cases, dyspnea.

MINERALS

Minerals are essential for many of the body's musculoskeletal, cardiovascular, immune, and nervous system functions. Some experts list 70 major and trace minerals as essential for health. Some of the major minerals are calcium, potassium, manganese, chloride, magnesium, phosphorus, and sodium. Excess minerals are normally excreted through the urine and feces, however, many diseases can cause mineral imbalances that result in excess or deficiency. The functions of some of the minerals are described in the following paragraphs.

Calcium deficiency can be caused by not ingesting enough calcium, by a malfunctioning parathyroid gland, by inadequate Vitamin D, by poor intestinal absorption, or by liver or kidney disease. A calcium deficiency first causes the body to pull calcium from the bones to maintain the delicate calcium blood balance. When calcium is pulled from the bones, they become weaker and more porous. Severe calcium deficiency causes muscle weakness and cramping (tetany), depression, exhaustion, and irregular heartbeat. Calcium is vital to the formation of strong bones and teeth, a regular heartbeat, normal muscle contraction, blood clotting, and the transmission of nerve impulses. Good sources of calcium include dairy products, orange juice fortified with calcium, collard greens, sardines, tahini, bok choy, kale, broccoli, tofu, and corn tortillas (see box about calcium requirements and sources).

Potassium deficiency can be caused by inadequate intake, use of laxatives or diuretics (including many blood pressure medications), vomiting, and diarrhea. Symptoms include muscle weakness and, potentially, heart failure. Potassium helps the body maintain stable blood pressure, transfer nutrients into the cells, and transmit electrochemical impulses. Good sources of potassium include dairy foods, fish, fruits, legumes, meat, poultry, vegetables, nuts, and whole grains.

Magnesium deficiency can be caused by inadequate intake, chronic diarrhea, consumption of alcohol, diuretics, and large amounts of fats and foods that are high in oxalic acid (such as almonds, chard, spinach, cocoa, rhubarb, and tea), which interferes with magnesium absorption. However, magnesium is so widely distributed in foods that deficiency is rare. It is abundant in whole grains, fruits, and vegetables. Magnesium helps to regulate body temperature, neuromuscular contraction, and synthesis of protein. Symptoms of deficiency are similar to those produced by calcium deficiency, including severe muscle contractions, exhaustion, and depression.

Iron deficiency can be caused by intestinal bleeding, excessive menstrual bleeding, insufficient hydrochloric acid in the stomach, prolonged use of antacids, ulcers, excess coffee or tea intake, and prolonged illnesses. Iron deficiency also contributes to *anemia* (see *Specific Conditions*). Iron is essential for the production of hemoglobin, as well as many enzymes. It is important for immune health and energy production. Symptoms of deficiency are brittle hair, hair loss, nails that are spoon-shaped or have ridges running lengthwise, fatigue, pallor, and dizziness. Iron is abundant in eggs, fish, liver, meat, poultry, green leafy vegetables, raisins, prunes, soybeans, seaweeds, whole grains, and enriched breads and cereals. Iron excess has been linked to higher risks for developing heart attacks and some cancers so, in general, healthy adults should not take iron supplements, unless they are pregnant, have had a large loss of blood, or are elderly.

Iodine is needed only in trace amounts, but it is essential to thyroxine synthesis by the thyroid gland (see chapter 9), helps to metabolize excess fat, and is important in physical and mental development. Deficiency most often results from inadequate intake. Good sources for iodine are iodized salt, seafood, salt-water fish, and seaweeds, including kelp, wakame, etc.

Zinc deficiency can contribute to poor wound healing, acne, white dots in the nailbeds, and a decreased sense of taste. Zinc is essential for the growth and function of the reproductive glands, maintenance of a healthy immune system, protein synthesis, collagen formation, and the healing of wounds. Good sources are fish, legumes, meats, poultry, seafood, seeds, and whole grains.

Copper is essential for normal development of red and white blood cells, bone, elastin, and collagen. It is involved in wound healing, energy production, hair and skin coloring, and taste sensitivity. Good sources are almonds, avocados, barley, beans, beets, broccoli, greens, lentils, liver, nuts, oranges, oats, raisins, seafood, and soybeans. It is not usually necessary to take copper supplements, and should be done with caution in small amounts, if at all.

ASSESSMENT: OBSERVATION AND PALPATION

Listen closely to the client's description of his/her health experience and read the intake form with your knowledge of diet and the gastrointestinal system in mind. Listen to any stories about eating patterns and/or gastrointestinal discomforts. Ask questions to clarify or add to the information the client gives. Observe the overall height, weight, and frame and the condition of the teeth, skin, hair, and nails.

Avoid abdominal palpation or bodywork when abdominal pain, discomfort, diarrhea, or inflammation are reported. Otherwise, when palpating the abdomen, hard stool may be detected anywhere within the intestines, and most frequently in the area of the descending colon (left side of the abdomen). Hard stool will feel firm and resistant, similar to the way a tumor might feel. An area where people often have a stool residue is at the ileo-cecal junction, on the abdomen's lower right quadrant. This area can benefit from massage within the client's comfort.

A particular and unique finding is *rebound tenderness*, which is tenderness felt at the end of deep palpation, as the hand is lifted off the area (and not felt when the hand is pressing the area). Presence of this finding may be indicative of appendicitis and the client should be referred to a physician for assessment.

GENERAL CONDITIONS RELATING TO THE GASTROINTESTINAL SYSTEM

The following are definitions and descriptions of general gastrointestinal findings. Information on more specific gastrointestinal disorders follows in the next section. As a general rule, refer clients with the following findings to a physician for assessment and diagnosis:

- history of persistent or recurring nausea or vomiting
- acute or persistent chronic abdominal pain
- rebound tenderness
- epigastric pain one to three hours after meals
- an unusually rigid or board-like abdomen
- blood in stools or vomit
- difficulty swallowing
- abdominal masses or nodules
- mouth, tongue, or lip lesions
- soft protrusions through the abdominal wall
- significant obesity or thinness
- chronic fatigue or lack of energy

SPECIFIC DIETARY AND GASTROINTESTINAL CONDITIONS

Diseases of the gastrointestinal tract are caused by a wide variety of factors. Tumors or malformations can produce obstruction, the mucous membrane lining can become inflamed and ulcerated, and cells can fail in their functions of secreting digestive juices or absorbing nutrients. Abdominal bodywork should always be avoided when pain, tenderness, or diarrhea are present.

Adhesions, abdominal: An adhesion is a fibrous band, usually caused by inflammation, trauma, and/or surgery, that holds parts together that are normally separated. Abdominal adhesions occur around and between loops of the intestine, sometimes causing partial or complete obstruction. When an obstruction blocks the intestine, the pressure inside the intestine compresses the local arteries and results in bowel ischemia. Bodywork is indicated locally only if no pain or tenderness are present.

Anorexia nervosa: This is a condition characterized by an extreme lack of eating, sometimes accompanied by voluntary vomiting, use of diuretics, or laxatives. It occurs most often in young women between the ages of 12 and 20, but it can also occur in young men and adults. The person usually has a problem with self-esteem and intense fear of becoming fat. She often sees herself as fat, even as she gets extremely thin. These are complicated situations that often require help from a mental health professional. Bodywork is indicated unless there is capillary fragility (a common condition, evidenced by bruising) or some other condition for which bodywork is contraindicated.

Appendicitis: This is inflammation of the appendix, which is located in the lower right abdomen. Signs and symptoms often begin with pain or discomfort in the umbilical area, followed by nausea, vomiting, swelling, and tension in the abdomen. The discomfort gradually moves to the lower right abdomen, and fever develops. A common sign is rebound tenderness (area hurts when palpated pressure is released). When severely inflamed, the appendix can burst, causing peritonitis, a serious bacterial infection that is potentially fatal if untreated.

Blood in a stool: This can be a sign of colon cancer, particularly if it is dark red. More common but less serious causes of rectal bleeding are hemorrhoids, anal fissures, and benign polyps. These typically cause small amounts of bright red blood. Bodywork is only contraindicated locally to the abdomen if pain, tenderness, or diarrhea are present, however the client should be referred to a physician for assessment.

Bulimia: This is a condition characterized by an insatiable appetite, followed by voluntary vomiting, fasting, or inducing diarrhea. Sometimes this is called a binge-purge cycle. It occurs most often in young women but can also occur in young men and adults. Like anorexia, the person usually has low self-esteem and an intense fear of becoming overweight. The binge-purge activity can lead to severe upper gastrointestinal damage. Bodywork is indicated unless there is capillary fragility or another condition for which bodywork is contraindicated.

Celiac Disease: This is a malabsorption syndrome characterized by diarrhea, malnutrition, abdominal pain, weight loss, bleeding tendency, and hypocalcemia. It is caused by a hypersensitivity to the protein in wheat, barley, rye, and oats. Bodywork is indicated for relaxation and body awareness but locally contraindicated to the abdomen if pain or tenderness are present.

Cholecystitis: This is inflammation of the gallbladder. It can be acute or chronic. In the acute form, the gallbladder swells and can decay or rupture. Symptoms include severe steady pain in the upper right abdomen area that refers to the right shoulder. There may also be fever, nausea, and weakness. In the chronic form, the gallbladder walls thicken and become scarred. Symptoms include intermittent upper right abdominal pain, nausea, vomiting, and intolerance of fatty foods. Bodywork is contraindicated to the abdomen whenever pain or tenderness are present.

Cholelithiasis (gallstones): Gallstones are solidified masses formed in the gallbladder or its ducts. The most common type is formed from cholesterol when the bile contains more cholesterol than can be kept in solution. Gallstones most often occur in women over forty who are overweight and have given birth to several children. Diabetes mellitus is also a risk factor. There may be few signs or symptoms until a gallstone enters the bile duct. Then there can be nausea and/or severe, intermittent abdominal pain that refers to the right scapula. Bodywork is indicated unless pain or tenderness are present, then avoid abdominal work and refer the client to a physician for assessment.

Cirrhosis: This is a generalized pathology of the liver with enlargement and infiltration of the lobes with fibrous tissue and nodules. These changes are accompanied by impaired liver function and can progress to complete liver failure. Symptoms include abdominal swelling, jaundice, weakness, weight loss, anorexia, nausea, and mild fever. As the disease progresses, the portal blood from the small intestines is forced to find new channels, causing the superficial abdominal veins to enlarge and causing hemorrhoids and esophageal varices. In the U.S. alcoholism is the main cause of cirrhosis. However, it can occur in people with no history of alcoholism. Other causes occur in relation to use of toxic substances, infectious hepatitis, metabolic disorders, heart disease, bile duct obstruction, or a complication of intestinal bypass surgery. Bodywork is contraindicated to the abdomen unless a physician has verified that the client can tolerate gentle work.

Colitis: This is a general term for inflammation of the colon. There are several types:

- *Traveler's diarrhea* is transmitted through contaminated water bearing *E. coli* bacteria or other pathogen.
- *Food poisoning* is usually caused by salmonella or shigella, which grow in warm moist conditions, especially in poultry, eggs, and dairy products.
- *Dysentery* can be caused by viral, bacterial, or parasitic pathogens and is highly contagious. Symptoms are abdominal pain and severe watery and/or bloody diarrhea.
- *Ulcerative colitis* is a general term with an unknown etiology that produces serious inflammation and ulceration of the bowel with watery stools, mucous, pus, fever, and potential for perforation and hemorrhage.
- *Irritable bowel syndrome* is a malfunction of the peristalsis in the large and small intestines. The cause is unknown, but it is affected by stress, food allergies, and drug allergies. Stools alternate between constipation and diarrhea, and the person may have bloating, gas, nausea, fatigue, and headache.

Bodywork is contraindicated to the abdomen for all types of colitis. Refer symptomatic clients to a physician for assessment.

Colon Cancer: This is very common in the U.S. and is related to risk factors of genetics, a high fat, low fiber diet; and/or chronic constipation. The size and location of the cancer will have a great effect on the symptoms the client experiences. Symptoms may be unnoticed until the cancer is advanced, but include: change in bowel habits or stool size, blood in stool, cramps, weakness, malaise, and weight loss. Colon cancer is especially prevalent in men over age 40. It is often curable if treated early (see *Chapter 12*).

Constipation: This is when stools are hard, dry, or difficult to pass. The most common cause is when a person does not eat a well-balanced diet, drink approximately one to two liters of fluids, perform a moderate amount of exercise each day, and/or heed her/his natural urge to defecate. Other common causes of constipation include intestinal obstruction, tumors, excessive use of laxatives, weakness (atonus) of intestinal smooth muscle, and use of certain drugs. A change in frequency of bowel movements can be a sign of serious intestinal or colonic disease. Always refer clients with such changes to a physician for assessment. Bodywork is locally beneficial to the abdomen for the condition of constipation unless pain or tenderness is present.

Crohn's Disease (Regional Enteritis; Regional Ileitis): This is inflammation of the small intestine (specifically the ileum), which becomes inflamed and ulcerates. The etiology is unknown, but research indicates that there is probably some genetic predisposition and that some infectious organism or something in the diet triggers the inflammatory process. The affected portion becomes thick, rigid, and edematous, and the passageway becomes progressively narrowed. The lymph glands enlarge, and the adjacent mesentery becomes thickened. Crohn's is most often found in the terminal end of the ileum, but it can spread to other parts of the bowel and to the cecum. Adhesions may form. Pain is centered around the umbilicus and right lower abdomen. The abdomen may swell, and there may be diarrhea alternating with constipation. Other symptoms include vomiting, abdominal cramps, and fever. Crohn's is a chronic illness with remissions and exacerbations. Avoid abdominal work unless the disease is in remission.

Diarrhea: This is when stools are frequent, unformed, and/or watery. The most common causes are excess fiber or spice in diet causing inflammation or irritation of the intestinal mucosa; gastrointestinal infection; certain drugs; and psychogenic (mental/emotional) factors. Bodywork is locally contraindicated to the abdomen in people who have had diarrhea that day. Refer clients who communicate distress or concern about their bowel movements to a physician or other qualified health care provider.

Diverticulitis: This is diverticulosis with inflammation. It can be acute or chronic. The acute form is an emergency, with symptoms and treatment similar to acute appendicitis. Symptoms of the chronic form include progressive constipation, recurring intermittent abdominal pain, and/or blood in stools. Sometimes diverticulitis leads to bacterial infection. Refer clients with any of these symptoms to a physician for assessment and avoid abdominal work.

Diverticulosis: This is a sac or pouch in the wall of the stomach, small intestine, or large intestine. Usually more than one will be present. The pouches can trap undigested material as it passes by, but they are usually asymptomatic unless they become inflamed (see diverticulitis). Bodywork is locally contraindicated only if pain or tenderness are present.

Esophageal Varices: This is varicose veins in the esophagus, and is associated with chronic alcoholism. There will usually be other physical dysfunctions occurring because of the alcoholism. Bodywork is locally contraindicated to the abdomen but otherwise is indicated for relaxation and body awareness if the physician verifies that there are no other problems that prevent the client from tolerating the stimulation.

Esophagitis: This is inflammation of the esophagus. It often occurs as a result of gastric reflux (flow of stomach contents into the esophagus), bulimia, or chronic vomiting from any cause. Bodywork is indicated for relaxation and body awareness. Advise symptomatic clients to consult a physician for assessment.

Gastritis: This is inflammation of the stomach. It can be acute or chronic. The etiology is unknown, but it seems to be associated with irritants, e.g., alcohol, aspirin, acidic or spicy food, stress, poisoning, and/or bacteria in the stomach. An excess or deficiency of hydrochloric acid is sometimes related. Symptoms include gastric pain or tenderness, nausea, vomiting, and atrophic or hypertrophic changes in the gastric mucosa. Bodywork is indicated for relaxation and body awareness. Avoid the gastric area if pain or tenderness are present.

Hepatitis: This is inflammation of the liver caused by a virus. There are three types, and all have similar symptoms, that include loss of appetite, fever, chills, nausea and vomiting, headache, tenderness in the liver area, jaundice, dark urine, and itching.

- *Hepatitis A*, formerly called infectious hepatitis, is transmitted via the oral route through food that is contaminated with fecal material, water, and under-cooked shellfish. Symptoms develop between two and six weeks after contact with the virus. It is communicable for one week before and two weeks after the onset of symptoms, usually affects children under the age of 15, and causes no permanent liver damage. Vaccination is available to prevent developing this disease.
- *Hepatitis B* is transmitted by blood and body fluids. Vaccination is available to prevent this disease.
- *Hepatitis C* is also transmitted by blood and body fluids. No vaccination is available in 1996, but one is expected in the next few years (also see chapter 8). Bodywork is locally contraindicated to the abdomen due to liver enlargement and fragility.

Hernia: This is a protrusion or projection of an organ or a part of an organ through the wall of the cavity that normally contains it. It is synonymous with the word "*rupture*." Common types of hernias include: *abdominal*, in which small intestine protrudes through the muscular abdominal wall; *femoral*, in which small intestine descends through the ring of femoral muscle; *hiatal*, in which the stomach protrudes upward through the opening of the diaphragm into the mediastinal cavity (see illustration); *incisional*, in which some soft tissue protrudes through a surgical scar; *inguinal*, in which the small intestine protrudes through the inguinal opening (these account for about 80% of all hernias); and *umbilical*, in which small intestine protrudes through the navel (this is seen mostly in children). *Hiatal hernia* can cause severe heartburn and difficulty in deep

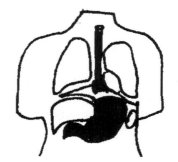

Illustration 61 Hiatal Hernia

breathing. Bodywork is contraindicated within an hour after a meal unless the client is positioned upright (such as seated). Prone and supine positions after a meal will aggravate the hiatal hernia condition. Massage is otherwise indicated for relaxation and body awareness.

Lactose Intolerance: This is an intolerance to milk, characterized by abdominal bloating, gas, nausea, constipation, and/or cramps after ingestion of dairy products. It is caused by a deficiency of the enzyme lactase, which is essential to the digestion of lactose (milk sugar) in the gastrointestinal tract. This deficiency can be present at birth or acquired as an adult. Bodywork is locally contraindicated only if abdominal pain or tenderness are present.

Liver Cancer: This is the most common gastrointestinal cancer and it is often a site of metastasis from other sites and so it is often fatal. Clients may have pain, nausea, vomiting, enlargement of the abdomen due to the presence of extra fluid, edema in the lower legs, and jaundice. They may itch severely and may have an unpleasant body odor that is not removed by bathing. Mental confusion may come and go, and eventually the person may slip into unconsciousness (see *Chapter 12*).

Malabsorption Syndrome: This is disordered or inadequate absorption of nutrients from the small intestine. The person eats, but the small intestine does not absorb the nutrients. It can be associated with or due to a number of diseases including those affecting the intestinal mucosa as infections, tropical sprue, gluten intolerance, pancreatic insufficiency, lactose intolerance, or the effects of surgery or antibiotic therapy. Bodywork is indicated for relaxation and body awareness. Avoid work to the abdomen if pain or tenderness are present.

Obesity is an abnormal amount of fat in the body. This term is usually used when a person's weight is 20% above average for his/her age, sex, and height. Obesity results from an imbalance between the calories ingested and the calories burned, but the underlying factors can be complex and difficult to treat. When obesity is severe, it can limit the person's ability to perform activities of daily living, including basic movements and respiration. Chronic obesity increases a person's risk for many illnesses and dysfunctions including cancer, heart disease, hypertension, dyspnea, arthritis, Type II diabetes, and stroke. However, recent studies are showing that carrying extra weight around the chest and abdomen creates more health risks than carrying extra weight on the hips and thighs.

Ostomies: An ostomy is a surgically created opening between a body cavity or passage and the body's surface. The two most common types are: 1) *Colostomy*, which is an ostomy through the abdominal wall into the colon, which diverts the feces into a bag that is worn on the abdomen and emptied as necessary, and 2) *Ileostomy*, which is an ostomy through the abdominal wall into the ileum, which diverts liquid feces into a bag that is worn on the abdomen and emptied as needed. In some cases, people with colostomies are able to train their colon to empty only at a predictable time of the day, and are thus able to not wear a bag. Bodywork is indicated for people with colostomies and ileostomies unless contraindicated by another condition. Abdominal work should be discussed with the client before it is given. Most people with colostomies are well-informed about their conditions and can direct their bodywork in that area.

Pancreatic Cancer: This is the second most common gastrointestinal cancer. It occurs more often in smokers and diabetics and is often fatal because it metastasizes quickly. Symptoms include abdominal pain, lack of appetite, jaundice, weight loss, weakness, fatigue, diarrhea, nausea and vomiting. Massage is contraindicated for the abdomen (see *Chapter 12*).

Pancreatitis: This is an inflammation of the pancreas, and can be acute or chronic. The acute form is usually associated with gallstones or alcoholism, both of which can lead to blockage of the pancreatic duct. Trapped pancreatic enzymes can digest the pancreas itself, leading to upper abdominal pain, hemorrhage, shock, and, eventually, death. In the chronic form, repeated attacks gradually cause scarring and decreased pancreatic function. Bodywork is locally contraindicated when pain or tenderness are present. Refer the symptomatic client to a physician for assessment.

Polyps: These are benign tumors with a stalk, or pedicle. They are commonly found in the rectum, but can be a risk factor for colon cancer. Polyps bleed easily, especially with the passage of hard or dry stool. Bodywork is indicated for relaxation and body awareness.

Stomatitis: This is a general term for inflammation of the mouth, and can include a white or beige plaque on the tongue (*thrush/candida*), small oval blisters or open spots (*canker sores*), *oral herpes* (*cold sores/fever blisters*), and *periodontal disease* (*gingivitis*). Candida and herpes are contagious, canker sores are caused by a hypersensitivity and influenced by vitamin C and/or B deficiency, and gingivitis is an inflammation and/or infection of the gums, caused by poor oral hygiene. Bodywork is locally contraindicated to the mouth. Advise symptomatic clients to consult a physician for assessment.

Ulcer: This is an open sore or lesion of the mucous membrane accompanied by sloughing of inflamed necrotic (dead) tissue. Ulcers of the stomach or duodenum are called *gastric, duodenal, or peptic ulcers*. Signs and symptoms include recurring gnawing or burning pain in the upper abdominal and low back areas. Symptoms can be either triggered or relieved by eating. Gastric ulcers sometimes start as gastritis, and often heal with antibiotic therapy, which reduces abnormal overgrowth of *Helicobacter pylori* bacteria. If the ulcer goes untreated, the erosion can develop completely through the wall (*perforate*) and empty food and digestive juices into the abdominal cavity, causing hemorrhage and/or *peritonitis* (serious abdominal infection). Bodywork is indicated for clients with ulcers, but locally contraindicated if pain or tenderness are present.

COMMON EFFECTS OF AGING ON THE GASTROINTESTINAL SYSTEM

In general, the gastrointestinal system often begins to weaken after the age of 70. This may be due to decreased nutrition and/or the accumulation of years of use. Common changes that occur include: loss of dental bone and gum tonicity, with more gum bleeding, weakening and/or loss of teeth; atrophy of gastrointestinal mucosal lining, with diminished production of digestive enzymes, hydrochloric acid, and intestinal absorption; hypotonicity of smooth muscle resulting in delayed stomach emptying and increased constipation and gas; increased difficulty in chewing and swallowing, with more energy needed to complete a meal; decreased senses of thirst, taste, and smell, resulting in decreased water intake and appetite. Because of all these changes, calorie, protein, vitamin, and mineral deficiencies are more common, which leads to capillary and bone fragility (easier bruising, bleeding, and fractures), anxiety, and lack of coordination. Another change is that, after age 25, the human metabolic rate usually decreases by about 1% per year, so a 70 year old has a 45% slower metabolic rate and requires 45% fewer calories. That means the calories eaten must be very high quality in order to provide all the essential nutrients.

CASE PRESENTATIONS

9/28/96: 29 yo male, competitive body builder, wants R arm pain relief

History: regional enteritis (Crohn's); arthritis R elbow

S: pain and stiffness in R elbow; pain comes & goes depending on the intensity of training; MD prescribed med for Crohn's but he doesn't take it because it negatively affects his ability to gain muscle mass; MD gave OK for massage, but to avoid abdomen.

O: no visible inflammation at R elbow; difficulty extending joint fully

A: Variety of methods, esp. compression & friction, to muscles of R arm, superior & inferior to elbow, and to the attachments of L elbow in effort to stimulate law of symmetry. Avoided abdomen. General relaxation & sports techniques to rest of body.

Outcome: Client said his elbow felt better & asked if I'd continue to work with him. Recommended he consider reducing his training to give his elbow time to heal & that he take his med for Crohn's.

STUDY QUESTIONS

Which parts of the above case presentations are subjective?
Which parts are objective?
What questions would you have asked that were not asked?
What bodywork techniques would you have done?
What referral(s)?
What other ways could the therapeutic outcome have been evaluated?
How might you have changed the format or way the cases were written?
What were the indications for massage/bodywork?
What were the contraindications?

REFERENCES

Fritz, S. (1995). Mosby's fundamentals of therapeutic massage. St. Louis: Mosby Lifeline.

Jarvis, C. (1992). Physical examination and health assessment. Philadelphia: W. B. Saunders Co.

Kapit, W. & Elson, L.M. (1977). The anatomy coloring book. NY: Harper & Row.

Kapit, W., Macey, R.I., & Meisami, E. (1987). The physiology coloring book. NY: Harper and Row.

Malasanos, L., Barkauskas, V., & Stoltenberg-Allen, K. (1990). Health assessment. St. Louis, MO: C.V. Mosby Co.

Mulvihill, M.L. (1995). Human diseases: A systemic approach (4th ed.) Norwalk, CT: Appleton & Lange.

Newton, D. (1995). Pathology for massage therapists. Portland, OR: Simran Publications.

Sameulson, P. (1994). Pathophysiology for massage: The travel guide. Overland Park, KS: Mid-America Handbooks, Inc.

Thomas, C.L. (1989). Taber's cyclopedic medical dictionary (16th ed.). Philadelphia: F.A. Davis Co.

CHAPTER REVIEW

1. _____ is the process by which food is broken down and converted into absorbable forms.

2. _____ is an involuntary reflexive movement produced by distention of the walls of the tube.

3. The _____ is a saclike pouch where the food is moistened and mixed.

4. The greatest amount of digestion occurs in about the first 10 inches of the small intestine, called the _____.

5. _____ is produced in the liver and stored in the gallbladder.

6. _____ stimulates peristalsis, is an antiseptic, is a laxative, and breaks down fats into smaller units.

7. The greatest amount of nutrient absorption occurs in the _____ _____ of the gastrointestinal tract.

8. The purpose of the _____ is to absorb water and minerals.

9. The _____ is a tight muscular sphincter at the end of the gastrointestinal tube that opens externally.

10. The _____ performs many vital jobs including immunologic, metabolic, coagulation, and digestive functions.

11. The major groups of nutrients are (7) _____ _____

12. The 4 fat-soluble vitamins are _____

13. The 7 water-soluble vitamins are _____

14. Most of the _____ vitamins are required for carbohydrate metabolism and nerve function.

15. We need approximately _____ liters of fresh, pure water daily.

16. The average American diet provides only about half the recommendation for _____.

17. _____ deficiency first causes the body to pull this mineral from the bones to maintain its blood level.

18. Caloric needs increase with _____ and decrease with _____.

19. _____ is what makes up most of the atherosclerotic plaques that block arteries.

20. Refer clients with the following gastrointestinal findings to a physician: _____

_____

_____

_____

21. _____ are solidified masses, formed in the gallbladder or its ducts.

22. _____ is inflammation of the colon.

23. Pouching in the walls of the small intestine is called _____

24. _____ has 3 main forms, all of which are viral and have symptoms of loss of appetite, fever, chills, nausea and vomiting, headache, tenderness in the liver area, jaundice, dark urine and itching.

25. _____ is a protrusion or projection of an organ or a part of an organ through the wall of the cavity that normally contains it.

26. _____ results from an imbalance between the calories ingested and the calories burned.

27. A _____ is an ostomy through the abdominal wall, into the colon, which diverts the feces into a bag that is worn on the abdomen and emptied as necessary.

28. An _____ is an open sore or lesion of the mucous membrane accompanied by sloughing of inflamed necrotic (dead) tissue.

ANSWERS TO CHAPTER REVIEW

1. digestion

2. peristalsis

3. stomach

4. duodenum

5. bile

6. bile

7. small intestine

8. colon or large intestine

9. anus

10. liver

11. protein, carbohydrate, fat, vitamins, minerals, water, fiber

12. A,D,E,K

13. C, B1, B2, B3, B6, B12, and folic acid

14. B

15. 1 1/2, or 1 to 2

16. fiber

17. calcium

18. pregnancy, lactation, trauma, stress, exercise, and certain illnesses; a sedentary lifestyle, age, and certain illnesses

19. cholesterol

20. history of persistent or recurring nausea or vomiting
    acute or persistent chronic abdominal pain
    rebound tenderness
    epigastric pain one to three hours after meals
    an unusually rigid or board-like abdomen
    blood in stools or vomit
    difficulty swallowing
    abdominal masses or nodules
    mouth, tongue, or lip lesions
    soft protrusions through the abdominal wall
    significant obesity or thinness
    chronic fatigue or lack of energy

21. gallstones

22. colitis

23. diverticulosis

24. hepatitis

25. hernia

26. obesity

27. colostomy

28. ulcer

Chapter 11, Part 1

GENITO-URINARY SYSTEM

ANATOMY AND PHYSIOLOGY REVIEW

The term *genito-* refers to the internal and external reproductive organs. The term *urinary* refers to the organs that make, contain, or secrete urine. Therefore, the genito-urinary system consists of the kidneys, ureters, urinary bladder, and urethra; ovaries, uterus, vagina, and vulva in the case of females; testes, prostate, and penis in the case of males. The breasts are not part of this system, but it serves the purposes of this chapter to include them.

Normally, people have two bean-shaped *kidneys*, located in the posterior abdominal cavity, one on each side of the spine. In rare cases, some people are born with only one functioning kidney, and others sometimes lose a kidney during their lifetime through infection or failure. The kidneys' primary jobs are to make urine and help regulate the fluid, acid-base, and electrolyte (mineral salts) content of the blood. These are essential to total body function and health. Each kidney is surrounded by fatty tissue that protects and cushions the kidney and a tough fascial mesh that holds the kidney in place.

The *nephron* is the functional unit of the kidney. Each kidney has about one million nephrons whose job is to filter waste products from the blood, reabsorb the water and nutrients that the body still needs, and secrete the excess substances as urine. The concave border of each kidney faces the spine and has an opening in its center where a ureter exits. The *ureters* are thin hollow tubes that carry the urine away from the kidney to the bladder where it is collected and stored until it is released through a single hollow tube called the *urethra*.

The formation of *urine* is a continuous process, day and night. The normal amount of urine varies between 1000 and 2000 ml daily, depending on fluid intake, diet, exercise, environmental and body temperature, age, and other factors. In healthy people, urine is transparent or slightly cloudy, yellow or light amber colored, with a peculiar but not offensive odor. Ingesting asparagus, saffron, or mint/menthol can temporarily alter the odor. Normal urine is 95% water and 5% solids.

The urinary *bladder* is a membranous sac that receives the urine from the ureters and stores it until voluntary release through the urethra. The bladder is connected to the umbilicus by the median umbilical ligament and supported in other directions by various other ligaments. The walls of the bladder consist of an inner mucous layer of epithelium, a middle layer of smooth muscle, and an outer layer of tough fibrous tissue. In health, the adult bladder holds about 500 ml (1/2 liter) or more. A pair of sphincter muscles, one at the bladder neck and one a few centimeters distal to the first muscle, respond to voluntary control to hold or release the bladder's contents.

The female reproductive system consists of the ovaries, fallopian tubes, uterus, vagina, and vulva. The *ovaries* are two small almond-shaped glands, one on each side of the abdominal cavity, that are attached to the uterus and the pelvis by ligaments and that lie very close to the open end of the fallopian tube. The ovaries have two main functions: to produce hormones (particularly estrogen and progesterone) and to produce eggs (ovum). Each ovary contains thousands of undeveloped eggs awaiting their turn to be ovulated and sent into the fallopian tubes. Normally, one egg is ovulated each month as a part of the hormonal cycle of menstruation. The ovaries' hormones are responsible for the development and maintenance of female sex characteristics, preparation of the uterus for pregnancy, and development of the mammary glands in the breast.

The *uterus* is a hollow pear-shaped organ lined with a mucous membrane (called the *endometrium*) and located in the mid-pelvis, approximately halfway between the sacrum and the pubic bone. It is supported by the pelvic diaphragm, supplemented by two broad ligaments, two round ligaments, and two uterosacral ligaments as well as other lesser ligaments. The largest part of the uterus is made up of thick longitudinal and circular musculature. The walls of the uterus normally lie in contact with each other, but can easily expand with the presence of a fetus.

The mouth, or *cervix*, of the uterus connects and opens into the *vagina*, which is a musculo-membranous tube that forms the passageway between the uterus and the vulva. The bladder lies anterior to the uterus and the rectum lies directly posterior. The walls of the vagina are lined with mucous membrane and normally lie in contact with each other but can easily expand during sexual penetration.

The *vulva* is the exterior female genitalia and consists of two layers of labia, the clitoris, the vaginal opening, and the glands inside the opening that secrete lubricating mucous.

Menstruation is the periodic discharge of a bloody fluid from the uterus, occurring at more or less regular, monthly intervals from about the age of 13 (the menarche, or beginning of regular menstruation) until about the age of 50 (the climacteric, or ending of regular menstruation). The discharge contains normal and clotted red blood cells, disintegrated endometrial cells, and glandular secretions. Menstruation stops when an ovulated egg has been fertilized by a sperm and does not begin again until sometime after the pregnancy ends. Lactation (milk production) often delays the resumption of regular menstrual periods. Normal age of menstrual onset ranges from 9 to 17 years of age. Average length of flow is 4 to 5 days, with the normal range being from 3 to 7 days. Average length of time from one month's first day of flow to the next first day is 27 - 28 days, and "normal" range from 18 - 40 days.

Pregnancy is the condition of carrying a developing embryo in the uterus. Signs and symptoms include missing a menstrual period, nausea and vomiting, increased appetite, darkened pigmentation around the nipple, and frequent urination. The normal pregnancy lasts 280 days, or about 9 months and one week. The nine month pregnancy is categorized into thirds (trimesters), each lasting three months.

Common, normal changes that occur during pregnancy include: increased reflection on life, relationships, and one's abilities; mood swings; breast enlargement and tenderness; progressive abdominal distention, with a two to three pound weight gain per month (up to 30 lb total gain); nausea and/or vomiting during the first trimester; increased heart rate and blood volume with unchanged blood pressure; softening and increased mobility of pelvic and sacro-iliac joints; backache and slower, more deliberate ambulation; tendency toward constipation, and, during late pregnancy, limited expansion of lungs with dyspnea on exertion, non-pitting edema in feet and lower legs, and more frequent urination.

There are a number of *indications for massage in pregnancy*:

> •supports the work of the heart, by encouraging venous return
> • contributes to parasympathetic activation
> • temporarily relieves stress on weight-bearing joints, lumbar and cervical joints, and overall musculo-fascial structures
> • develops sensory awareness
> • offers emotional support and physical nurturing
> • provides woman with models of gentle, loving touch that she can repeat with her baby

For *contraindications for massage in pregnancy*, see page 221.

Menopause is the complete cessation of menstruation and occurs naturally between the ages of 40 and 55, with 50% of women experiencing it by age 50, and 72% by age 52. In the U.S., menopause is often brought on surgically by the removal of the ovaries. In those cases, if the woman does not receive prescription hormones, she immediately experiences all the changes that normally occur over the course of one to three years. The symptoms of menopause commonly include: progressively decreased flow each month and/or irregular flowing; nervousness; hot flashes (some women call these "power surges"); chills, excitability, fatigue, apathy, depression, elation, insomnia, dizziness, headaches, numbness, tingling, and muscle aches. Under natural menopause conditions, these symptoms can range from hardly noticeable to severely disturbing and may last from a few months to a few years. Officially, menopause is not reached until one year after the woman's last menstrual period. The period of time during which this change is going on is called the *climacteric*. Bodywork is indicated during the climacteric, with local contraindications only when the client has sharp, progressive, or persistent pain in the abdomen.

The male reproductive system consists of the testes, epididymis, vas deferens, seminal vesicle, prostate gland, and penis. The *testes* are two small oval glands, located and suspended inside the scrotum by the spermatic cord. Their two main functions are to produce a hormone (testosterone) and to produce sperm cells. *Sperm cells* are produced inside the testes' tubules, and sent through straight ducts into a plexus, then into the epididymis.

The *epididymis* is a small oblong body that rests on and beside the posterior surface of the testes. It constitutes the first part of the excretory duct of each testis. During sexual excitement, sperm move into the *vas deferens*, which is an extension of the urethra, and pick up fluids from the *seminal vesicles, prostate gland,* and *bulbourethral glands.* The *prostate gland* surrounds the neck of the bladder where it joins the urethra. It is partly muscular and partly glandular with ducts opening into the urethra. *Ejaculation* is a reflex phenomenon in which the semen (sperm cells and fluids) are ejected through the penis via the urethra. The average ejaculation contains between 120 and 750 million sperm.

The human *breasts* are located in the upper anterior portion of the chest, exterior to the pectoralis muscles. Each breast is made of fatty (adipose) tissue that contains mammary glands. The mammary glands consist of 15 to 20 lobes of glandular tissue that are capable of producing milk when stimulated by sucking and the hormones associated with pregnancy. The milk drains through a duct system and exits through openings in the tip of the nipple. Female breast tissue normally swells a few days before a menstrual flow and may become slightly tender. Also, during the first 6 to 12 weeks of pregnancy, the female breasts will swell and become tender. Male breasts can also swell, and do so, slightly, as men age, and in conjunction with certain illnesses. This condition is called *gynecomastia.*

ASSESSMENT: OBSERVATION AND PALPATION

According to all professional and State codes of ethics, bodywork is locally contraindicated on the genitalia and female breasts. However, it is still important that bodyworkers listen closely to their clients' descriptions of health experiences with their knowledge of genetics and the genito-urinary system in mind, so that appropriate referrals can be made, when necessary. Particularly listen for reports of groin, genital, flank, or abdominal pain; painful urination (dysuria); unusual urine color, amount, frequency, or odor; edema; unexplained weight changes; skin changes; genital inflammation; discharges, or masses.

In addition, be aware that vaginal bleeding after menopause may be due to endometrial cancer, vaginal cancer, or recurrence of monthly menstruation from hormone (estrogen) replacement therapy. Painless bleeding into the urine can be an early sign of kidney or bladder tumor. A kidney stone or bladder infection can also produce blood in the urine, but there will be mild to severe pain, accompanied by an urgency to urinate.

GENERAL CONDITIONS RELATING TO GENITO-URINARY SYSTEM

The following are definitions and descriptions of general genito-urinary findings. Information on more specific disorders follows in the next section. As a general rule, refer clients with the following findings to a physician for assessment and diagnosis:

- history of unusual genito-urinary or inguinal pain
- unusual discharge or secretions from genitals or breasts

- genital, inguinal, or breast nodules or masses
- genital, inguinal, or breast rashes, inflammation, or itching
- changes in urinary color, amounts, frequency, or odor
- unexplained sudden weight gain; edema
- unusual menstrual flow or pain (for that individual)
- skin abnormalities
- low back pain with fever or malaise
- tenderness or swelling in the costovertebral region (where the lowest rib and its vertebrae join)

SPECIFIC GENITO-URINARY CONDITIONS

According to all professional and State codes of ethics, bodywork is locally contraindicated on the genitalia and breasts. Therefore, the following information is given only as a general reference to help bodyworkers better understand clients' health conditions, and so that bodyworkers can better listen, offer emotional support, and give referrals, when indicated. Also, it should be noted that genital secretions/discharges can transmit any of a number of infectious diseases, so bodyworkers are cautioned to handle linens with care to prevent direct contact. Systemic contraindications are specifically noted where indicated.

Benign Prostatic Hypertrophy (BPH): This is a progressive enlargement of the prostate gland, which is a common condition in men over age 50. BPH can cause difficulty in starting urination, and obstruction of the urethra, which results in a decrease in the urine stream. Refer symptomatic clients to a physician for assessment. Bodywork is indicated for relaxation and general body awareness.

Bladder Infection (Cystitis): This is inflammation of the bladder, usually occurring in conjunction with a urinary tract infection that starts in the urethra. Cystitis can be acute, with frequent and painful or burning urination, or chronic, in which it is secondary to some other problem, such as a structural defect, obstruction, or calculi (stone). *Interstitial cystitis* involves inflammation and irritation of the bladder wall. The etiology is unknown. Bodywork is indicated for relaxation and general body awareness.

Bladder Cancer: This occurs more often in older men and is thought to be associated with occupational exposures to chemicals. See discussion in Chapter 12 about bodywork for people with cancers.

Breast Cancer: In the U.S., this is the leading cause of cancer in women, and approximately one in eleven women will develop it. It begins with a microscopically small, painless tumor that gradually grows until it is palpable. It usually begins as a moveable mass and progresses into one that is immovable. Risk factors in order of importance include: family history of breast cancer; client had no childbirth or experienced first pregnancy after age 30; history of chronic breast disease; exposure to radiation during adolescence, and obesity. Breast cancer is often curable if treated early, however, many women are afraid to check their breasts so the cancer grows undetected. A combination of monthly self-exams, yearly exams by a physician, and periodic mammograms has been found to be the best approach to early detection. If clients talk with you about their fears regarding self-exam or mammography, encourage them to get more information and, if possible, to begin as much of the early detection monitoring process as they can. Education for performing self-exams is readily available at public health departments, physicians' offices, and many other health organizations. Mastectomy is the removal of the breast, nearby lymph nodes, and in some cases, some of the muscle tissue beneath the breast. Before you give massage/bodywork to a person who has had breast cancer or a mastectomy, ask her to tell you what tissues were removed, how long ago the surgery was, etc. If she is not sure, consult with her physician before working on the area (see *Chapter 12* about bodywork for people with cancers).

Cervical Cancer: This is the cancer that can be detected by the Pap test. It occurs most often in middle-age and is one of the leading causes of cancer death in women. Early detection is the best predictor for survival. Risk factors include: the initiation of intercourse at an early age, multiple sex partners, and genital herpes or warts. Symptoms include unusual bleeding and painful intercourse (see *Chapter 12* about bodywork for people with cancers).

Chlamydia: This is the most common sexually transmitted disease (STD) in the U.S. It is a bacterial infection, transmitted through genital secretions, that can result in infertility in males and females. The symptoms are similar to gonorrhea's symptoms, and, like gonorrhea, it is often symptomless in women. Men usually have burning during urination and a clear or pus-like discharge. Symptoms usually appear 5 to 10 days after exposure. Untreated symptoms can lead to the same serious complications as gonorrhea, including blindness in newborns. Chlamydia is curable by taking antibiotics. Bodywork is indicated for relaxation and general body awareness. Genital secretions may be infectious.

Cramps (Dysmenorrhea): This is painful menstruation. Approximately 50% of menstruating women experience dysmenorrhea, and about 5% are incapacitated for several days during each menstrual period. There are several types, but two main ones. In primary dysmenorrhea, the pain begins just before or at the onset of menarche, is spasmodic, and located in the lower abdomen, sometimes radiating to the back and/or thighs. Some women also experience nausea, vomiting, diarrhea, headache, and dizziness lasting from a few hours to several days. These symptoms usually decrease or disappear after the first childbirth, and also decrease with age. In secondary dysmenorrhea, the pain is similar, but it usually begins later in life and is associated with a history of pelvic inflammatory disease (PID), use of an IUD (intra-uterine device), endometriosis, or fertility problems. Sometimes direct pressure to the sacrum and/or iliac crest can relieve an episode of primary dysmenorrhea. Otherwise, advise symptomatic clients to consult with a health care practitioner for assessment and treatment. Bodywork is indicated for relaxation and general body awareness.

Eclampsia (Toxemia): This is a very serious, often fatal, complication of pregnancy characterized by coma and/or convulsive seizures that can occur between the 20th week of pregnancy (about 5 months) and the first week after childbirth. It develops in about 1 out of 200 women with *pre-eclampsia*, which is much less severe, but which warrants close monitoring of blood pressure, urine output, and weight in order to prevent progression. The etiology is unknown, however, it occurs more often in first pregnancies and in women who have pre-existing hypertension and/or kidney dysfunction. Symptoms of *pre-eclampsia* include headache, abnormally high blood pressure, systemic edema , and protein in the urine. Refer symptomatic clients to their physician for assessment. Bodywork is systemically contraindicated without physician's approval.

Endometritis: Inflammation or infection of the endometrium, usually produced by bacteria such as staphylococci, E. coli, or gonococci. It can be acute, subacute, or chronic. The subacute and chronic types are the result of repeated acute episodes. Symptoms include low back and/or low abdominal pain, dysmenorrhea, constipation and sterility. In the chronic form, there is a scant blood-tinged vaginal discharge. Bodywork is locally contraindicated in the presence of abdominal pain or known infection.

Endometriosis: This is a condition where the lining of the uterus (endometrium) has migrated outside the uterus and attached to the ovaries, fallopian tubes, or various sites in the abdomen, causing significant pain at the site. Bodywork is locally contraindicated in the presence of abdominal pain.

Enlarged Prostate (see *Benign Prostatic Hypertrophy*)

*Fibrocystic Breasts (*also called *Mammary Dysplasia):* This is a non-specific diagnosis for palpable, non-cancerous lumps in the breasts. It is usually associated with pain and tenderness that fluctuates with the menstrual cycle and becomes progressively worse until it disappears after menopause. It is estimated that at least 50% of menstruating women have palpable lumps in the breasts caused by this condition. According to some authorities, women with fibrocystic breast disease have a slightly greater risk of developing breast cancer. In general, reducing caffeine and fat intake can decrease symptoms. Bodywork is indicated for relaxation and general body awareness.

Fibroids, Uterine: This is a benign, fibrous, encapsulated connective tissue tumor with an irregular shape and slow growth. These tumors rarely cause symptoms before the age of 30, and symptoms depend on the location of the fibroid. They can range in size from a few millimeters in diameter to large enough to fill the entire abdomen and can be single or multiple. They may cause the abdomen to be tender to deep palpation and are susceptible to infection and degenerative changes. Bodywork is indicated for relaxation and general body awareness. Avoid abdominal work if it is uncomfortable for the client.

Gonorrhea: This is a specific, contagious bacterial infection (STD) of the genital mucous membrane that can occur in both sexes and is transmitted by genital secretions. Symptoms are more evident in men and include yellow discharge from the penis, slow, difficult and painful urination, and sometimes pain or swelling in the penile tissue. In women, symptoms often are not noticed. If they are noticed, they can include urethral or vaginal discharge, painful or frequent urination, and/or lower abdominal pain. Untreated gonorrhea will result in sterility, pelvic inflammatory disease (PID), and blindness in newborns. It can be cured with antibiotics. Bodywork is indicated for relaxation and general body awareness. Genital secretions may be infectious.

Herpes, Genital: This is a viral infection of the genital and/or anorectal skin and mucous membranes. It is spread by sexual or any direct contact. About 4 to 7 days after exposure to the virus, a small cluster of blisters appears. The blisters may be very painful and itchy and gradually turn into open ulcers with red, inflamed tissue around them. Some people also experience swollen lymph nodes, fever, and flu-like symptoms. The ulcers and their drainage are highly contagious. The ulcers can heal without treatment in about 10 days, but the virus stays inside the body. Episodes often recur periodically. Bodywork is indicated for relaxation and general body awareness. Genital secretions may be infectious.

Kidney Stone (Renal calculi): This is an abnormal, very dense rocklike formation of mineral salts in the kidney(s). There are many risk factors for making kidney stones: heredity; gender and age (men between the ages of 20 and 50 have the greatest rate of stones); hyperparathyroidism; injury to the kidney; diet; hyperthyroidism; a low water intake; chronic urinary tract infections; certain medications, and having given birth recently. Many times the etiology is unknown. Symptoms include sudden, severe pain as the body tries to pass the stone from the kidney, through the ureter and/or through the urethra; potential blockage of the urine flow from the kidney; fever, chills, and blood in the urine. Bodywork is systemically contraindicated, and symptomatic clients should be encouraged to seek professional assessment as the prognosis is very serious if the stone blocks release of urine.

Kidney Infection (Nephritis): This is a general term for any infectious kidney disorder, most often caused by a urinary tract infection that began in the urethra and progressed upward to the kidney. Symptoms include back pain, fever, malaise, and/or painful urination. If untreated, kidney failure can result. Bodywork is systemically contraindicated.

Kidney (Renal) Failure: This is a general term for diminished function of the kidney in which the kidney is less able to remove wastes and toxins from the blood. It can be acute and temporary, or it may progress to the complete loss of kidney function. This is the cause for *renal dialysis* and kidney transplants. The six warning signs of kidney disease are: high blood pressure; puffiness around the eyes and edema in the hands and feet; pain in the kidney area; difficulty urinating or burning during urination; passage of bloody or cola-colored urine; and more frequent urination. Kidney failure can be caused by chronic hypertension, poorly managed diabetes, and/or chronic kidney infections. People with any type of kidney failure, and their bodyworker, should consult with the treating physician *before* beginning any bodywork to determine if the person can tolerate the work and if there are any specific contraindications.

Miscarriage: This is the lay term for termination of pregnancy any time before the fetus is able to live outside the uterus. The most common cause is some genetic defect in the fetus. Symptoms include vaginal bleeding and severe cramps, followed by the expulsion of the fetus, and then lessened bleeding can continue for several days. Clients who have experienced miscarriage need to be assessed by a qualified professional as soon as possible afterwards and need sensitive emotional support for a period of time, sometimes many months, afterward. Avoid abdominal bodywork until all bleeding has ceased. Otherwise, bodywork is indicated for relaxation, general body awareness, and nurturance.

Ovarian Cyst: This is a fluid-filled sac that develops in the ovary, consisting of one or more chambers. Although not cancerous, the cyst may burst, twist, or have other difficulties that can cause pain, pressure, hemorrhage, or gangrene. Avoid abdominal bodywork in clients with ovarian cysts. Otherwise, bodywork is indicated for relaxation and general body awareness.

Ovarian Cancer: This is often a fatal cancer, causing more deaths than uterine and cervical cancer combined. Women who have not given birth are at higher risk. Symptoms include pain and irregular periods. Avoid abdominal bodywork. See information in Chapter 12 on bodywork for people with cancers.

PID (Pelvic Inflammatory Disease): This is any bacterial infection in the pelvis, although it is most frequently caused by Chlamydia or Gonorrhea. PID usually starts in the vagina and/or cervix and progressively ascends into the uterus, fallopian tubes, and broad ligaments. Symptoms include a muco-purulent vaginal discharge, painful urination, abdominal pain, and sometimes rectal pain, nausea, and vomiting. Abdominal adhesions and infertility can result, but early treatment with antibiotics can reduce that potential. Avoid abdominal bodywork. Otherwise, bodywork is indicated for relaxation and general body awareness.

PMS (Premenstrual Syndrome): This is a syndrome that occurs several days prior to the onset of menstruation characterized by one or more of the following symptoms: irritability, emotional tension, anxiety, mood swings, depression, headache, breast tenderness with or without swelling, and water retention. Most or all of these symptoms subside when the menstrual flow begins. Approximately 40% of American women have PMS in varying degrees at some time in their lives. The etiology is unclear but is thought to be related to the changes in estrogen and progesterone levels at that point in the menstrual cycle. Some factors that have reduced or eliminated symptoms include: reducing salt intake; moderate exercise 4 times per week; reducing caffeine and sugar intake; bringing body weight to 15 pounds or less over what is ideal for ones height and age, and reducing general stress. Bodywork is indicated for relaxation, nurturance, and general body awareness. Refer clients who experience severe or disabling symptoms to a physician for assessment.

Polycystic Kidney Disease: This is an inherited condition in which the kidney tissue is replaced by grape-like clusters of cysts. The etiology is unknown. As the cysts grow in size, they compress and destroy healthy kidney tissue, kidney stones can form, kidney function deteriorates, and the kidneys become more susceptible to infection. Kidney failure often occurs within 5 to 15 years after the first symptoms. Symptoms may include: a dull or sharp pain in the lower back; blood in the urine; frequent urinary tract infections; high blood pressure; enlarged kidneys; and decreased kidney function. There is presently no curative medical treatment other than simple things to protect the kidneys and keep them healthy such as drinking lots of water. Bodywork is indicated for relaxation, nurturance, and general body awareness, but systemically contraindicated during times of systemic edema, bloody urine, or acute kidney pain.

Pregnancy: (Also read the information about pregnancy on page 214.) During the third trimester, it is particularly important that effleurage on the legs be done only in the direction toward the heart. Avoid enlarged or varicose veins. Special positioning, either on the side or with full body cushioning, is needed during the third trimester to prevent pressure on the abdomen. Deep abdominal bodywork is contraindicated throughout pregnancy, and deep or stretching bodywork on the hip and pelvic joints is contraindicated after the first trimester. Some women will find stretching exercises during pregnancy to be beneficial, but this does not mean that bodyworkers should add more stretch to the hip and pelvic joints. Pressure points reflexive to the uterus and ovaries should be avoided. Women experiencing the following complications in their pregnancies should consult with their primary healthcare practitioner and provide you with a written release before you give them bodywork:

- being over 35 or under 20 years old
- expecting multiple births (twins, triplets, etc.)
- gestational or other types of diabetes
- hypertension (high blood pressure)
- heart disease
- kidney disease
- phlebitis
- any other types of known complications

Massage is systemically contraindicated for women who are experiencing any of the following signs and symptoms. Advise them to consult a physician immediately:

- bloody vaginal discharge
- severe intermittent, and/or moderate continual abdominal pains
- sudden gush of water or any leakage of vaginal fluid
- systemic edema and/or pitting edema in legs
- severe persistent headaches
- chill and/or fever over 100 degrees
- blurred vision and/or seeing spots
- increased and unusual thirst with reduced urination
- frequent urination with burning sensation

Prostate Cancer: In the U.S., this is the second most common cancer occurring in men (after lung cancer), and its incidence is increasing. The etiology is unknown, but known risk factors include: genetics, high dietary fat, exposure to viruses, radiation, and/or industrial or agricultural chemicals. Usually, there are no symptoms until the cancer is advanced, however, a periodic palpation of the prostate by a physician and a blood test can provide early detection. Prognosis is usually good with early detection and treatment (see *Chapter 12* about bodywork for people with cancers).

Prostatitis: This is a general term meaning inflammation of the prostate gland. It can be acute or chronic. Symptoms of acute prostatitis include discomfort and/or pain in the perineal area, frequent urination, and, if severe, fever, malaise, chills, and vomiting. Chronic prostatitis occurs because of chronic bacterial infection. Symptoms tend to be milder than in the acute form, but still include fever, pain, and painful urination. Bodywork is indicated for relaxation and general body awareness.

Syphilis: This is a bacterial infection, transmitted by sexual contact and/or direct contact with genital discharges. This organism can enter through unbroken skin or mucous membrane. Its first signs are a small red papule that changes into a small ulcer and then into a hard chancre sore. If untreated, further lesions develop that can involve any organ or tissue, with remissions and exacerbations as it progresses over time toward death due to cardiovascular and central nervous system damage. Untreated syphilis can also cause birth defects or fetal death. Early detection and antibiotic treatment are available at many public health clinics and private physician's offices. Bodywork is indicated for relaxation and general body awareness. Genital secretions may be infectious.

Testicular Cancer: This is a fairly rare cancer found usually in young men and characterized by a painless swelling in the testicles. Early detection and treatment are essential to survival as this cancer can metastasize quickly. See discussion in Chapter 12 about bodywork for people with cancers.

Toxemia of Pregnancy: This is an outdated term for pregnancy-induced hypertension (see *Eclampsia)*.

Ectopic ("Tubal") Pregnancy: This is a pregnancy in which the ovum is fertilized and develops outside the uterus, most commonly in the abdominal cavity near the ovary or in the fallopian tube. This occurs in approximately 1% of pregnancies. It is characterized by severe abdominal pain. If it progresses and ruptures, it can cause hemorrhage and possibly death. Refer symptomatic clients to a physician for assessment. Bodywork is locally contraindicated to the abdomen.

Urethritis: This is a general term meaning inflammation of the urethra. It can be caused by using bubble baths and other chemicals that irritate the urethral opening, by the friction of wearing tight clothing, or by bacteria. About 50% of cases in adults is attributable to Chlamydia or gonorrhea and, if so, genital secretions may be infectious. Refer symptomatic clients to a physician for assessment. Bodywork is indicated for relaxation and general body awareness.

Vaginitis: This is a general term meaning inflammation of the vagina. It can be caused by any of a number of different infectious pathogens (bacteria, protozoas, fungi, and viruses), chemical irritations, neoplasms in the cervix or vagina, severe vitamin A deficiency, lack of bathing, and/or presence or use of foreign objects. Symptoms include purulent vaginal discharge that is sometimes odorous and/or stained with blood. Often there is also itching of the vulva and/or perineum, burning, and increased frequency of urination. Refer symptomatic clients to a physician for assessment. Bodywork is indicated for relaxation and general body awareness. Genital secretions may be infectious.

Chapter 11, Part 2

GENETIC CONDITIONS

ANATOMY AND PHYSIOLOGY REVIEW

A *gene* is the basic unit of *heredity*, or, what is inherited from one's biological parents. Genes are found in the nucleus of each living cell. During growth and repair, the cell's *DNA* (which is organized into *chromosomes*) doubles and divides, with each new cell getting identical, complete chromosomes. Each chromosome contains thousands of genes, and each gene has a code to make one protein that contributes in its own way to the structure, development and growth of the body. Genes are self-producing, ultra-microscopic structures, and each one occupies a unique and precise location on a chromosome.

Humans generally have *23 pairs of chromosomes*, with 22 pairs being autosomes and the last pair being the sex chromosomes (meaning that they determine if the person has male or female anatomy). Generally, males have XY sex chromosomes and females have XX sex chromosomes. The male Y chromosome does not have the additional genetic material that is carried on the section that would make the Y into an X.

Each person inherits one chromosome in each pair from each parent. Hereditary traits are determined by the two genes located in the exact same position on any pair of chromosomes. In each pair, some genes are *dominant* and others are *recessive*. For example, the gene for brown eyes is dominant over the gene for blue eyes which is recessive. This means that if a person inherits the gene for brown eyes from one parent and the gene for blue eyes from the other parent, the person will probably have brown eyes. Traits caused by recessive genes will only occur when the person has inherited the gene from BOTH parents, unless the recessive gene is carried on the X (female) sex chromosome, and inherited by a male offspring.

Sometimes disorders occur because of unusual genetic transfers from parents to their off-spring. There are two main categories of genetic disorders: gene mutations and whole chromosome disorders. The word mutation means change, and the *gene mutation disorders* occur when single genes have been changed in some way, so that they can not make their normal protein. This can be caused by a virus, chemical agent, and/or radiation. The result can be so slight that it is unnoticed, or it can cause dysfunction (such as cystic fibrosis or sickle cell anemia), or death and spontaneous abortion. In *whole chromosome disorders*, either a section of chromosome is missing, or the person has an abnormal number of chromosomes. The result is unique physical development, such as occurs in Down Syndrome or hermaphroditism. Common genetic disorders will be discussed individually in the *Conditions* section.

SPECIFIC HEREDITARY CONDITIONS

Albinism: This is a non-pathological, partial or total absence of pigment in the skin, hair, and eyes caused by mutation of a recessive gene. It is frequently accompanied by astigmatism, visual hypersensitivity to light (photophobia), and involuntary eye movements. People with albinism must be extraordinarily protective of sun exposure because they have no melanin to protect them. They are therefore more at risk for skin cancer and sun injury to the retina. Bodywork is indicated, but be aware that the client may have sensitive skin and may want to provide his/her own oil.

"Color Blindness" (Color Deficiency): This is a non-pathological absence or defect in the perception of colors, and the preferred term is the second one listed. It is caused by a gene mutation on one of the sex chromosomes. In most cases, the person is deficient in perceiving either red, green, or blue. In rare cases, all colors are perceived as shades of gray. Bodywork is indicated unless some other condition exists for which it would be contraindicated.

Cystic Fibrosis (CF): This is a disease of the exocrine glands affecting the pancreas, respiratory system, and sweat glands in the axillae and groin. It is caused by mutation of a recessive gene and is the most common of that type of disorder, occurring in approximately 1 in 2,000 white infants, being most common in those of Northern European ancestry. CF usually begins in infancy and is characterized by chronic respiratory infection due to the very thick, copious mucous made by the lungs; pancreatic insufficiency, and increased electrolytes (minerals) in the sweat. Prognosis is often poor, although many people live to adulthood and experience a decrease in symptoms. Tapotement on the chest and back with the head positioned lower than the waist is one of the primary treatments in facilitating mucous drainage from the lungs and is often taught to the child's parents. Bodywork is indicated for general relaxation and body awareness, and, in the case of minors, with parental consent and presence.

Down Syndrome: This is a form of unusual mental and physical development, caused by the presence of an extra 21st chromosome. Characteristics include: sloping forehead, small ear canals, gray or very light yellow spots at the edge of the iris, short broad hands with a single crease across the palm, a flat nose, low-set ears, and a generally dwarfed stature. Women more often give birth to a child with this syndrome when they are over 40 years old. Bodywork is indicated but may need to be kept to a short time to accommodate a client's attention span.

Hemophilia: This is a blood disease characterized by greatly prolonged bleeding time because the blood does not clot. It is caused by a recessive gene mutation on a sex chromosome, and is usually transmitted by the mother to her son. There are two types, A and B, and each are caused by a deficiency in a different plasma factor. There is no cure at this time, although emergency treatments are available to stop bleeding episodes. People with hemophilia must be careful to avoid injuries, including cuts, scrapes, and bruises. Bodywork is systemically contraindicated unless a physician verifies that the person's tissues can tolerate the work.

Hermaphroditism: This is a condition in which both ovarian and testicular tissue exist in the same person and is caused by an unusual formation of the sex chromosomes. Although rare, it occurs in many forms and has been kept a highly secret diagnosis, with some individuals never even being told about their own condition. In most cases in the U.S., one set of tissues is selected to be made dominant, and the secondary tissues are surgically removed early in childhood. Currently, many survivors of those surgeries are identifying themselves and networking for support of their unique issues. Bodywork is indicated unless some other condition exists for which it would be contraindicated.

PKU (Phenylketonuria): This is a condition where the body fails to oxidize a certain amino acid (phenylalanine) into tyrosine and is caused by a mutant recessive gene. If the disorder is not treated very soon after birth, brain damage will occur when the infant ingests milk. Most States require PKU tests at birth. Prognosis is excellent if treatment is started early. In the U.S. the incidence is approximately 1 in 40,000 births. Symptoms include tremors, spasticity, convulsions, hyperactivity, unusual hand posturing, and offensive odor in the sweat and urine. Bodywork is contraindicated until the condition is treated.

Sickle Cell Anemia: This is a chronic form of anemia in which abnormally shaped (curved, like a sickle) red blood cells are present. It is caused by mutation of a recessive gene and occurs most often in persons with African or Mediterranean ancestry. Approximately 8% of African-Americans carry the gene, and one in 400 African-American children are born with sickle cell anemia. The sickle-shaped blood cells interfere with oxygen transport and obstruct capillary blood flow, often causing pain. Acute episodes can last from hours to days and produce severe pain and low-grade fever. Pain occurs most commonly in the bones (especially the long bones and those in the back), joints, chest, and abdomen, and may be provoked by infection, dehydration, hypoxia, or by nothing noticeable. Symptoms can exacerbate to the point of crisis, especially when the environmental oxygen is decreased, such as in flying or visiting elevated locations. Non-healing ulcers over the lower tibia are common. Strokes, blindness, and chronic damage to vital organs, such as the heart and liver, often end in death between ages 20 and 40. There is no specific curative medical treatment at this time, but there are supportive approaches available. Bodywork is contraindicated without the physician's verification that the client's tissues can tolerate the work.

COMMON EFFECTS OF AGING ON THE GENITO-URINARY SYSTEM

Between the ages of 25 and 75, the renal blood flow decreases by about 53%, and the glomerular filtration rate decreases by about 50%. This contributes to urinary retention, infection, pain, decreased excretion of toxic substances, and anxiety. There is a systemic weakening of the muscles that contributes to decreased abdominal muscle and bladder tone, which increases the risk of incontinence; in women, there is atrophy of the ovaries with a decrease in vaginal and urethral elasticity and secretions, resulting in increased susceptibility to vaginal and urethral infections; in men, there is enlargement of the prostate gland, resulting in urinary frequency and urgency, and atrophy of the testes with a decrease in testosterone and sperm, contributing to decreased libido and reduced volume of seminal fluid.

CASE PRESENTATIONS

3/11/96: 33 yo woman with pelvic and L buttock pain since 1989

Goal: Relief of L buttock pain, radiating into L leg

History: Has been to neurologist, orthopedic surgeon, Mayo clinic, & chiropractor, but has no diagnosis or relief. Ruptured disc was ruled out. Has tried physical therapy and acupuncture. Medical diagnosis of abdominal problem is endometriosis and had laser surgery for that three yrs ago, without reduction of pain. Symptoms started after a car accident in 1989.

S: Is in constant, severe L leg pain: sharp & shooting, increasing with fatigue, stress, exercise, standing, and sitting for long periods. Is often sick with colds, flu, etc. Rates L leg pain at 10 on 0-10 scale. Related some recent stressful events in her life.

O: Walked into office independently, without any limp or assistive device. Color good. No visible marks or bruises. Breathing normally. L calf, quads, & hamstrings tight, especially medially, with several tender areas. Trapezius tight and tender along tip of scapula. Abdomen tender to gentle pressure.

Intuitive: Felt there was a connection between knot on traps and the sacrum, which had more energy than I usually notice. Felt drawn to tie the two areas together, & felt a line connecting the areas to the L ankle.

A: Effleurage & petrissage to arms, legs, shoulders, back & neck Light effleurage to abdomen. Focused on L leg and traps. Encouraged client to reduce amount of time sitting or standing, by taking short stretch breaks. Suggested she explore emotional facets of her pain and offered a referral.

Outcome: L leg pain rated at 5

P: Says will get bodywork 1-2x/month and will explore emotional aspects in relation to her pain on her own.

STUDY QUESTIONS

Which parts of the above case presentations are subjective?
Which parts are objective?
What questions would you have asked that were not asked?
What bodywork techniques would you have done?
What referral(s)?
What other ways could the therapeutic outcome have been evaluated?
How might you have changed the format or way the cases were written?
What were the indications for massage/bodywork?
What were the contraindications?

REFERENCES

Fritz, S. (1995). Mosby's fundamentals of therapeutic massage. St. Louis: Mosby Lifeline.

Jarvis, C. (1992). Physical examination and health assessment. Philadelphia: W. B. Saunders Co.

Kapit, W. and Elson, L.M. (1977). The anatomy coloring book. NY: Harper and Row.

Kapit, W., Macey, R.I., & Meisami, E. (1987). The physiology coloring book. NY: Harper & Row.

Malasanos, L., Barkauskas, V., & Stoltenberg-Allen, K. (1990). Health assessment. St. Louis, MO: C.V. Mosby Co.

Mulvihill, M.L. (1995). Human diseases: A systemic approach (4th ed.) Norwalk, CT: Appleton & Lange.

Newton, D. (1995). Pathology for massage therapists. Portland, OR: Simran Publications.

Sameulson, P. (1994). Pathophysiology for massage: The travel guide. Overland Park, KS: Mid-America Handbooks, Inc.

Thomas, C.L. (1989). Taber's cyclopedic medical dictionary (16th ed.). Philadelphia: F.A. Davis Co.

CHAPTER REVIEW

1. The kidneys' primary jobs are to _____

_____

2. The _____ is the functional unit of the kidney.

3. The nephrons' jobs are to _____

_____

4. The _____ are thin hollow tubes that carry the urine away from the kidney, to the bladder, where it is collected and stored until it is released through a single hollow tube called the _____.

5. The _____ is a membranous sac that receives the urine from the ureters and stores it until voluntary release.

6. The ovaries have two main functions: _____

7. The _____ is a hollow pear-shaped organ, lined with a mucous membrane called the _____.

8. The mouth, or _____, of the uterus connects and opens into the _____

_____

9. The _____ is the exterior female genitalia.

10. The common, normal changes that occur during pregnancy include: _____

_____

_____

_____

_____

11. Bodywork contraindications during pregnancy include

    a)_____ after the first trimester,

    b)_____ during the third trimester, and

    c)_____ throughout the entire pregnancy.

12. Officially, _____ is not reached until one year after the woman's last menstrual period.

13. The two main functions of the _____ are to produce a hormone (testosterone) and to produce sperm cells.

14. In males, the _____ surrounds the neck of the bladder, where it joins the urethra.

15. A _____ is the basic unit of heredity.

16. Humans normally have _____ pairs of chromosomes, with the last pair being the sex chromosomes.

17. According to all professional and State codes of ethics, bodywork is locally contraindicated on the _____.

18. In general, refer clients with the following genito-urinary symptoms to a physician: _____

    _____

    _____

    _____

    _____

    _____

    _____

    _____

    _____

19. Genital secretions/discharges can transmit any of a number of infectious diseases, so bodyworkers are cautioned to: _____

    _____

20. Bodywork is systemically contraindicated without physician's approval in the following genito-urinary conditions: _____

21. Bodywork is systemically contraindicated without physician's approval in the following genetic/hereditary conditions: _____

    _____

    _____

    _____

ANSWERS TO CHAPTER REVIEW

1. make urine and help regulate the fluid, acid-base, and electrolyte (mineral salts) content of the blood

2. nephron

3. filter waste products from the blood, reabsorb the water and nutrients that the body still needs, and secrete the excess substances as urine

4. ureters; urethra

5. urinary bladder

6. to produce hormones and to produce eggs

7. uterus; endometrium

8. cervix; vagina

9. vulva

10. increased reflection on life, relationships, and one's abilities; mood swings; breast enlargement and tenderness; progressive abdominal distention, with a two to three pound weight gain per month (up to 30 lb total gain); increased heart rate and blood volume with unchanged blood pressure; softening and increased mobility of pelvic and sacroiliac joints; backache and slower, more deliberate ambulation; tendency toward constipation, and, during late pregnancy, limited expansion of lungs with dyspnea on exertion; and more frequent urination

11. a) deep or stretching work on the hip and pelvic joints
    b) effleurage on the legs away from the heart; avoid enlarged or varicose veins; special positioning, either on the side or with full body cushions
    c) deep abdominal bodywork

12. menopause

13. testes

14. prostate gland

15. gene

16. 23

17. genitalia and breasts

18. history of unusual genital, inguinal, or nipple discharge
    genital, inguinal, or breast nodules or masses
    genital, inguinal, or breast rashes, inflammation, or itching
    changes in urinary color, amounts, frequency or odor
    unexplained sudden weight gain; edema
    unusual menstrual flow or pain (for that individual)
    skin abnormalities
    low back pain with fever or malaise
    tenderness or swelling in the costovertebral region

19. handle linens with care to prevent direct contact

20. pre-eclampsia; kidney failure

21. hemophilia; sickle cell anemia

Chapter 12, Part 1
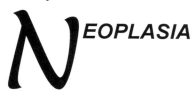
NEOPLASIA

ANATOMY AND PHYSIOLOGY REVIEW

The discovery of a lump or mass can be frightening because we first think of the possibility of cancer. The word *neoplasia* means the development of new and abnormal tissue formation(s), including *tumors*, and changes in blood and lymph cells. Strictly defined, "tumor" means abnormal swelling or enlargement. However, the term "tumor" is often used in place of "neoplasm" or "cancer", perhaps because it may sound less frightening. Neoplastic cells and tissues are often named for their major cell type, with the suffix "-oma" (which means tumor) at the end. For example: a muscle tumor is a myoma, a fatty tumor is a lipoma, and lymph cell neoplasia is lymphoma. The medical study of (*neoplasms*) is called *oncology*. Neoplasms serve no useful function but grow at the expense of the healthy organism and are categorized as *benign* or *malignant*.

Benign neoplasms are relatively harmless and tend to grow slowly. Benign neoplastic cells usually resemble the cells of the tissue in which they are growing. For example, benign skeletal muscle tumors tend to be formed from skeletal muscle cells and can be easily identified as such under a microscope. This trait of being easily recognizable is called *well-differentiated*. In other words, benign tumor cells are an easily-recognizable mutation of the host tissue. Benign neoplasms are usually enclosed by a fibrous capsule that prevents them from spreading into surrounding tissue, and they are usually not harmful unless their growth puts pressure on neighboring vital organs or causes hypersecretion of a gland.

Malignant neoplasms comprise what is commonly called *cancer*. At this time, cancer is the second leading cause of death in adults in U.S. Malignant neoplasms generally grow rapidly, and their cells are usually *poorly differentiated* (meaning they do not resemble the cells of the tissue in which they are growing). Malignant cells can have very unusual shapes, sizes, and nuclei, and they often *metastasize*, which means they spread from one part of the body to another.

There are three major classifications of malignant neoplasms: *carcinomas* are the most common and affect the epithelial tissue, such as the skin and mucous membrane, and the glandular tissue, such as the breast, prostate, liver, and pancreas. Carcinomas metastasize through the lymph vessel system, destroying healthy tissue in each new site. *Sarcomas* affect the connective tissues, such as bone, muscle, and cartilage. Sarcomas are less common but spread more rapidly, spreading mainly through the blood vessel system. Neoplasms of the circulatory system are the third category, and include leukemias and lymphomas.

Different cancers probably have different causes, however, in most cancers the etiology is unknown. Some people experience *remission*, in which their cancer stops growing and may even disappear. So far, research has not identified why this happens, although many theories are proposed. What we do know is that there are many probable contributors to cancer development, there are many early screening and diagnostic tests, and the success rate of cancer treatments is improving daily.

CANCER DEVELOPMENT

In general, cancer is thought to develop in three stages: initiation, promotion, and progression. In the *initiation* stage, there is a genetic cell change (mutation), caused by contact with some chemical, radiation, and/or viral stressor. In many cases, the person's immune system may neutralize and eliminate the mutated cells at this stage, as it does foreign materials and pathogens. In certain breast cancers, researchers have identified a particular gene, inherited by a small percentage of women, that seems to be more susceptible to mutation than normal.

During the *promotion* stage, the mutated cells grow and resemble benign neoplasms, which can then either regress back into normal-appearing tissue or can develop into cancer. Sometimes the person's immune system neutralizes and eliminates the growth at this stage. Removing or avoiding the stressor (chemical, radiation, and/or virus) at this stage can also sometimes prevent further development into cancer.

Within the *progression* stage, the tumor starts as *pre-cancerous*. In the pre-cancerous stage, the tumor cells can be watched for further development, or they can be removed easily. Sometimes these cancers are called "in situ", which means "in position" or "localized". The next step in progression is that the tumor becomes malignant, and begins to invade the underlying tissues with crab-like fingers. When this occurs, complete surgical removal of all cancer cells is more difficult, and so surgery is usually supplemented with chemotherapy, radiation, or both. If the cancer metastasizes, treatments are less likely to facilitate a cure and the overall survival rate is much lower. However, each person has unique strengths, resources, and circumstances. Many people with metastasized cancers have been able to heal themselves, with help from a variety of standard and alternative approaches. For more information about this topic, read Hirshberg & Barasch, 1995 (see *Further Resources*).

Most cancers are found during the progression stage. Many levels of screening techniques are now available to help people assess themselves. Screenings are not meant to diagnose. They are meant to identify who has risk factors or symptoms that warrant more in-depth assessment by a physician. Self-examinations of the skin, breasts, bowel habits, and so on, are the first level of screening. Mammograms, x-rays, certain blood and stool tests, and physician palpations are the next level. When a tumor is identified that shows characteristics that may be cancerous, a *biopsy* is usually done, which means a small sample is removed and examined under a microscope. A definite cancer diagnosis is not made until this last step.

Pathologists have developed a system of grading tumor cells removed for biopsy. The cells are judged according to their appearance. Grade 1 tumor cells are well-differentiated; grade 2 and 3 cells are moderately or poorly differentiated, and grade 4 cells are so undifferentiated that their tissue origin can not be recognized. Survival rates are most favorable for people with grade 1 tumors, and least favorable for people with grade 4.

CANCER PREVENTION

The sites where most fatal cancers develop are the lungs (#1), breast (#2), and colon (#3). Many cancers can be prevented by making healthy life-style choices. Cigarette smoking and use of other tobacco products contributes to about one-third of all cancers. In fact, cigarette smoking is the single most preventable cause of major diseases in adults, including cancer, heart disease, chronic bronchitis, and emphysema.

Diet and nutrition also play a significant role in reducing the risk of cancer. Diets low in fiber and high in fat, additives and preservatives increase the risk of cancers, especially in cancers of the breast, lung and colon. The following are common, basic dietary recommendations for preventing cancer:

- eat less than 30% of your daily calories as fat
- drink no more than one or two alcoholic drinks daily
- avoid charbroiled, smoked, and salted foods
- maintain your ideal weight
- eat at least five servings of fruits and vegetables daily, preferably ripened on the plant with a minimum of contamination with pesticide or herbicide. Especially include:

    - apricots, peaches, carrots, spinach, asparagus, squash, and sweet potatoes, spinach, kale, broccoli, and other dark green vegetables for vitamin A
    - oranges, lemons, grapefruit, strawberries, tomatoes, cabbage for vitamin C
    - vegetable oils for vitamin E
    - fresh vegetables and fruits of all kinds, whole grain breads and cereals, nuts, beans, peas for fiber

The American Cancer Society recommends these additional preventative measures:

- Do not smoke or chew tobacco.
- Protect the skin during sun exposure.
- Minimize exposure to x-rays.
- Minimize exposure to chemicals, including asbestos, nickel compounds, aniline dyes, arsenic, chromium, vinyl chloride, benzene, petroleum products, cleaning solvents, paint thinners, etc.
- Avoid heavily polluted air.
- Perform cancer screens and self-exams yearly for the mouth, colon, rectum, cervix, prostate, testes, and skin.
- Have a physical check-up by a physician every 2-3 years after age 40, and every 1-2 years after age 50.

General, long-term, unrelieved stress increases cancer risk by keeping the sympathetic nervous system turned on and the immune system suppressed by the body's cortisol. A history of early sexual intercourse (before complete maturation of the reproductive system, at about 18), early first pregnancy, multiple pregnancies, multiple sex partners, and having sexually transmitted diseases are all factors that increase a woman's risk for cervical cancer. Unprotected sun exposure, certain hormonal factors, exposure to hazardous chemicals, chronic irritation or inflammation, and advancing age increase the risk of cancers.

CANCER SIGNS AND SYMPTOMS

The signs and symptoms of cancer vary with the site. Pain is usually NOT an early sign of cancer. Pain usually only occurs in the later stages, when the tumor has grown large enough to obstruct a passageway or put pressure on adjacent nerve endings. The American Cancer Society has compiled a list of seven early warning signs of cancer, and the first letter of each word spells the word *CAUTION*.

- *C*hange in bowel or bladder habits
- *A* sore that does not heal
- *U*nusual bleeding or discharge
- *T*hickening or lump in breast or elsewhere
- *I*ndigestion or difficulty in swallowing
- *O*bvious change in wart or mole
- *N*agging cough or hoarseness

ASSESSMENT: OBSERVATION AND PALPATION

The signs and symptoms of various cancers depend on the body system involved. Sometimes tumors have no signs or symptoms until they have grown for years and are large enough to block or press on nearby vital tissues. Listen closely to the client's description of his/her health experience and read the intake form with your knowledge of neoplasia and/or the terminal phase of life in mind. Ask questions to clarify or add to the information the client gives. Observe for the seven warning signs of cancer (see above), the ABCDs of melanoma (see page 69), and any other deviations from health. Refer symptomatic clients to a physician for assessment.

COMMON NEOPLASTIC CONDITIONS

BENIGN NEOPLASMS

Adenoma: This is a benign tumor of glandular tissue, and often develops in the breast, thyroid gland, or mucous glands of the intestinal tract. A benign tumor in a gland can cause oversecretion of its hormone, often with very serious side effects. Bodywork is locally contraindicated.

Angioma: This is a benign tumor composed of blood vessels or lymph vessels, however, since lymph vessels are colorless, they are rarely seen. Angiomas are one type of benign tumor that is not encapsulated, which accounts for their typical "port-wine stain" appearance. Laser technology is very effective in erasing these. Bodywork is locally contraindicated.

Lipoma: This is a soft, fatty benign tumor that develops in the fat (adipose) tissue, most commonly in the neck, back, and buttocks, but can occur anywhere there is fat. Bodywork is locally contraindicated.

Myoma: This is a benign tumor of the muscle tissue. These usually develop in smooth or involuntary muscle; rarely in skeletal muscle. Myomas of the uterus are called fibroids. Bodywork is locally contraindicated to the abdomen in the presence of pain.

Nevus: This is the common mole, and, like the angioma, it is not encapsulated. Moles contain melanin and are congenital but may not appear until later in life, usually enlarging at puberty. This benign tumor can progress into malignant melanoma, which is a very deadly cancer. Always tell a client if you notice changes in a mole from one visit to the next (see *malignant melanoma*). Bodywork is locally contraindicated.

Papilloma (or Polyp): This is a benign tumor that starts with a fixed base and then grows a stalk. The common wart is a benign tumor of the keratin cells. Other examples of polyps occur in the uterus and intestines. Polyps can become irritated and bleed, and, in some cases, can progress into cancer. Bodywork is locally contraindicated.

Teratoma (or Dermoid Cyst): This is a unique benign tumor of the ovary. Lining this cyst is epidermis, skin with hair, sweat glands, and oil, and sometimes even teeth. Teratomas probably originate from a primitive cell that has the potential to develop into several different cells, but for some reason that development is altered. Sometimes these cysts can cause acute abdominal pain. Surgical removal is often necessary. Bodywork is locally contraindicated to the abdomen.

MALIGNANT NEOPLASMS

Many bodyworkers have been taught that the presence of any malignant (cancerous) condition is a contraindication for work. This may or may not be true. Research has been showing that informed, caring touch can have a positive effect on the immune system. Theoretically, this can positively affect cancer prevention and, perhaps, cancer neutralization.

At this time, there is no research, that I am aware of, indicating that bodywork causes cancer to spread. True, bodywork tends to increase circulation, but so does exercise or a hot shower, and those are not contraindicated. Without much research on the effects of bodywork on humans to inform us, we are left to make our own individual and collective judgments. My opinion is that bodyworkers follow these steps:

- advise clients with cancer symptoms to consult with their physician for assessment and diagnosis of what is going on;
- inform clients that there is some controversy as to whether bodywork is systemically contraindicated or not;
- encourage the client to ask his/her physician if s/he knows of any compelling reason to justify systemic contraindication in this client's case. If not, and the client wants to proceed, then
- provide bodywork with a local contraindication to avoid the cancerous area(s), keep in mind the principles of health and pathology described in this and other professional resources, and
- collectively support individuals and groups who scientifically explore the effects of bodywork on people with cancer.

Further, if a client is undergoing radiation, chemotherapy, or any other anti-neoplastic treatment, bodywork can often help reduce the client's pain, nausea, fatigue, insomnia, and apprehension. The client and bodyworker are advised to consult with the physician to collaboratively identify any contraindications or modifications that might be needed, and to keep the physician informed of the benefits that the bodywork is giving the client, if any. In the case of chemotherapy, Chamness suggests that bodyworkers wear gloves to prevent absorbing the toxic chemicals into their own skin when working with a client within 72 hours after a chemotherapy treatment (see *References*).

For information about the different types of malignancies, refer to each individual body system, described in earlier chapters, with the following addition:

Kaposi's Sarcoma (KS): This cancer is extremely rare in people who do not have AIDS. Lesions can range from a small plaque or nodule the size of an insect bite to much larger sizes. Lesions can be located internally, where they are not seen, as well as appear externally, on the skin. Skin lesions can be flat and smooth (plaques) or raised and nodular, and are a reddish-blue or reddish-purple color, just under the skin, usually on the lower extremities. Kaposi's skin lesions can change from day to day. Bodywork is locally contraindicated wherever lesions are present and systemically contraindicated for deep work or deep pressure.

Chapter 12, Part 2

BODYWORK FOR PEOPLE WHO HAVE A TERMINAL ILLNESS

When cancer or any other life-threatening disease has progressed to the point where physicians and/or other healers do not expect a cure, the person enters what can be called his/her terminal, or final, phase of life. Although we are all "terminal," in that we all will die, the words "terminal illness" commonly refer to a prognosis of six to twelve months. People who have been struggling with severe symptoms for months or years, and who have been told there are no further treatment options, can experience many overwhelming emotions.

Dr. Elizabeth Kubler-Ross, Dr. Bernie Segal, Stephen Levine, and many others have written extensively and movingly about living and being supported in this last phase of life. According to Dr. Kubler-Ross, dying persons and their loved ones typically progress through five reactions: denial, anger, bargaining, depression, and acceptance. Originally thought to be an orderly progression, we now know that people can feel more than one response at the same time, can move back and forth among these feelings, and may not have time to work through all of them. It is ideal that everyone comes to peaceful acceptance of their own or a loved one's death, but it is not always the case.

In your local community, a great resource for care, comfort, education and support is the Hospice. Hospices are staffed by dedicated nurses, physicians, social workers, and volunteers who have learned how to ease suffering and honor the last phase of life with dignity. Hospices provide palliative care, that is, care directed toward reducing the dying person's distressing symptoms without expectation of cure and supporting his/her comfort and communication with significant others. Caring, nurturing, supportive touch can profound support to people who are preparing to die and to the people who love them and are preparing for the loss. Most hospices value this, are happy to have volunteer bodyworkers on the team, and will provide training and support.

When working with people who have a terminal illness, the goals are to relax, nurture, comfort, and provide a safe space. The goals are not to fix, cure or remove lactic acid or toxins. Deep tissue massage is contraindicated because it is too invasive and may damage fragile tissues or upset delicate homeostasis (Chapman, 1996).

It is important to remember the same essential components that you use in all bodywork: 1) permission must be obtained before touching, and 2) the effectiveness of the work depends on the caring, sensitivity, and compassion that you give. If the person is unconscious or confused enough that s/he is unable to give you consent, it is important that you get consent from his/her primary caregiver, who is usually a husband, wife, child, or close friend. As you initiate the touching, watch closely for non-verbal signs that indicate whether the person is opening and relaxing to your touch or is withdrawing or tensing. Some clues to watch for include the person's breathing, muscle tension, body movements, and eye contact if any is present.

People who have a terminal illness are similar to "healthy" people in many ways and are different in some significant ways, too. The similarities are:

- We all have had different experiences regarding touching and being touched. Some were positive and some were not.
- We all have had cultural messages about who can touch us and what it means when they do.
- We all have a certain amount of mental/spiritual/emotional/physical tension that manifests in tight muscles, shallow breathing, and anxiety.
- When our skin is dry, a natural oil, like sesame or canola, is the best choice for lubricating it. Sometimes people prefer particular lotions or oils, so it is good to ask about that.
- We all like warmth. Warm your hands at the sink, if they are cold, before beginning the touching. You can also warm the oil or lotion in a pan of hot water.
- We all need to be positioned comfortably. That includes both the giver and the receiver of massage.
- We all need to be protected from infectious diseases, so the giver must always wash his/her hands both before and after the work.

The significant differences include:

- Skin is more fragile, due to immobility, poorer circulation, and poorer nutrition. Bruising, shearing, and skin tearing can occur with minimal pressure.
- Feet, legs, and other areas may have edema. Where edema is present, use only the lightest strokes and stroke toward the heart.
- Extremities are often cold and may be mottled. Soft tissues (muscles, fasciae, tendons, and ligaments) may be stiff or hard. If so, use a slow pace in your techniques, especially in effleurage and petrissage, and stay in an area for at least a minute or longer, to facilitate a gradual warming and softening in the tissue.
- Stimulation from friction, pressure, tapotement, fragrances, and talking can be overwhelming. It is often best to use little or none of these things.
- The person's energy is often low and is best conserved for the most important uses. In these cases, even gentle massage can wear a person out, and it is best to work only 20 minutes or less, depending on the person's tolerance. Stop if the person is getting tired.
- Research tells us that even when people appear to be unconscious, they may still be able to hear and feel, and therefore benefit by caring words and touch or be hurt by uncaring actions, as well.

From my experience, as well as many others who have given caring touch to people who were dying, the four most effective places to touch for comforting are:

- hands and feet (including wrists and ankles)
- head (forehead, scalp, temples and jaw)
- neck and shoulders
- low back (lumbar and sacral areas)

Most recipients of terminal, comforting massage will be lying in bed or seated in a chair. When in bed, a side-lying position can facilitate reaching the low back, and pillows in front of the person can give him/her a safe and supported feeling. If the person is very thin, placing a pillow between the knees also increases his/her comfort.

CASE PRESENTATIONS

10/11/96: 54 yo woman w/metastatic breast cancer. Goal: relax

History: referred by Hospice; MD approved w/out restriction; having anxiety, insomnia, lack of appetite, and pain in chest and back; taking narcotic meds by prescription; using oxygen intermittently to decrease dyspnea

S: rates intermittent, aching back pain at 4-5 and constant dull and pressure-like chest pain at 3-4 on 0-10 scale

O: appears pale and very thin; skin thin w/ bruises on arms; cervicals, traps, erectors, levator scapulae, & rhomboids all hypertonic, with many tender points

A: work was provided in her bed and lasted approx. 20 min; used light effleurage, petrissage, and pressure point approaches to areas described above, plus hands, feet, scalp, temples, jaw, and low back (lumbar). Extra care given to not exert too much pressure or stretching to fragile skin.

Outcome: rates back pain at 0; chest pain at 1.

Follow-up call to caregiver the next day: Says client slept well that night and feels bodywork is the reason.

STUDY QUESTIONS

Which parts of the above case presentations are subjective?
Which parts are objective?
What questions would you have asked that were not asked?
What bodywork techniques would you have done?
What referral(s)?
What other ways could the therapeutic outcome have been evaluated?
How might you have changed the format or way the cases were written?
What are the indications for massage/bodywork?
What are the contraindications?

FURTHER RESOURCES

Cheryl C. Chapman, RN, NCTMB, Director of Professional Massage Therapy, Short Hills, NJ, (201) 912-9060. Cheryl's full-time bodywork practice is devoted to people with cancer, HIV/AIDS, and other serious illnesses.

Program Planetree
621 Sansome Street
San Francisco, CA 94111
(415) 956-4215

Hirshberg, C. & Barasch, M.I. (1995). Remarkable recovery: What extraordinary healings tell us about getting well and staying well. Institute of Noetic Sciences: 1-800-383-1586.

REFERENCES

Chamness, A. (1996). Breast cancer and massage therapy. Massage Therapy Journal, Winter, 44-46.

Chapman, C. (1996). The forbidden client: Cancer/HIV/AIDS. Nurse's Touch, 2(2), 10; 21.

Curties, D. (1994). Could massage therapy promote cancer metastasis? Journal of Soft Tissue Manipulation, April-May.

Dunn, T. & Williams, M. (1989). Massage therapy guidelines for hospital and home care. San Francisco: Planetree Program.

Fritz, S. (1995). Mosby's fundamentals of therapeutic massage. St. Louis: Mosby Lifeline.

MacDonald, G. (1995). Massage for cancer patients: A review of nursing research. Massage Therapy Journal, Summer, 53-56.

Mulvihill, M.L. (1995). Human diseases: A systemic approach (4th ed.) Norwalk, CT: Appleton & Lange.

Newton, D. (1995). Pathology for massage therapists. Portland, OR: Simran Publications.

Sameulson, P. (1994). Pathophysiology for massage: The travel guide. Overland Park, KS: Mid-America Handbooks, Inc.

Thomas, C.L. (1989). Taber's cyclopedic medical dictionary (16th ed.). Philadelphia: F.A. Davis Co..

CHAPTER REVIEW

1. The development of new and abnormal tissue formation(s) is called _____

2. _____ tumors are relatively harmless and tend to grow slowly.

3. _____ tumors grow more rapidly and can invade underlying tissues or metastasize.

4. _____ are the most common malignant tumors and effect the epithelial tissue and the glandular tissue.

5. _____ are less common malignant tumors and effect the muscle, bone, and connective tissues.

6. Metastasizing cancers spread through the _____ and _____ vessels.

7. Cancer is thought to grow in three stages: _____ _____, and _____.

8. Most cancers are found during the _____ stage.

9. Survival rates are best for people with grade _____ tumors and worst for people with grade _____ tumors.

10. Many cancers can be prevented by _____

11. _____ is the single most preventable cause of cancer, heart disease, chronic bronchitis, and emphysema.

12. The seven warning signals of cancer are: _____
_____
_____

13. Dying persons and their loved ones typically progress through five reactions: _____
_____
_____

ANSWERS TO CHAPTER REVIEW

1. neoplasia

2. benign

3. malignant

4. carcinomas

5. sarcomas

6. blood and lymph vessels

7. initiation, promotion, progression

8. progression

9. 1; 4

10. making healthy lifestyle choices

11. cigarette smoking

12. Change in bowel or bladder habits; A sore that does not heal; Unusual bleeding or discharge; Thickening or lump in breast or elsewhere; Indigestion or difficulty in swallowing; Obvious change in wart or mole; Nagging cough or hoarsenes

13. denial, anger, bargaining, depression, and acceptance

Appendix

Table of Contents

Code of Ethics for Massage Therapists

This Code of Ethics is a summary statement of the standards by which massage therapists agree to conduct their practices and is a declaration of the general principals of acceptable, ethical, professional behavior.

Massage Therapists shall:

• Have a sincere commitment to provide the highest quality care to those who seek their professional service.

• Perform only those services for which they are qualified and represent their education, certifications, professional affiliations, and other qualifications honestly.

• Acknowledge the inherent worth and individuality of each person and, therefore, do not unjustly discriminate against clients or colleagues and work to eliminate prejudices in the profession.

• Strive for professional excellence through regular assessment of personal strengths, limitations and effectiveness and by continued education and training.

• Actively support the profession through participation in local, state, and national organizations which promote high standards of practice of massage therapy.

• Work in their communities toward the understanding and acceptance of massage therapy as a valuable health service, abide by all laws governing massage practice and work for the repeal or revision of laws detrimental to the legitimate practice of massage therapy.

• Acknowledge the confidential nature of the professional relationship with a client and respect each client's right to privacy.

• Respect all ethical health care practitioners and work together amicably to promote health and natural healing.

• Conduct their business and professional activities with honesty and integrity and project a professional image in all aspects of their practices.

• Accept the responsibility to self, clients and associates to maintain physical, mental and emotional well-being.

• Respect the integrity of each person and, therefore, do not engage in any sexual conduct or sexual activities involving their clients.

Used with permission of American Massage Therapy Association™, © copyright 1995. For further information on joining the AMTA, call 847-864-0123.

Words *with* Dignity

By using words with dignity, we encourage equality for everyone

Words with Dignity	Avoid these words
person with a disability/disabled	cripple/handicapped/handicap/invalid (literally, *invalid* means "not valid")
person who has/person with (e.g. person who has cerebral palsy)	victim/afflicted with (e.g. victim of cerebral palsy)
uses a wheelchair	restricted, confined to a wheelchair/wheelchair bound (the chair enables mobility. Without the chair, the person is confined to bed)
non-disabled	normal (referring to non-disabled persons as "normal" insinuates that people with disabilities are abnormal)
deaf/does not voice for themselves/nonvocal	deaf mute/deaf and dumb
disabled since birth/born with	birth defect
psychiatric history/psychiatric disability/ emotional disorder/mental illness	crazy/insane/lunatic/mental patient/wacko
epilepsy/seizures	fits
learning disability/mental retardation/ developmental delay/ADD/ADHD	slow/retard/lazy/stupid/underachiever

*O*ther terms which should be avoided because they have negative connotations and tend to *evoke pity and fear* include:

abnormal	handi-capable	moron	spastic
burden	incapacitated	palsied	stricken with
condition	imbecile	pathetic	suffer
deformed	maniac	physically challenged	tragedy
differently abled	maimed	pitiful	unfortunate
disfigured	madman	poor	victim

*P*referred terminology

blind (no visual capability)
legally blind/low vision (some visual capability)
hearing loss/hard of hearing (some hearing capability)
hemiplegia (paralysis of one side of the body)
paraplegia (loss of function in lower body only)
quadriplegia (paralysis of both arms and legs)
residual limb (post-amputation of a limb)

PARAQUAD
Independence for People with Disabilities

*311 North Lindbergh Boulevard • St. Louis, Missouri 63141 • (314) 567-1558 voice • 567-5222 TTY • 567-1559 fax
website: http://www.paraquad.org • e-mail: paraquad@paraquad.org*

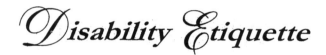

Disability Etiquette

Basic guidelines

- Make reference to the person first then the disability. Say "a person with a disability" rather than "a disabled person." However, the latter is acceptable in the interest of conserving print space or saving announcing time.

- The term "handicapped" comes from the image of a person standing on the corner with a cap in hand, begging for money. People with disabilities do not want to be the recipients of charity or pity. They want to participate equally with the rest of the community. A disability is a functional limitation that interferes with a person's ability to walk, hear, talk, learn, etc. Use "handicap" to describe a situation or barrier imposed by society, the environment or oneself.

- If the disability isn't germane to the story or conversation, don't mention it.

- Remember, a person who has a disability isn't necessarily chronically sick or unhealthy. He or she is often just disabled.

- A person is not a condition, so avoid describing a person as such. Don't present someone as "an epileptic" or "a post polio". Instead, say "a person with epilepsy" or "a person who has had polio."

Common courtesies

- Don't feel obligated to act as a caregiver to people with disabilities. Offer assistance, but **wait** until your offer is accepted **before** you help. Listen to any instructions the person may give.

- Leaning on a person's wheelchair is similar to leaning or hanging on a person. It is considered annoying and rude. The chair is a part of one's personal body space. Don't hang on it!

- Share the same social courtesies with people with disabilities that you would share with someone else. If you shake hands with people you meet, offer your hand to everyone you meet, regardless of disability. If the person is unable to shake your hand, he or she will tell you.

- When offering assistance to a person with a visual impairment, allow that person to take your arm. This will enable you to guide, rather than propel or lead the person. Use specific directions, such as "left one-hundred feet" or right two yards," when directing a person with a visual impairment.

- When planning events which involve persons with disabilities, consider their needs before choosing a location. Even if people with disabilities will not attend, select an accessible spot. You wouldn't think of holding an event where other minorities could not attend, so don't exclude people with disabilities.

Conversation

- When speaking about people with disabilities, emphasize achievements, abilities and individual qualities. Portray them as they are in real life: as parents, employees, business owners, etc.

- When talking to a person who has a physical disability, speak directly to that person, not through a companion. For people who communicate through sign language, speak to them, not to the interpreter.

- Relax. Don't be embarrassed if you use common expressions such as "See ya later" or "Gotta run."

- To get the attention of a person who has a hearing loss, tap them on the shoulder or wave. Look directly at the person and speak clearly, slowly and expressively to establish if they read lips. Not all people with hearing loss can read lips. Those who do rely on facial expressions and body language for understanding. Stay in the light and keep food, hands and other objects away from your mouth. Shouting won't help. Written notes will. Use an interpreter if possible.

- When talking to a person in a wheelchair for more than a few minutes, place yourself at eye level with that person. This will spare both of you a sore neck.

- When greeting a person with severe loss of vision, always identify yourself and others. For example say, "On my right is John Smith." Remember to identify persons to whom you are speaking. Speak in a normal tone of voice and indicate when the conversation is over. Let them know when you move from one place to another."

PARAQUAD
Independence for people with Disabilities

311 North Lindbergh Boulevard • St. Louis, Missouri 63141 • (314) 567-1558 voice • 567-5222 TTY • 567-1559 fax
website: http://www.paraquad.org • e-mail: paraquad@paraquad.org

Sample Syllabus: 50-Hour Pathology Course

Instructor

Name _____

Please reach me through the _____ Program office.

Course Description

Pathology is the study of the nature of diseases and the structural and functional changes produced by them. Therapeutic massage therapists are ethically and legally responsible for recognizing clients' deviations from normal health, knowing if massage is indicated or contraindicated, and, if contraindicated, referring the client to the appropriate health practitioner. Expertise in these areas requires lifelong learning. The purpose of this course is to help the beginning massage student form a knowledge base upon which s/he can begin to practice. Total class time is 49 hours, plus one additional hour of credit is given for the independent study case preparation to be done by the student outside of class, for a total of 50 course hours.

Course Objectives

Upon successful completion of this course, the student will be able to:

1. perform a basic health assessment, including health history, observation and palpation
2. identify at least 50 common abnormal assessment findings
3. recognize massage indications and contraindications for common health conditions
4. make referrals to other health professionals, when necessary
5. evaluate therapeutic outcomes

Grading: Pass/Fail

In order to pass this course, the student must:

1. attend classes according to school policy
2. score at least 70% correct on the final exam
3. average at least 70% on the weekly chapter tests
4. pass the independent study case presentation
5. present a brief summary of least one article, related to the course, from a professional massage book or journal
6. actively listen and share in class discussions

Textbooks

Required: Recognizing Health & Illness: Pathology for Massage Therapists/Bodyworkers by Burch
Suggested: Mosby's Fundamentals of Massage by Fritz, Job's Body by Juhan, Physiology Coloring Book by Kapit, Macey & Meisami, Merck Manual by Merck, Sharp & Dohme.

Content Outline

Class 1　Intro to course, learning contracts, resources etc.
Human health, disability & illness

Class 2　Assessing health conditions, including:
　　　Health history, observation & palpation
　　　The client's goal(s)
　　　Indications & contraindications
　　　Making referrals
　　　Evaluating therapeutic outcomes

Class 3　Effects of stress & aging
Emotional conditions

Class 4　Integumentary system
Inflammation & repair

Class 5　Musculoskeletal system, part I

Class 6　Musculoskeletal system, part II

Class 7　Nervous system

Class 8　Cardiovascular system

Class 9　Immune system
Respiratory system

Class 10　Endocrine system
Digestive system

Class 11　Urinary, and Reproductive systems
Hereditary conditions
Neoplasia

Class 12　Bodywork for terminally ill persons
Independent case study presentations, to include:
　　　Basic health assessment, including health history,
　　　　　observation with subjective and objective information,
　　　　　and palpation.
　　　Client goals.
　　　Abnormal assessment findings.
　　　Massage indications and contraindications.
　　　Referrals to other health professionals, when necessary.
　　　Evaluation of therapeutic outcomes.

Class 13　Review for final exam

Class 14　Final exam
Course evaluation
Celebration of completion!

Project Outline

In this project, each student is required to select an actual client's case to present to the class. Keeping all identifying information confidential, the student performs an assessment, massage/bodywork session, outcome evaluation, and referral (if applicable) and presents a verbal five to ten minute summary of that experience to the class. The student also completes a brief written summary, which is given to the instructor (see next page).

Essential components of this project include:

> Basic health assessment:
> > health history
> > observation with subjective and objective information
>
> Client goals
> Abnormal assessment findings
> Massage indications and contraindications
> Referrals to other health professionals, when necessary
> Evaluation of therapeutic outcomes.

I graded these projects as Pass/Fail, with a "Pass" grade given when the student completed the project with all essential components in place.

CASE PRESENTATION by: _____ Date _____

1. Assessment info:
   History

   Observations
   (Subjective)

   (Objective)

2. Client goals:

3. Abnormal findings:

4. Indications:

5. Contraindications:

6. Application:

7. Referrals:

8. Evaluation:

Sample Syllabus: 3-Hour Communicable Disease Class

Program: Massage Therapy

Course: Communicable Disease   3 hours

Instructor: Name _____

Please reach me through the _____ Program office.

Course Description: Through lecture and discussion, students will be able to:
1) identify names and modes of transmission of common communicable diseases
2) understand how to prevent disease transmission in a massage practice.

Prerequisites: None

Grading: Pass/Fail

In order to pass this course, the student must score at least 70% correct on the exam.

Content Outline:

Introductions of instructor and students

Definitions of terms

Names, symptoms & modes of transmission of these common communicable diseases:
Common colds & flu
Hepatitis A & B
HIV
Staphylococcus
Skin & nail fungi
Herpes
Pediculosis
TB
Pneumonia

Prevention of disease transmission in massage practice, including:
Handwashing
Universal precautions
Disinfection of linens & equipment

Review

Exam

Evaluation of course

Materials: Instructor handouts

Glossary

abuse anything that hurts oneself or others mentally, emotionally, spiritually or physically

acute illness an illness that develops quickly and potentially corrects quickly

afferent nerves carry stimuli from the senses to the spinal cord and brain; also called sensory nerves

aggression striking out at someone or something to get rid of pain or to defend oneself; generally stimulated by frustration, which is a form of anger

aging becoming older; maturing

airborne route a path for communicable disease transmission; pathogens enter the body through breathing

allergen a type of antigen; causes allergic reaction; examples are certain drugs, pollen, dust, animal dandruff, fur, feathers, insect bites and stings, eggs, chocolate, milk, wheat, seafood and citrus fruits

allergy an abnormal reaction of tissues to an antigen; often includes the release of histamine from injured cells.

anorexia lack of appetite

antibody protein substances carried in the blood and developed in response to an antigen; the body's efforts to neutralize an antigen

antigen a protein or polysaccharide substance on the surface of a pathogen or other substance; antigens stimulate the body to produce antibodies

anxiety feeling great apprehension, uneasiness and agitation; can range from simple restlessness and irritability to an extreme feeling of powerlessness and panic.

acute anxiety is also known as a **panic attack**. In this situation, the feelings are very strong and accelerate quickly.

chronic anxiety is more generalized, less intense, and lasts in varying degrees for a month or more.

apathy lack of interest or enthusiasm in life

assessment the collection and interpretation of information provided by the client, any referring health professionals, and your own observation. It usually includes looking, listening, and feeling in a continual and ongoing process to identify deviations from normal wellness.

autoimmune disease caused by antigens attacking the person's own cells, e.g. rheumatoid arthritis, lupus, etc.

autonomic nervous system (ANS) made up of the sympathetic and parasympathetic systems, which control the fight or flight and relaxation responses of the smooth muscles, the cardiac muscle and the glands

bacteria primitive cells without nuclei that secrete toxins that damage body tissues; they become parasites inside cells or form colonies that disrupt normal body function; they thrive in warm, dark, moist places and can usually be killed by antibiotics, disinfectants, sunlight, and dryness

benign relatively harmless and slow-growing tumor tissue; usually enclosed in a fibrous capsule that prevents them from spreading to surrounding tissues

bipolar affective disorder severe mood swings ranging from an unusual high to depression;

also known as manic/depression

blood and body fluids the most likely vehicles for transmission of serious communicable diseases; includes blood, semen, vaginal fluid, urine, feces, vomit, nasal and lung secretions, saliva, breast milk, and wound discharges (tears and perspiration are not considered carriers of significant pathogens)

blood pressure the pressure exerted by the blood on a blood vessel wall; highest at the moment when the ventricles contract and lowest when the ventricles relax; a healthy adult blood pressure averages between 140 and 100 for the highest (top) number and between 90 and 60 for the lowest (bottom) number; expressed as a ratio, e.g. 120/80

body the physical material facet including cells, fluids, organs and systems. A factory for body maintenance and repair, heating, cooling, using fuel, and taking in input through the senses. Carries out the directions of the mind as influenced by the spirit and emotion.

body/mind a condensed term for the whole mind/body/spirit/ emotion person

bursae sacs or cavities in the connective tissue, usually near a joint

central nervous system (CNS) the brain and spinal cord and their coverings

chronic illness develops gradually and can last a long time, sometimes for the rest of the person's life. If an illness
lasts for 6 months or more, its generally considered chronic.

clubbing enlarged finger or toe tips caused by chronic oxygen deprivation

collaboration working together; cooperating with or assisting one another

communicable disease a contagious disease; caused by pathogens that are easily spread

connective tissues fascia, joint cartilage, bursa, tendon and ligament

contamination process by which an object or an area becomes inhabited by pathogens

contraindication any persuasive reason to avoid the action under consideration

conversion a somatoform disorder; the person has a hysterical reaction to an emotional event or trauma and physical symptoms emerge

contracture an abnormal shortening of fascia, muscle, tendon and/or ligament tissue, and occurs when a body area is paralyzed, as in stroke or spinal injury

crepitation a grating, clicking or crackling sound heard on movement of joints, usually due to roughness and irregularities on the articulating surfaces

cyanosis (blueness) due to the presence of deoxygenated blood and excess carbon dioxide; a progression of pallor; indicates severe lack of oxygen

defense mechanism a mental process (often unconscious) that helps us deal with situations that are painful or that we feel anxious about

denial refusing to believe the truth about a situation, event or person

depression feeling sad, pessimistic, dejected or discouraged; becomes considered a mental illness if it lasts more than two months

diagnosis naming a disease or illness; can only be performed by a licensed physician (MD, DO, ND or chiropractor) or nurse practitioner

direct contact route a path of communicable disease transference by touching or being touched by contaminated fluids or objects

disability limited function in any aspect of the body/mind. Many disabilities are "invisible."

disease a lack of ease; any group of symptoms distinct from normal health conditions; impaired performance of any vital function

disinfection destruction of most or all living pathogens on inanimate objects

dissociation a symptom, not a specific illness; includes the separation of whole segments of the personality (as in multiple personality disorder), the separation of distinct mental processes (as in schizophrenia), or the separation of one's awareness from one's body and physical sensations (as in PTSD)

dysfunctional something that does not help us function in life and gives many negative consequences

dyspnea shortness of breath; difficult breathing

edema swelling; can be localized or systemic; the most common locations for edema are the feet and lower legs

efferent nerves carry stimuli from the brain and/or spinal cord to the muscles; also called motor nerves

emotion Energy in motion. An intangible facet consisting of four basic emotions: glad (happy), mad (anger), sad, and afraid. Physical tension decreases when emotions are released. Creativity is emotion directed by spirit and mind.

erythema (redness) caused by vasodilatation, usually as a result of inflammation or infection; also can be caused by friction, heat, cold, pressure or radiation

etiology the cause of a condition or disease

evaluation determining the value or effectiveness

fascia a fibrous membrane that unites the skin with the underlying tissue and covers, supports, and separates the muscles

fatigue constant feeling of tiredness

functional something that helps us function in life without too many negative consequences

fungi plant-like organisms without chlorophyll that thrive in warm, dark, moist conditions; they often live on the skin or mucous membranes

health history a record of past health events, including past illnesses, accidents, and surgeries

health a condition in which all functions of the body/mind are normally active

homeostasis the state of relative constancy or balance in the body's internal environment

hypertonicity excessive muscle tone or tension

hypervigilence being overly concerned and overly attentive to one's inner state or outer environment

hypochondriasis a somatoform disorder; a person has a heightened awareness of their body and an abnormal fear of disease

hypotonicity deficiency of muscle tone; weak, limp or flaccid

hypoxia significant reduction in a cell's oxygen supply

idiopathic the cause, or etiology, is unknown

immune having or producing antibodies

immune system one of the body systems; monitors for foreign bodies and neutralizes them if possible

immunity being protected by antibodies from a disease; this occurs after a person is exposed to a pathogen, is immunized or vaccinated; is generally increased by massage, rest, relaxation, laughter, good nutrition, pure water, comfortable temperatures, and regular exercise; generally decreased by sugar, caffeine, stress, grief, and isolation

indication any persuasive reason to do the action under consideration

infection the presence and replication of pathogens in or on the body; the most common symptoms of systemic infection are fever, chills, fatigue and pain

inflammation normal mechanism that usually facilitates recovery from infection or injury and includes pain, heat, redness and swelling

intact skin having no open areas; prevents pathogens from entering the body

insomnia not being able to sleep when you feel tired

ischemia a local and temporary lack deficiency of blood supply, usually due to obstruction of circulation

jaundice (yellowness) can be present in the sclera of the eyes, the skin and/or urine; indicates an excess of bilirubin in the blood

local contraindications relate to a specific area of the body; bodywork can be given except for the specific problem area

localized pain pain confined to one site of origin

local massage bodywork done directly on the physical area of concern

malignant usually also called "cancerous"; tissue that grows rapidly and often metastasize

malnutrition "bad nutrition"; includes both deficiencies and excesses of dietary components such as proteins, fats, sugars/starches, vitamins and minerals

metastasize spread from one part of the body to another

mind an intangible facet that analyzes things, organizes data, asks questions, seeks answers, makes decisions. Directs vehicle (body), decides/chooses how to express emotion and spirit.

motor nerves carry stimuli from the brain and/or spinal cord to the muscles; also called efferent nerves

mucous membranes the thin, fragile tissues that line most of the body's openings and passages; they protect the body by secreting mucus, which keeps the tissues moist and elastic and contains antibacterial, antiviral, antifungal chemicals

multiple personality disorder a fairly rare condition in which the person exhibits two or more distinct personalities. Generally each personality is unaware of the others and has its own identity, its own age, its own likes and dislikes, and in some cases, its own distinct illnesses that the other personality(s) don't have.

nutrition all the processes involved in taking in and utilizing food; includes ingestion, digestion, absorption and metabolism

objective something that can be seen, touched, and measured by an observer, e.g. a wart

observation watching and inspecting carefully, with attention to detail

obsessive/compulsive disorder (OCD) consists of two different dimensions: **Obsession** is having uncontrollable thoughts over and over again. **Compulsion** is having an uncontrollable urge to act upon the obsessive thoughts.

open skin areas breaks in the continuum of skin or mucous membrane, including rashes, cuts, scrapes, hangnails, etc.

oral route a path of communicable disease transference through eating or drinking contaminated foods or fluids

pain the sensory and emotional experience associated with actual or potential tissue damage

pallor (paleness) usually indicates a moderate lack of oxygen and is most often caused by oxygen deficiency or vasoconstriction due to stress, disease or cold temperature

palpation the process of examining the body by applying one's hands to the body surface

paranoia feelings of persecution that are unsupported by actual evidence, and results in unreasonable fears that someone or something is going to do them harm

parasites organisms that feed off another animal's tissue, such as worms, insects or amoebas

parasympathetic nervous system activated by periods of rest or nurturance; commonly called the relaxation response; conserves and replenishes energy

pathogens organisms (some can be seen with the naked eye and some can't) that can injure cells; includes viruses, bacteria, parasites and fungi

pathology the study of the nature of diseases and the structural and functional changes produced by them

peripheral nervous system (PNS) the cranial and spinal nerves and their ganglions; carries nerve impulses between the central nervous system (CNS) and the muscles, glands, skin and other organs

peristalsis an involuntary reflexive wavelike movement stimulated by distention of the walls of the gastrointestinal tube; this wave consists of contraction of the circular smooth muscle above the distention and relaxation and opening of the area immediately distal to the distention, which moves the contents of the tube forward in the tube

pitting edema a type of edema pits or indentations are formed in the area when the skin is pressed gently with the fingertips

poorly differentiated cancer cells that don't resemble the cells of the tissue in which they are growing

post traumatic stress disorder (PTSD) initially the person represses the memories of traumatic experience(s) and then has anxiety, hypervigilence and sleep problems, alternating with emotional or physical numbness. There may also be unexplained rage, guilt, depression, phobias and suicidal thoughts.

projected pain pain perceived in the tissue distal to a compressed nerve

projection blaming others for one's own problems or difficulties

proprioceptors sensory receptors in the muscles and connective tissues that give the person kinesthetic information about position, movement, pressure, tension, stretch and balance

psychogenic pain a somatoform disorder; a person feels pain but there is no diagnosable reason for the pain

radiating pain pain that diffuses out and around its site of origin or travels along a nerve

range of motion (ROM) the range of movement of a joint

rationalization trying to justify what happens, by blaming it on circumstances

referral a recommendation that the client seek the advice of another health care practitioner

referred pain pain that is felt in an area distant from the site of its origin; often originates in an organ that receives innervation from the same segment of the spinal cord as the muscular or connective tissue area where the pain is felt

reflex a specific, purposeful and predictable involuntary neuromuscular response to a stimulus

reflux backward flow

regression behaving in ways that are less mature than the person is normally capable of

repression putting one's feelings or thoughts out of one's mind because they are unpleasant or painful

risk factors conditions that make a negative event more likely, but do not necessarily constitute the cause. Major categories of risk factors for illnesses include: genetics, age, lifestyle, stress, environment, and pre-existing illnesses.

schizophrenia an inability to distinguish reality from fantasy. The person generally has decreased ability to think, plan and relate normally and may hear or see things that you don't hear or see (hallucinations)

sensory nerves carry sensory information (sensations) to the brain and/or spinal cord; also called afferent nerves

sexual abuse any unwanted or inappropriate sexual contact, either verbal or physical, between two or more people, that's intended as an act of control, power, rage, violence and intimidation, with sex as a weapon

sign evidence of illness that an observer can see, e.g. bruise

spasm sudden involuntary muscle contraction

somatic nervous system (SNS) the nerves of the joints and skeletal muscles

somatization a somatoform disorder; the person feels physically ill but has no diagnosable disease

somatoform disorder occurs when the person is trying to resolve some inner mental or emotional conflict, but they aren't able to do it directly, so they unconsciously create physical signs or symptoms of illness.

spirit An intangible facet. The drive to grow, learn, and experience life. Is often sensed as a connection with a higher power. Contains the pattern of our wholeness. Considered by many to be the 'breath of life' that animates the body and underlies mind and emotion.

state dependent memory memories are stored in the body as well as the mind

sterilization destruction of all living organisms on inanimate objects; not usually required in massage therapy settings

stress any factor that causes tension. Changes in routine and/or factors that require a person to adapt are common stressors.

subjective something known only by the subject, e.g. a feeling.

suicide killing oneself

sympathetic nervous system activated for energy production; commonly called the fight or flight response

symptom evidence of illness that an observer can't see; must be reported by the client, e.g. pain

syndrome a group of different signs and symptoms, assumed to have a common cause

systemic pertaining to the body as a whole, rather than to its one of its parts

systemic contraindication prevents all bodywork to the client; requires the attention of a physician to assess the client's condition and determine if bodywork would be safe or not.

therapeutic outcome the effect your bodywork has on the client

thixotropy a substance that becomes more fluid when it's moved and/or heated and more solid when it's cool or sits undisturbed

treatment procedures done to alleviate symptoms or cure an illness

universal precautions procedures set forth by the CDC to prevent the spread of serious communicable diseases

varicose veins enlarged, swollen or twisted veins; most often occur in the feet and legs, but can occur in almost any part of the body; local massage is contraindicated

viruses protein capsules made of DNA or RNA. They invade healthy cells and replicate there. Viruses can lie dormant for years until conditions support their activation, and are unaffected by antibiotics. They enter the body through the respiratory system, open skin, and breaks in the mucous membranes.

well-differentiated cancer cells easily recognizable as similar to the cells of the tissue in which they are growing

Index

Gene mutation disorders 225
Generalized tonic-clonic seizure 115
Genito 213
Gestational diabetes 182
Gigantism 184
Gingivitis 208
Gloves 150
Glucagon 178
Glucose 197
Goiter 183
Gonorrhea 219
Gout 89
Granulation 72
Graves' disease 185
Ground substance 77
Gynecomastia 216

H

Hand washing 149
Hay fever 170
Head lice 64
Headaches 112
Health 15
Health history 20
Heart 123
   attack 132
   murmur 132
Helicobacter pylori bacteria 208
Hemolytic anemia 129
Hemophilia 132, 226
Hemorrhage 111
Hemorrhagic anemia 130
Hepatitis 153, 154, 206
Heredity 225
Hermaphroditism 226
Hernia 206
Herniated disc 88, 89
Herpes 154, 220
High cholesterol 132
Histmine 146
HIV 154
Hives 64
Hodgkin's disease 133
Homeostasis 17
Hormones 175
Hydrocortisone 177
Hyperadrenalism 183
Hyperglycemia 181
Hyperparathyroidism 184
Hyperpituitarism 184
Hypersecretion 180
Hypertension (high blood pressure) 133
Hyperthyroidism 185

Hypertonicity 85
Hypervigilance 42
Hypoadrenalism 184
Hypochondriasis 47
Hypoglycemia 181, 184
Hypoparathyroidism 184
Hypopituitarism 185
Hyposecretion 180
Hypotension (low blood pressure) 133
Hypothalamus 175, 176
Hypothyroidism 185
Hypotonicity 85
Hypoxia 37

I

Idiopathic 18
Ileocecal valve 193
Ileostomy 207
Ileum 193
Immune 143, 144
Immune response 144
Immune system hypersensitivity 37
Immunity 144
Impaired glucose tolerance 182
Impetigo 62
Indication 25
Indications for masssage in pregnancy 215
Infection 148
Infectious 61
Infectious hepatitis 153
Infective arthritis 86
Inflammation 71
Influenza 153, 166
Inhalation 164
Initiation 234
Insoluble fiber 197
Insomnia 116
Insulin 178
   reaction 181
   shock 181
Integument 57
Intermittent claudication 133
Interstitial cystitis 217
Intractable 108
Intractable pain 109
Iodine 201
Iron deficiency 201
Iron deficiency anemia 129
Irritable bowel syndrome 204
Ischemia 81, 124

J

Jaundice 58, 127

Continuing Education Test: Recognizing Health and Illness
by Sharon Burch RN, MSN, CNS, ARNP, NCTMB

The following test is approved by both the National Certification Board
of Therapeutic Massage/Bodywork (provider #054616-00) and
the Kansas State Board of Nursing (provider #LT0187-0772)
for **15 Continuing Education Credits**.

If you want to receive credit for reading this book, simply complete the following
open-book test and mail it with your check or money order to:

Health Positive!, 1510 E. 1584 Rd., Lawrence, KS 66046-9273
Phone 785.843.5884, Fax 785.841.1761, E-mail 4health@idir.net

The cost is $50.00 for 15 CE credits from either Board and an additional $5.00
if you want another 15 CE credits from the second Board.

Please allow 3 to 4 weeks for your test to be processed and your certificate(s)
mailed to you. If you need the certificate(s) in less time, let me know
and we can discuss additional costs for Express Service.

NAME _____ PHONE _____ DATE _____

ADDRESS_____ CITY _____ STATE ____ ZIP _____

PAYMENT ENCLOSED: (circle one) $50 OR $55

TYPE OF CE CREDIT DESIRED: (circle 1 or both) NCBTMB   KS Board of Nursing

MASSAGE/BODYWORK LICENSE NUMBER: _____ EXP DATE _____

NURSING LICENSE NUMBER: _____ EXP DATE _____

MULTIPLE CHOICE
WRITE THE ONE <u>BEST</u> ANSWER TO EACH QUESTION IN THE SPACE PROVIDED

_____ 1. Which factor DECREASES the body's immunity to communicable diseases?
      a. stress
      b. laughter
      c. adequate rest
      d. caring, respectful touch

_____ 2. One of the basic components of a health <u>history</u> is:
      a. explanation of your prices
      b. past surgeries, illnesses or injuries
      c. confidentiality of client's concerns
      d. qualifications of the therapist

_____ 3. One of the basic components of an <u>assessment</u> is to:
    a. correct the client's problem
    b. ask about the present problem or concern
    c. evaluate the outcome of the session
    d. refer client to another health practitioner

_____ 4. You have just finished giving a therapeutic massage. To evaluate the therapeutic outcome objectively, you:
    a. assume it was a good massage if client doesn't complain
    b. ask client to compare this massage to the last one
    c. ask client to let you know if they need any more work
    d. compare client's range of motion to an earlier range

_____ 5. The massage therapist refers the client for further evaluation if a mole has this characteristic:
    a. asymmetry
    b. irregular borders
    c. more than one color
    d. all of the above

_____ 6. During assessment, the massage therapist asks the client to describe any pain according to its:
    a. location, intensity, size, & duration
    b. quality, location, intensity & comfort
    c. intensity, location, quality & duration
    d. duration, character, type & quality

_____ 7. A massage therapist does not work on intoxicated persons because:
    a. the person will not respect your opinion
    b. the person's awareness will be cloudy
    c. the therapist is liable if the person injures himself after the massage
    d. it is illegal to massage intoxicated persons

_____ 8. The first symptoms of heart attack usually include:
    a. pallor & pain in the chest
    b. loss of consciousness
    c. difficulty breathing
    d. dizziness when standing

_____ 9. Appropriate intervention for a massage client with degenerative disc disease includes:
    a. instructing client to bend or twist past comfort
    b. hard pressure on or near the spine
    c. effleurage on the trapezius
    d. manipulations of the vertebrae

MATCHING (ONLY ONE ANSWER PER BLANK)

MATCH THE CARDIOVASCULAR TERM TO ITS DEFINITION:

10.	_____ angina	a. weakened heart beat & poor circulation
11.	_____ stroke	b. temporary heart pain without damage
12. ·	_____ heart attack	c. chronic elevation of blood pressure
13.	_____ CHF	d. irreversible damage to heart muscle
14.	_____ embolus	e. blood clot attached to vein wall
15.	_____ hypertension	f. inflammation of vein
16.	_____ phlebitis	g. abnormally dilated vein
17.	_____ thrombus	h. blood clot floating freely in vein
18.	_____ stasis ulcer	i. disrupted blood flow in the brain
19.	_____ varicose	j. skin breakdown at or above ankle

MATCH THE DISEASE WITH ITS DEFINITION OR SYMPTOMS:

20.	_____ lymphoma	a. benign neoplasm of melanocytes
21.	_____ dermatitis	b. infected nodule or pustule
22.	_____ abscess/boil	c. cancer of the lymph system
23.	_____ psoriasis	d. skin inflammation caused by contact with a substance the person is allergic to
24.	_____ mole/nevus	e. non-contagious skin disease where cells are replaced in 4 days instead of 28

MATCH THE MUSCULOSKELETAL DISORDER WITH ITS DEFINITION OR SYMPTOM:

25.	_____ gout	a. joint pain & deformity, starts in 30s-40s
26.	_____ osteoarthritis	b. progressive spinal curvature
27.	_____ osteoporosis	c. caused by excess urate crystals in joints
28.	_____ Rheumatoid arthr.	d. joint cartilage is worn away
29.	_____ scoliosis	e. bone is absorbed faster than its replaced
30.	_____ strain	f. progressive destruction of myelin sheaths
31.	_____ fibromyalgia	g. compressed nerve, causing leg pain
32.	_____ sprain	h. cervical sprain
33.	_____ multiple sclerosis	i. predictable tender points, fatigue
34.	_____ whiplash	j. ligament injury with joint pain & swelling from wrenching or twisting.
35.	_____ sciatica	k. muscle &/or tendon injury from over-stretching; "pulled muscles"

TRUE OR FALSE: WRITE "T" OR "F" IN EACH BLANK

36. _____ When a client indicates he/she is experiencing a body memory of a past trauma, the massage therapist should ignore it and keep working, so as to not embarrass the client.

37. _____ Even though you tell the client to let you know when your work is uncomfortable, the clients with low self-esteem or dissociation from their bodies might not tell you.

38. _____Massage is contraindicated for clients with multiple sclerosis.

39. _____Massage is contraindicated for clients with chronic anxiety.

40. _____Insomnia & difficulties concentrating are common symptoms of depression.

41. _____Researchers estimate 1 in 12 adults in the U.S. have been sexually abused.

42. _____Survivors of sexual abuse experience long lasting mental & emotional trauma
         similar to that experienced by survivors of war, torture, and concentration camps.

43. _____Symptoms of anxiety can range from restlessness & irritability to extreme feelings
         of powerlessness and panic.

44. _____Paranoia & hallucinations are common symptoms of schizophrenia.

45. _____It's important to tell the diabetic client about any sore on his/her feet.

46. _____Massage can offer abuse survivors a safe way of being in touch with their bodies
         and being in control.

47. _____In working with survivors, treatment mistakes most often occur when the therapist
         works too deeply or inadvertently violates a boundary.

48. _____Cyanosis is the term for yellow discoloration of the skin & mucous membranes.

49. _____Homan's sign is characterized by pain in the calf when the foot is plantar flexed.

50. _____Tuberculosis is transmitted by droplets in the air.

MULTIPLE CHOICE

WRITE THE ONE <u>BEST</u> ANSWER TO EACH QUESTION IN THE SPACE PROVIDED

_____ 51. Veins carry the blood:
         a. to the heart
         b. away from the heart
         c. to the lungs
         d. to the brain

_____ 52. Tiredness, blue fingernails &/or lips, anxiety, irritability, and confusion are signs of:
         a. too much oxygen
         b. too little oxygen
         c. overmedication
         d. diabetic coma

_____ 53. Some people know when they will have a seizure by experiencing a smell or
         sensation. This is known as a/an:
         a. intuition
         b. precognition
         c. recognition
         d. aura

_____ 54. The seizure where there is a stiffness of the total body, followed by a jerking action
         of the muscles is known as a:
         a. petit mal
         b. grand mal
         c. Jacksonian
         d. psychomotor

_____ 55. In an emergency, what branch of the nervous system is stimulated to redistribute
         blood to where its needed most?
         a. automatic
         b. sympathetic
         c. cardiovascular
         d. parasympathetic

_____ 56. Massage would be contraindicated when pulse rate is:
         a. greater than 100/minute
         b. greater than 80/minute
         c. less than 100/minute
         d. less than 80/minute

_____ 57. Massage would be contraindicated when B/P is:
         a. diastolic less than 90
         b. diastolic more than 110
         c. systolic less than 120
         d. systolic more than 140

_____ 58. _____ is a yellow or orange coloration of the skin & sclera.
         a. cyanosis
         b. erythema
         c. jaundice
         d. pallor

_____ 59. _____ dilates small blood vessels in an allergic reaction, so that circulation
         is increased to that area.
         a. cortisone
         b. histamine
         c. antihistamine
         d. glucose

_____ 60. _____ softens connective tissues & suppresses the immune system while it decreases inflammation.
   a. cortisone
   b. histamine
   c. antihistamine
   d. glucose

_____ 61. Which of the following could be transmitted from client to massage therapist?
   a. melanoma
   b. staph
   c. contact dermatitis
   d. psoriasis

_____ 62. Which of the following is NOT considered contagious?
   a. herpes simplex (cold sores)
   b. conjunctivitis (pink eye)
   c. verruca vulgaris (warts)
   d. urticaria (hives)

_____ 63. A client stumbles while walking to your office. When she arrives, her left ankle is slightly swollen and painful to walk on. All of the following are appropriate massage interventions EXCEPT:
   a. rest & ice
   b. compression & elevation
   c. referral to a physician
   d. massage & range of motion

_____ 64. All of the following are considered endangerment sites for sustained deep pressure or pounding EXCEPT:
   a. anterior triangle in neck
   b. lateral ulnar epicondyle
   c. iliac crest
   d. twelfth rib, dorsal body

_____ 65. When working of a 68 year-old woman's legs, the massage therapist notices her fingertips are leaving slight indentations in the tissue. This is called _____ and the therapist should ___.
   a. pitting edema; stop working and refer her to a doctor
   b. pitting edema; avoid the area and refer her to a doctor
   c. renal failure; recommend a low salt diet
   d. CHF; recommend diuretics

_____ 66. The neuron that carries impulses toward the CNS is:
   a. interneuron
   b. efferent
   c. sensory
   d. motor

_____ 67. A 56 year-old man complains of chest pain during his massage, and he says "I probably just ate too much." You should:
  a. continue until his pain stops
  b. call his doctor or 911
  c. help him sit up and observe for changes
  d. continue unless his pain gets worse

_____ 68. The predicted outcome of a disease is the _____.
  a. diagnosis
  b. prognosis
  c. pathology
  d. remission

_____ 69. Hardening of the arteries is _____.
  a. arteriosclerosis
  b. atherosclerosis
  c. aneurysm
  d. phlebitis

_____ 70. Acute inflammation begins _____ after injury & lasts _____.
  a. immediately; 3-4 days
  b. in 24-48 hrs; 3-4 days
  c. immediately; 24-48 hrs
  d. in 24-48 hrs; 24-48 hrs

_____ 71. Chronically inflamed tissue tends to feel more _____ than normal tissue.
  a. dense, hot & more mobile
  b. dense, cool & less mobile
  c. thin, hot & more mobile
  d. thin, cool & less mobile

FILL IN THE BLANKS:

The 4 indicators of acute inflammation are:
  72. _____
  73. _____
  74. _____
  75. _____

WRITE THE CORRECT INITIAL IN THE BLANK IN PARTS I AND II.

I. Skin Cancers: S/squamous cell

                          B/basal cell

                          M/malignant melanoma

76. _____ most common skin cancer
77. _____ most dangerous & least common skin cancer
78. _____ small reddish brown plaque with firm elevated margins & scaly surface
79. _____ metastasizes rapidly
80. _____ small, firm raised nodule develops into ulcerated crater
81. _____ ABCD signs

II. Skin Disorders: C/contagious

                          N/non-contagious

82. _____ dermatitis
83. _____ ringworm
84. _____ athlete's foot
85. _____ yeast infection
86. _____ rosacea
87. _____ scleroderma
88. _____ scabies
89. _____ lice
90. _____ psoriasis
91. _____ shingles (oozing)

MULTIPLE CHOICE

WRITE THE ONE <u>BEST</u> ANSWER TO EACH QUESTION IN THE SPACE PROVIDED

_____ 92. The fat soluble vitamins are the ones most likely to be toxic, and include:
      a. A, B, E & C
      b. A, D, E & K
      c. A, C, E & D
      d. A, C, E & K

_____ 93. A client you've never met before arrives for an appointment and describes sharp, stabbing abdominal pain off & on for the past few hours. Your best approach is:
      a. ask client to rate pain from 0 to 10
      b. ask what relieves and worsens pain
      c. refer client to physician before you'll massage
      d. refer client to physician after you massage

_____ 94. A 24 year-old woman comes for massage monthly. She is thin, has dry hair and skin, several bruises on her arms and legs, talks about food a lot, and apologizes for her "fat" tummy. Which is the most therapeutic assessment and approach?
   a. Possible abuse. Call a protective agency.
   b. Possibly undernourished. Recommend a nutritionist.
   c. Low self-esteem. Recommend affirmations.
   d. Possible anorexia. Tell her what you see. Refer for help.

_____ 95. A massage therapist accidentally touches a client's blood when the client has a nosebleed. The therapist has no open areas on his hands. He immediately washes his hands thoroughly, but is still at risk for:
   a. HIV
   b. hepatitis A
   c. syphilis
   d. none of the above

_____ 96. Which of the following is part of our immune system?
   a. antigen
   b. antibiotic
   c. antibody
   d. adhesion

_____ 97. Pathogens are:
   a. viruses
   b. bacteria
   c. parasites
   d. all of the above

_____ 98. When part of the large intestine is removed and the remainder is fixed so that feces exit the body from the abdomen, it's called:
   a. an ileostomy
   b. a colostomy
   c. a urinary bypass
   d. an appendectomy

_____ 99. Which is an early warning sign of cancer?
   a. sudden hair loss
   b. dizziness when standing
   c. a sore that doesn't heal
   d. a change in personality

_____ 100. All of the following are contagious EXCEPT:
   a. tuberculosis
   b. upper respiratory infections
   c. hepatitis
   d. colitis

Recognizing Health and Illness
Pathology for Massage Therapists and Bodyworkers

Order Form for Additional Books

Name _____

School or business name, if applicable _____

Street address _____

City/State/Zip _____

Phone _____ Fax _____ E-Mail _____

Number of books ordered: _____ (1-4 books)   @ $45.00 each = $_____
                                _____ (5-10 books)   @ $35.00 each = $_____
                                _____ (11 or more)   @ $25.00 each = $_____
Add shipping and handling @ $5.00 first book and $1.00 each additional $_____
                                                        Total $_____

Enclose a check or money order made payable to:
   Health Positive!, Dept. B, 25603 Loring Road, Lawrence, KS 66044-7128.

Prices may change.
For more information, call 785-843-5884, fax 785-841-1761, or e-mail *4health@idir.net.*

Local Contraindications for Bodywork

(Often OK to proceed after consulting with the physician)
*Usually contraindicated, regardless of physician consultation

BY DIAGNOSIS

Abscess*
Acne
Angiomas*
Ankylosing spondylitis
Arthritis, acutely inflamed*
Athlete's foot*
Bell's palsy
Boils*
Bruises*
Bursitis, acute*
Candida albicans*
Carpal tunnel syndrome
Celiac disease, when acute*
Cellulitis*
Cholecystitis*
Cirrhosis (to the abdomen)*
Crohn's disease, when acute*
Decubitus ulcers (bedsores)*
Diarrhea (to abdomen)*
Diverticulitis (to abdomen)*
Edema, pitting*
Fractures
Goiter (to the anterior neck)
Gout, acute*
Graves' disease (hyperthyroidism)
Hepatitis (to abdomen)*
Hernia*
Herpes simplex (cold sores; fever blisters)*
Hyperthyroidism (Graves' disease)
Infection, in any area*
Inflammation, in any area*
Lipomas
Mononucleosis (to the abdomen)
Nodules, in any area*
Osgood-Schlatter disease*
Paget's disease
Pancreatitis (to abdomen)*
Pitting edema*
Psoriasis (if inflamed or tender*)
Rashes*
Ringworm*
Rosacea*
Sciatica

BY DIAGNOSIS (cont'd.)

Sebaceous cyst*
Shingles*
Skin lesions*
Sprain, first 48 hrs.*
Strain, first 48 hrs.*
Surgical incisions, fresh*
Tendinitis, acute*
Thrombophlebitis*
Thrombus*
Tinea (ringworm, athlete's foot, etc.)*
Trigeminal neuralgia*
Tumors, benign*
Tumors, malignant*
Varicose veins*
Warts*
Whiplash, after acute stage
Yeast infection*

BY SYMPTOM[1]

Pain, acute, in any area*
Unusual swelling
Unusually hot areas
Unusual redness
Excessively scaly skin
Bleeding*
Cyanosis in nails, hands or feet
Swollen lymph nodes
Abdominal tenderness
Numbness, in any area
Twitching, in any area
Unusual drainage or discharge*
Mood changes: irritable, withdrawn, sullen, depressed, aggressive, abusive, anxious, or demanding[2]

[1] Refer the client to a physician for assessment of the symptom.
[2] Set the boundaries you need and then refer client to a mental health professional.

Systemic Contraindications for Bodywork
(Often OK to proceed after consulting with the physician)
*Usually contraindicated, regardless of physician consultation

BY DIAGNOSIS

Addison's disease
Anemia, aplastic
Aneurysm
Anxiety, acute
Arthritis, infective*
Brain injuries
Bronchiectasis*
Cushing's syndrome*
Dementia, acute
Hemophilia
Hepatitis
Hodgkin's disease
Hyper-parathyroidism
Hypertension over 160/90
Hypo-parathyroidism
Intoxication (drugs or alcohol)*
Joint dislocations*
Kyphosis w/ functional limitation
Leukemia
Lice*
Meningitis
Multiple sclerosis
Muscular dystrophy
Non-Hodgkin's lymphoma*
Osteomyelitis*
Osteoporosis
Panic attack (acute)*
Paranoia, acute*
Pneumonia, with fever*
Rheumatic heart disease
Scabies*
Schizophrenia, dissociated*
Scleroderma
Scoliosis w/ functional limitation
Spinal cord injuries
Thrombocytopenia
Tuberculosis
Whiplash, acute stage*

BY SYMPTOM[1]

Sudden loss of strength
Cool, moist, clammy skin
Jaundice (skin yellowing)
Rapid, labored breathing
Grimacing when breathing
Pale or blue lips
Nausea or vomiting
Unusually slow responses
Sudden loss of memory, confusion, or
    difficulty following directions[3]
Chest pain, acute or radiating[2]
Severe abdominal pain[3]
Fever
Cannot awaken client[2]
Acute panic attack[3]
Pain, intractable

[1]Refer the client to a physician for assessment of the symptom.
[2]Call 911.
[3]Call someone to come and help the client get to a physician.